Home, Health & Garden

PROBLEM SOLVER

2007

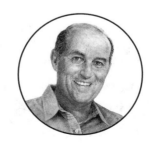

www.jerrybaker.com

Other Jerry Baker Good Gardening Series™ books:

Secrets from the Jerry Baker Test Gardens
Jerry Baker's All-American Lawns
Jerry Baker's Backyard Bird Feeding Bonanza
Jerry Baker's Bug Off!
Jerry Baker's Terrific Garden Tonics!
Jerry Baker's Year-Round Bloomers
Jerry Baker's Giant Book of Garden Solutions
Jerry Baker's Flower Garden Problem Solver
Jerry Baker's Perfect Perennials!
Jerry Baker's Backyard Problem Solver
Jerry Baker's Green Grass Magic
Jerry Baker's Terrific Tomatoes Sensational Spuds,
    and Mouth-Watering Melons
Jerry Baker's Great Green Book of Garden Secrets

Other Jerry Baker Good Health Series™ books:

Jerry Baker's Nature's Best Miracle Medicines
Jerry Baker's Supermarket Super Remedies
Jerry Baker's The New Healing Foods
Jerry Baker's Cut Your Health Care Bills in Half!
Jerry Baker's Amazing Antidotes
Jerry Baker's Anti-Pain Plan
Jerry Baker's Homemade Health
Jerry Baker's Oddball Ointments, Powerful Potions
    & Fabulous Folk Remedies
Jerry Baker's Kitchen Counter Cures

Other Jerry Baker Good Home Series™ books:

Grandma Putt's Old-Time Vinegar, Garlic,
    Baking Soda, and 101 more Problem Solvers
Jerry Baker's Supermarket Super Products!
Jerry Baker's It Pays to Be Cheap!

To order any of the above, or for more information on Jerry Baker's *amazing* home, health, and garden tips, tricks, and tonics, please write to:

**Jerry Baker, P.O. Box 1001
Wixom, MI 48393**

Or, visit Jerry Baker on the World Wide Web at:

www.jerrybaker.com

Home, Health & Garden

PROBLEM SOLVER

2007

by Jerry Baker

Published by American Master Products, Inc.

Executive Editor: Kim Adam Gasior
Managing Editor: Cheryl Winters-Tetreau
Production Editor: Stacy Mulka
Interior Design and Layout: Sandy Freeman
Cover Design: Kitty Pierce Mace
Indexer: Nanette Bendyna
Special Thanks: Tom Donnelly and Sally Seabury

Publisher's Cataloging-in-Publication
(Provided by Quality Books, Inc.)

Baker, Jerry.
    Jerry Baker's home, health & garden problem solver 2007.
    p. cm. -- (Jerry Baker's good home series)
    Home, health and garden problem solver.
    Includes index.

    1. Home economics. 2. Health. 3. Gardening. I. Title. II. Title: Home, health & garden problem solver 2007. III. Title: Home, health and garden problem solver 2007.

    TX158.B298 2006   640
                QBI05-600053

Printed in the United States of America
2 4 6 8 10 9 7 5 3 1 hardcover

To: The thousands of folks who
I've met over the years in my travels
across the good ol' U.S. of A.—thanks
for all of your wonderful tips, tricks,
and tonics that got the old wheels a spinnin'.
I couldn't have done it without you.
And you, too, Grandma Putt!

Contents

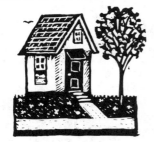
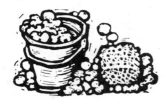

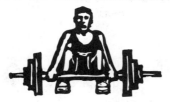
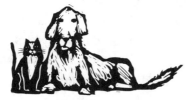
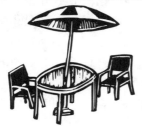
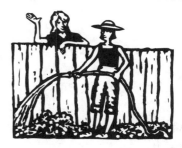

Howdy, Folks!

For over 40 years now, I've been sharing my unique home, health, and garden tips, tricks, and tonics with folks all across America. And during that time, lots of other folks have contacted me with their own neat ideas and home solutions. So I've been diligently jotting them all down—with an eye toward using them someday.

Well, there's no time like the present, so I spent the better part of the past year sifting through all the hints, helpers, suggestions, and secrets I'd gathered over the years. I discovered that I had a virtual treasure-trove of home, health, and garden solutions right at my fingertips. I knew right away that I just couldn't keep these incredible tips under my hat any longer, so I decided to put together a terrific new book containing the most ingenious problem solvers I could find.

Believe you me—it took a lot of hard work to choose the best of the best, but I'm proud to say I've done it, and the result is this very book you're holding in your hands. It's packed full of the best-kept problem-solving secrets I've used for many, many years, plus hundreds of new ones you've never heard of before.

This book is a gold mine of fast, fun, and easy ways for you to work out all sorts of trouble with your home, health, or yard—using common, household products you've already got lying around the house. Plus, you'll save loads of time, money, and effort in the process. We've included hundreds of my personal favorite remedies and terrific tips and tricks from folks all over the U. S. of A., and, of course, oodles of tried-and-true solutions passed down to me from my Grandma Putt.

Let me tell you a little about

my Grandma Putt. Every single day with her was a lesson in frugality and what she called good, old-fashioned horse sense. Because of her years of wisdom, she always seemed to know exactly what to do when something went wrong. She wasn't a know-it-all; she just knew a good idea when she heard one.

Growing up, I learned tons of problem-solving secrets from Grandma Putt—secrets using common, everyday household products to make things last or make 'em like new. No matter what the situation was, she made do with what she had. As a result, I learned how to be thrifty, resourceful, and self-sufficient. In fact, the very same lessons I learned from her all those years ago still serve me well today.

You know, it seems to me that these

What a Great Idea!

While working on this book, whenever I came across a really great idea, I put it in a special box like this one. So look for my Eureka! boxes where you'll learn all kinds of fun, yet practical stuff, like these tips on how to use baking soda:

☞ Soothe a bug bite or sting by applying a paste of baking soda and water to the area.

☞ To really clean tile surfaces, make a thick paste of baking soda and water, and spread it on. Let stand for a half hour, then wipe clean.

☞ Get your rain-soaked dog smelling sweet again by sprinkling him with baking soda, then toweling him down and brushing him out.

For more wild and wonderful uses for all kinds of household stuff, turn to page 327.

days, whenever folks want to get something done, they either drive all over the place or are quick to call an "expert" to take care of it for them. But that's not my style. Why run around, when in all likelihood, you already have what you need to fix the problem? For instance, there's the laundry additive in your kitchen cupboard that'll make your next load of whites even brighter than bleach. Then there's the item in your medicine chest that'll remove stubborn stains from the bathroom sink. And, oh yes, don't forget the secret concoction in your garage that'll keep your kitchen appliances sparkling like new. Want to know what they are? Would you believe lemon juice, hydrogen peroxide, and car polish?

One of Grandma Putt's favorite sayings was that an ounce of prevention is worth a pound of cure, and I couldn't agree with her more. Throughout this book, you'll find some great ideas about preventive maintenance, from easy, common stuff (like keeping cabbage from stinking up your kitchen when you boil it and keeping your closets from getting too cluttered) to being prepared for more serious emergencies, such as what to do if there's a fire in your home.

And as the seasons change, so do the problems you face and the chores that need to be done around the house. So, I've also included some terrific tips for all seasons, from making your spring cleaning a snap to taking care of those summertime mosquito blues (with a secret ingredient from your kitchen); from cleaning those autumn leaves out of your gutters (with a homemade scraper) to winterizing your air conditioner so that it'll run like a champ next summer. There are even hints on how to cure what ails you with common household products. And don't forget about the terrific tips that'll turn any old yard into a picture-perfect paradise.

> *Mid pleasures and palaces though we may roam, Be it ever so humble, there's no place like home.*
>
> JOHN HOWARD PAYNE

I've got to tell you, folks, I could go on and on...this book was loads of fun to write, and I hope you'll find it just as entertaining to read. Toward that end, I've included a few fascinating historical facts, some clever quotable quotes, and of course, lots of lists, schedules, and recipes—in fact, I've thrown in just about everything but the kitchen sink!

So the next time you're trying to get a busted light bulb out of the socket without electrocuting yourself, or you're figuring out how to keep your dog from barking up a storm, open up this book, and you're sure to find answers to these and hundreds more questions at your fingertips. I guarantee that they'll be interesting, amusing, practical...and sometimes all three at once. If they are, then I hope you'll think to yourself, 'why that ol' Jerry Baker, he really does know a thing or two about solving life's everyday problems.' That, my friends, would be the kindest compliment you could ever pay me.

Jerry Baker

CHAPTER 1

Home Sweet Home

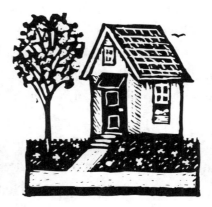

Your home is your castle, isn't it? And even if you live in a teeny, tiny one-bedroom house, what a castle it is! There's so much to maintain, fix, think about, and even plan.

In this chapter, I'm going to walk you through some of the simple repairs you may be faced with during the year. You'll learn how to straighten the "fins" on your air conditioner (I'll even tell you what the heck those fins are and what they do); how to fix that leaky faucet (even if you've never held a wrench before); and how to get a broken light bulb out of the socket. You'll learn how to hang a picture, too (it's *not* just banging a nail into the wall).

Decorating is part of what makes your house a home; it's adding your own personal stamp to the blueprint. So, to help you on that front, I've gathered up some of my favorite decorating tips and hints (including many I learned from my dear, old Grandma Putt). And if you like to shop at tag sales and antique shops, well, you've come to the right place. I'll let you in on my golden rules for getting the best deals in town. Once you get that flea market find back home, I'll give you a few tips that will make refinishing it a snap.

But wait! There's even more! When was the last time you got stuck in the dark when the power went off? Kind of a pain in the neck, huh? Well, I've put together some information I think everyone should have about being prepared for emergencies. Read it now, and you'll save yourself some irritation (and maybe worse) when nature doesn't cooperate with your plans.

Minor Repairs: Just Fix It!

My Grandma Putt was certainly a lady, but that didn't stop her from making repairs around the house. That's one thing I learned from her: It's important to be self-reliant. And besides, why pay someone else a pretty penny when you can fix it just as well yourself? Now, some of what I'm going to tell you is pretty simple, but I'm also going to spend a bit more time explaining how to make repairs like fixing a leaky faucet, just to make sure it's completely clear.

Taking Care of Your Air Conditioner

Is there anything better than walking into a nice cool room on a hot, sultry summer day? I don't think so. Here are some ways to keep your air conditioner up and running.

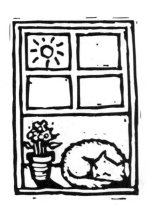

◆ FRESH AIR

One of the easiest, but most essential steps you can take to keep your air conditioner in tip-top shape is to change the filter. While some units have filters that you simply slide out of the front of the unit, others have filters that are inside the front panel, which you will need to remove (it's usually held in place by clips or plastic tabs). Replace the filter with foam material that you can buy really inexpensively at the hardware store. But don't throw away that old filter—use it as a template for making the new one.

How often should you change the filter? Under normal circumstances, once a season should do it. But folks who have allergies or pets in the house may want to change it twice a season. Let the condition of the filter be your guide.

◆ UNDERCOVER AIR CONDITIONER

Sure, air conditioners are made to hang outside your window or wall all year long. But yours will last a lot longer if you protect it during the cold weather. Now, you could buy a fancy cover from the home-supply store, but a heavy-duty plastic garbage bag will work just as well, and hey, it's a whole lot cheaper. Simply secure it to the outside of the air conditioner's case with duct tape, and remove it when the weather heats up (and it's time to cool down).

> *Keep strong, if possible.*
> *In any case, keep cool.*
>
> BASIL HENRY LIDDELL HART

◆ AN INTERNAL COVER-UP

If you can't reach the outside of the air conditioner to cover it because it's mounted too high, or if you can't remove it from the window, protect it from the inside. Remove the screws along the bottom of the air conditioner, then slide out the chassis without removing the entire unit. Cover the compressor and coils with a plastic garbage bag, and slide the chassis back into its case. Then wrap the plug in masking tape, or place a piece of tape over the switch to remind you to remove the bag before you use the air conditioner again.

When you remove the plastic from the chassis, this is also a great time to vacuum out the inside of the machine before the start of the season. A clean machine will run more smoothly.

◆ THE STRAIGHT INFO ON FINS

Air conditioners cool a room by removing heat from it. That heat has to go somewhere, or the machine will overheat. Usually, the heat is exhausted out the back of the air conditioner and out of your home. But if the soft aluminum "fins" on the back of your unit get bent together or are damaged, this seriously cuts down on the machine's cooling efficiency. In simple terms, the heat can't leave the air conditioner—or your room.

You can restore your air conditioner to tip-top form by straightening out those fins. The professionals use a tool called a "fin comb," which you can get rather cheaply at some hardware stores. But you don't need a special tool (or a pro) to do the job. Carefully use the blade of a slot-tipped screwdriver or a knife, and gently open up the flattened fins. Don't worry about making them perfect. Just look at the undamaged areas and imitate that spacing.

Jerry's Basic Tool Kit: Part I

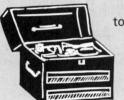

I've collected lots of tools over the years; some that I use all of the time, and some I hardly use at all. But if I were to start from scratch (knowing what I know today, of course) these are the first tools I'd buy just to keep pace with the household repairs.

☑ **Awl.** Useful for starting pilot holes for screws and screw-eyes.

☑ **Medium-duty claw hammer** (about 13 ounces). To drive a nail—or remove one, for that matter. The claw on the back of the hammer can also serve as a light-duty pry bar.

☑ **Slip-joint pliers.** These will help you get a grip on a nut, and I don't mean the next-door neighbor who always borrows your tools!

☑ **Long-nose or needle-nose pliers.** Especially helpful for holding a small nail for hammering, keeping your fingers a safe distance away.

Like anything else, when shopping for tools, you can spend a little or a lot, but you usually get what you pay for. A well-made tool may be expensive, but properly taken care of and used as it was designed, it will last several lifetimes. The moral of the story is to buy within your budget, and upgrade when you can.

Radiators: When the Heat is On

I'm a little like Pavlov's dog, you know, the pooch that gets hungry when he hears a bell ring? Well, whenever I hear the radiator start to ping and clang, I start to get warm. You see, I know that the steam or hot water is circulating through the system, and it's just a matter of time before the air warms up. But I also know that some folks' heating systems, especially the cast-iron radiator type, make more noise than they ought to. If yours falls into that category, read on, my friends.

◆ IN HOT WATER, OR ALL STEAMED UP?

Before you try some of my suggestions for keeping the noise level down when the heat is up, you need to know if you have a hot-water or steam system. If you don't know for sure, examine the radiator. Both hot-water and steam radiators have the same three parts, but the hot-water kind has one more.

1. The largest part of a radiator is the main section. This could be two or more tubes, and these make up the bulk of the heating area.

2. Then there's an intake valve. That's the do-hickey with the plastic handle on the side that you open and close to make it hotter or cooler.

3. Finally, most cast-iron radiators have an air vent. That's the bullet-shaped appendage that sometimes whistles and sputters when the heat is on. It's there to release excess air that builds up in the system. And that excess air is often the source of the loud clanking noise.

If your radiator has one more part—a bleeder valve—you'll know you've got a hot-water system. The bleeder valve looks like a little faucet that's missing its handle, and only hot-water systems have a bleeder valve.

◆ LET IT BLEED

To quiet down that hot-water radiator, you need to release or "bleed" the trapped air that's knocking around inside. You do this by opening the bleeder valve. In some models, the valve can be opened with just a screwdriver, but many require a special "key." If you don't already have a key, look for one at your local hardware store. They don't cost much, and they come in very handy

The Good Ol' Days

One of my favorite pastimes is sitting down with a mug of hot cocoa and leafing through all of the old-time books, magazines, and almanacs that Grandma Putt collected. Most times I get some good advice and information that I can use today. Every once in awhile, I find something that makes me smile at the ingenuity of our forefathers (and mothers!).

One of my favorite books is called *Handy Farm Devices and How to Make Them,* by an old-timer named Rolfe Cobleigh. First published in 1909 (and republished in 1996), it's filled with instructions about how to make dozens of time- and money-saving devices for farmers and homesteaders. My two favorites? Would you believe a sheep-powered (you read that right) machine that separates cream from milk and a dog-powered water pump? That's right!

when you need to bleed the radiators.

Take a few precautions before you begin. Remember that there's hot water in the radiator (about 180°F) so you may want to wear a pair of work gloves to protect your hands from sputtering hot water. Also, keep a small pot handy to catch any water that gets released.

With the intake valve closed, open the bleeder valve (remember: lefty loosey, righty tighty—just like the intake valve) with the pot under it. Keep the valve open until a steady stream of water comes out, then close it up again. Do this at the start of the heating season to each of your radiators, and you'll enjoy a more quiet winter. Now that was easy, wasn't it?

◆ YOU'VE GOT CLANK, CLANK—SHHHH—STEAM HEAT

OK. So you're sure you've got steam heat? Excess condensation is what causes knocking in this kind of radiator. After the steam enters and heats up the radiator (and your room), it cools down and returns to the boiler as water, usually through the same pipe it entered by. If that water has a hard time getting out, it rattles around, making noise. Sometimes that happens when the radiator is pitched away from the intake, causing the water to remain in the radiator.

You can fix this situation by raising the far side (opposite the side with the intake valve) of the radiator with small wooden blocks (½ to ¾ inch high should do) under the legs. Of course, you should do this when the heat isn't on, to avoid burning your hands.

Repairing Walls

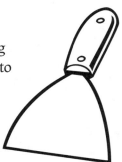

There's nothing more annoying than accidentally knocking a chip of paint out of the wall, or taking a picture down, only to find out that it was hiding a hole. But believe me, you don't have to be a master craftsman to repair minor cracks and holes in plaster and wallboard. Here's all you need to know.

◆ NEWFANGLED IS BETTER!

If you think I'm going to give you an old-fashioned tip for fixing cracks and holes that's been handed down for generations, this time you're wrong. With the invention of vinyl spackling compound—and you should always keep a small container on hand—anyone can repair a small crack or hole like a pro. You can apply it with a putty knife, or even a finger if the hole or crack is small. If your skin is sensitive, wear rubber gloves. Take a gander at the tips below for a few more points to keep in mind when you're working with Spackle.

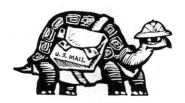

◆ GO SLOW

Remember that Spackle shrinks as it dries. So if you're filling a hole, don't expect to be finished in just one application. Apply some, and give it a chance to thoroughly dry before applying any more. You'll know it's dry when you can touch it without leaving an impression. Before repainting the area, allow about an hour (or more if the patch is large) for it to dry really well.

◆ THE HOLE STORY

If you're filling a small but deep hole, like the kind left by a plastic or lead anchor, fill it with a small piece of balled-up newspaper before spackling it. This will give the Spackle something to grab on to, and you won't use as much in the process.

◆ A LITTLE TOO MUCH IS OK

The final coat of Spackle should overflow the hole or crack by just a little bit. That way, you can sand down your patch to the same level as the wall. One way to get the last batch level is to wipe it with a clean, damp sponge, applying slight pressure to it.

Jerry's Basic Tool Kit: Part II

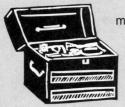

Here are some more tools in my ideal tool kit:

☑ **Screw-drivers.** As most folks know, there are two kinds of screws that you regularly come across: regular (slot) and Phillips-head (the one with the cross). So start off with a medium-sized screwdriver of each type. It's important to use the proper sized screwdriver to fit the screw; if you don't, you'll strip the head of the screw or break the tip of the tool. Don't be surprised if you need to go out and buy a size smaller or larger screwdriver.

☑ **Retractable metal tape measure.** A 16-foot model should serve most folks well for home use, but make sure the tape is at least ¾ inch wide, or it'll be too bendy to use when stretched out. And there's nothing worse than rasslin' with 12 feet of flimsy metal that's got a mind of its own.

☑ **Battery operated (cordless) drill** with drill and screwdriver bits. It's indispensable for home projects that require drilling and the multiple application of screws, like putting up shelves. There are many models on the market to fit most budgets. If you're looking to save money, buy a reconditioned model. It's as good as new, comes with a manufacturer's warranty, and best of all, will be about half the price of a brand-new one. Don't buy anything that bills itself solely as a "cordless screwdriver." It won't have nearly enough torque to drill holes. The standard assortment of bits sold in the hardware store can be used on wood, metal, and plastic, but buy masonry bits if you plan to drill through stone or plaster.

Thawing Frozen Pipes

Pipes that pass through an unheated basement or crawl space have a tendency to freeze up in the winter if they're not in use. A frozen pipe can burst if it doesn't get thawed out, and that can spell (expensive) trouble. Here's how you can avoid that costly (and very messy) scenario.

◆ RAG TIME

The simplest way to thaw frozen pipes is to place rags soaked in hot water over the them. This sounds simple enough, but remember, it only works when you have a water supply that's not frozen!

◆ TORCH SONG

Another method for thawing frozen pipes is to use a butane welder's torch on the pipe. I don't generally recommend this unless you're familiar with welding because you can do more harm than good. You could loosen welded joints or cause a buildup of steam to expand and burst the pipe. My advice? Don't use a torch unless you know what you're doing.

◆ THAR SHE BLOWS!

When you're thawing frozen pipes, you don't want to get the pipe too hot. A good rule of thumb is to never heat the pipe to more than your hand can stand. A hair dryer on a long extension cord can generate more than enough heat to thaw a blocked pipe, yet it won't overheat the pipe. You can also use a heating lamp (like the kind pet stores sell) or even your clothes iron to get things flowing.

Whatever method you choose, work from an open faucet toward the blockage so steam can escape, and also so you'll know when you've melted the ice.

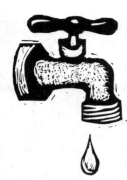

Fixin' Faucets: Water Torture

One thing that's as sure as you're reading this book is that faucets will leak and drip. It's a minor annoyance (that can waste lots of water) that we all have to deal with at one time or another. But don't worry, if you follow the tips below, you won't need to call a plumber to take care of it.

◆ WHATDOYOUCALLIT?

First, let's define our terms. To me, a drip is when water continues to seep out of the spout, even when the faucet is turned off. A leak is when the water flows from someplace it's not supposed to in the first place.

◆ DON'T FORGET YOUR RUBBERS

A faucet is 95 percent metal, usually brass covered with chrome. But it's the other 5 percent that you have to worry about—that's where the leaks and drips occur. There are usually two or three places where some kind of rubber or soft plastic gasket can be found, and depending on their function and appearance, they go by different names—like washer and O-ring. With a few exceptions, these are the only parts you'll ever need to replace, because they're the only ones that wear out. If you have a basic set of tools (see: "Jerry's Basic Tool Kit: Part III," at right), about the only special equipment you'll need is a replacement washer or O-ring, which can be easily purchased at your local hardware store.

◆ WASHER-WISE

Some sure signs that a washer needs to be replaced:

☑ You need to crank the handle so tight to keep the water from dripping that you need help turning it back on again.

☑ No matter how "open" the faucet is, only a trickle runs out.

◆ **SUSPICIOUS Os**

When should you suspect that an O-ring is the leaky culprit?
When the base of the faucet leaks where it meets the sink.

Jerry's Basic Tool Kit: Part III

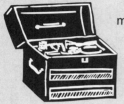

Here are a few more items to stock in your tool kit:

☑ **Assorted sandpaper and a sanding block.** You'll need lots of this stuff when you're refinishing furniture or repairing a crack in the wall.

☑ **Medium-sized adjustable wrench** (crescent wrench). These are good to have on hand when pliers aren't enough, like when you're repairing a leaky faucet.

☑ **Staple gun.** Just the thing you need when reupholstering that old sofa.

☑ **Putty (spackle) knives.** 2- and 4-inch sizes are handy. Flexible metal knives are best, but inexpensive plastic ones work well enough.

☑ **Heavy-duty scissors.** Use these mostly to keep you from ruining your good fabric or office scissors.

☑ **One set of Allen wrenches** (sometimes called hex keys). Certain screws are neither slot nor Philips-head, and that is where these six-sided wrenches come in handy. Setscrews on doorknobs often require one of these.

☑ **Paintbrushes.** Get natural bristle if you plan on using oil-based paints and varnishes, otherwise synthetic brushes will do. Be sure to clean them before storing them away.

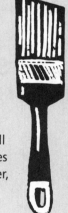

☑ **Household (white) glue or wood glue.** This will hold most any porous surfaces together, from wood to paper, and best of all, it cleans up with water.

☑ **Small container of Spackle.** For quick touch-ups of cracks and holes in plaster and wallboard.

☑ **Old candle stub or piece of sealing wax.** Use this for lubricating balky screws.

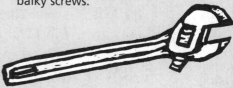

Quick Fix for a Drip

That drip, drip, drip keeping you up at night? Here's a simple way to temporarily stifle the waterworks—at least long enough to get some sleep! Stuff a piece of string or a rag up into the faucet, or drape it over the faucet in such a way that the drip runs down the string or cloth and into the sink silently. Make sure the string or rag is long enough to reach from the spout to the basin. Now go back to bed and it'll still be there to fix in the morning.

◆ GETTING STARTED

Once you've seen where the water leaks or drips from, leave the faucet turned on, and shut off the water from the shut-off valve, usually found under the sink. Once the water stops flowing, it's safe to take the faucet apart.

◆ BREAK IT DOWN

Not all faucets are identical, but most disassemble in the same general way: First, remove the handle. In many faucets, a decorative plastic cap hides the setscrew that holds the handle in place. It's on top, usually marked with an H or a C. Pop that out with a thin knife blade or your fingers.

The setscrew on most faucet handles can be removed with a Phillips-head screwdriver, but some handles, like the ones on some single-lever styles, require an Allen wrench or hex key to remove. If you don't already have one, a set of hexagonal wrenches are inexpensive and available at your local hardware store. They're easier than easy to use and are also handy to have for other repair jobs around the house. (See "Jerry's Basic Tool Kit: Part III" on page 11.)

◆ FOR ONE-ARMED FAUCETS

Some hardware stores sell repair kits for specific models of single-lever faucets. These kits include a special tool for removing the handle as well as all the necessary washers and O-rings.

◆ GET A GRIP ON THE PACKING NUT

Once the handle is removed, you'll see a part called the packing nut. This has at least two (and as many as six) flat sides, so it can be turned with a pair of adjustable pliers or a crescent wrench. Loosen this part by turning it to the left. Then unscrew the whole thing, lifting it up and out of the body of the faucet.

> *Remember:*
> *Lefty loosey,*
> *righty tighty*

◆ WASHER THIS

The washer responsible for stopping drips is usually on the bottom of the stem assembly you just removed, and it is held in place by another screw. If it needs to be replaced, it'll be pretty obvious by the condition it's in—it will most likely be very flat and badly worn. Carefully remove the screw that holds the washer, noting how it all fits together.

Take the washer to the hardware store when you buy a replacement. Some stores sell a pack of assorted washers, while others will sell you only the replacements you need. I prefer to buy just the kind I need, although I'll buy a few extra and keep a spare or two around.

Don't be surprised if the new washer looks a little different from the old one. The old one has probably been flattened by use, while the new one will have a flat side and a rounded side. Install the new washer with the rounded side up. Then throw away the old washer so it doesn't end up in your tool kit.

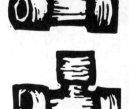

◆ HOT STUFF

It never fails—it always seems that the faucet's hot water washers wear out first. I'm not sure why, but an old friend who is a plumber once pointed that out to me, and I've noticed it ever since. It's kind of like Murphy's Law.

◆ A WASHER OF A DIFFERENT KIND

For single-lever faucets, the washers look a little different; they're more barrel shaped and usually come with a spring. Each model faucet has a slightly different setup, and since you might be buying the parts before you take the handle off (you may need to get the special wrench to remove the setscrew), it's a good idea to tell the folks at the hardware store what model faucet you have or, if possible, bring a picture along with you.

Once you have all your parts, reassemble the stem assembly and handle in reverse order, turn the water back on, and your drip will be gone!

◆ OH NO, YOU NEED AN O-RING

If it's a leak you're after, look at the O-rings. They look more like rubber bands than donuts, and they're thinner than washers. They're found at any joint in the faucet; for instance, the place where the stem assembly meets the rest of the faucet, or where the aerator screws onto the end of the spout. You can purchase O-rings at the hardware store, too—just make sure to bring the old one with you. Replace it and reassemble the handle, and your leak will be a thing of the past.

Sharpening Knives

I remember Grandma Putt saying, "Dull knives for dim cooks." And I now say: dangerous ones, too. It's important to know how to keep good knives sharp—and safe. A sharp knife handled carefully slices with ease. On the other hand, a dull knife requires more effort to use, and that means there's more of a chance the knife can slip and you'll get cut. Here's how to keep knives sharp and ready to slice.

◆ STONE IT!

The first thing you need to keep your knives sharp is a sharpening stone. Most hardware stores carry them in a variety of sizes and grades. A medium-grit stone, at least 3 inches long (though ideally the same length as your longest knife) is best. Sharpening stones can be expensive, but inexpensive ones can work well, too, so buy whatever fits into your budget. If you have a good set of kitchen knives, think of a sharpening stone as a solid investment in their future.

◆ STEADY AS SHE GOES

It's not hard to use a sharpening stone, and when you buy yours, it should come with directions. Here's my technique:

1. Place the sharpening stone on a sturdy, flat surface like a workbench or kitchen table.

2. Starting on one side, slide the blade forward, with the sharp edge away from you, as if you want to shave off a thin slice of the stone. Start from the base of the blade, near the handle, and work toward the point. Give the knife a few strokes this way, then flip it over and do the other side with the same amount of strokes. Repeat this a few times on both sides.

Some Sharp Ideas

If you don't have a sharpening stone handy, you can improvise by sharpening your knife on the unglazed under-side of a ceramic cup, or, if you're out in the garden, sharpen it on the underside of an unglazed terra-cotta flowerpot.

◆ WHAT'S YOUR ANGLE?

When sharpening a knife, the most important factor (aside from being careful) is to get the knife blade to meet the stone at the proper angle. The best angle for most knives is 11 degrees. Left your protractor in your high school locker? Here's how to get the proper angle:

☞ If you lay the knife flat on the stone it's at 0 degrees.

☞ If the blade is straight up and down, as if you were about to saw through the stone, it's at 90 degrees.

☞ A tilt halfway to the right or left is 45 degrees, half of that is 22 (or so) degrees, and half of that is 11 degrees. After you've done it a few times, you'll be able to eyeball the correct angle just about every time.

◆ WHET'S IN A NAME?

Sharpening stones are often called whetstones, but that doesn't mean they get wet. Some folks do like to use a drop or two of oil or even water to lubricate the stone while sharpening, but you don't need to. The word "whet" means to make sharp or keen by rubbing against something.

Miscellaneous Fixer-Uppers

Here are a couple of my favorite fix-it hints that just don't fit into any one category.

◆ DRIVE THAT NAIL!

One trick I use to keep from smashing my fingers when I'm trying to hammer in a small nail or tack is to push it through a piece of stiff paper or an old business card first. Then I use the paper like a handle and that lets me keep my fingers out of harm's way!

Squelch That Squeak

Here's a quick way to quiet a squeaky door hinge. Go to the medicine chest and grab the petroleum jelly. Take a fingertipful, and rub it into the noisy hinge, then open and close the door a few times to work the jelly in. Wipe off the excess with a cloth, and the squeak will be gone.

◆ SLIPPERY LITTLE DEVIL

Trying to get a screw through a piece of wood without splitting the wood? Don't curse, just try this old carpenter's trick: Rub the screw in a little wax from a candle stub (a piece of soap works just as well). That'll make the screw slip through the wood without causing any damage.

◆ DO THE POTATO TWIST

Here's an old-fashioned way to remove a broken light bulb that's still in the socket: *First, make sure the power is off.* No, I don't mean to call in an electrician, just make sure the switch is in the "off" position. Next, get a grip on the broken glass by pushing half of a raw potato or half an apple onto it, with the cut side up against the broken bulb. Now turn the potato or apple just as you would to unscrew a whole light bulb.

Once it's unscrewed, don't try to remove the broken bulb from the potato or apple—just throw it all in the trash.

◆ CRAY-ON, SCRATCH OFF

If you happen to put a slight scratch or nick in wood furniture or in a wood floor, don't worry. Just break out the crayons. Wax crayons work well because there are so many different colors, and you're almost certain to find a matching color. Once you find a perfect match, rub the crayon lightly into the scratch. Then buff the scratch (and the surrounding area of wood) with a clean, soft cloth. The scratch will disappear.

Decorating Around the House

I'll be the first person to admit that a lot of what I know about decorating I learned from Grandma Putt. So when I decided to include a section about home decorating, I went right back to my old photo albums, filled with pictures of the grand old house where she and Grandpa Putt lived. Then I pored over all the old almanacs and books that Grandma loved so well. It was about then that I realized that maybe I *did* know a thing or two about decorating. The fact of the matter is that we all do! Each of us has our own personal style and likes and dislikes. And decorating is simply incorporating who we are into our homes.

Getting Started

When it comes to decorating (or redecorating), how do you start? Well, even if you're moving into a brand-spankin' new house, my Grandma Putt would say not to do everything at once. Rather, slow down and take your time, adding elements that reflect who you are as you find them. Before you know it, you'll have your dream house!

But what if you're looking for a whole makeover for your, say, living room? Same thing; maybe you don't need to change everything. Perhaps all it'll take is rearranging something here, taking something away there, and adding a new item over there. Pretty soon, you've made the old homestead sparkle like new!

◆ HEAD FOR COVER!

Time for a new sofa? Maybe not. Perhaps all you need is a new slipcover. This is one of my favorite ways of updating the look of my living room while at the same time giving my sofa a longer life. This one I definitely learned from Grandma Putt, who always had a couple of sets of slipcovers stashed away in the linen cupboard. In fact, she had a different slipcover for each season! Now, mind you, she wasn't being frivolous—these slipcovers made her trusty sofa last for a good 25 years! (And of course, the slipcovers came off when "company" came over.)

Well, slipcovers aren't just a thing of the past. You can buy them all over these days, even in department stores. You can have one custom made (fancy), or you can buy one ready-made. But whichever option you choose, make sure to get something durable—chintz ain't the way to go, and neither is a leopard print! Imagine looking at those spots every day for two years! If you choose a slipcover in a neutral color, you can keep changing the accents (like pillows), which lets you update the look whenever you like.

◆ PILLOW TALK

If slipcovers don't appeal to you, or you just got a new sofa and you like it just fine, all you may need are a few well-placed accessories, like pillows. Make or buy new throw pillows or pillowcases to go over old pillows. You'd be surprised how these

Spruce Up Your Decor

Before you give up and hire an expensive interior designer, try any (or all) of these quick spruce-ups:

☑ **Rearrange the furniture.** Not only will it surprise the cat, but it can also make the room look totally different, even with the same old furniture!

☑ **Replace the curtains.** Curtains keep out prying eyes and add lots of character to a room. Try something different.

☑ **Change the lamp shades.** This minor replacement can make a big difference, not only in the look of the lamps when the lights are off, but in the look and feel of the room when the lights are on. Tiffany style shades are my favorites.

small wonders spruce up the look of a room.

Buy inexpensive solid-color pillows, and add some pizzazz to them by embellishing them with sewn-on buttons or bows. If your throw pillows don't get a lot of wear, try one of my favorite, crafty ways to decorate them: Buy (or make) covers with inexpensive, plain fabric, then decorate them with a little fabric paint. Make a freehand design or use stencils.

Painting Pointers

OK. So you've decided that taking minor redecorating action just wouldn't be enough to change your decor and you need to take a more drastic approach. It's time to bring out the heavy artillery: paint.

◆ COLOR MY WORLD

Now when I say, "paint the room," I don't mean to run out and buy a can of white paint and slap it on the walls. This is a decorating section, after all. What I am suggesting is that you try a little color. Now, if you're like most folks, you're afraid to use color in your home. That's why they stick to white. Don't get me wrong. White's nice. White's good. But white can create glare, give you a headache, and cause eyestrain. It can also seem sterile and uninviting.

Now, I'm not suggesting that you paint your living room walls red, either. All I'm saying is that painting a room is a relatively inexpensive way to change the way a room looks. It's also very effective. So why not try it?

S. O. S. or Save Old Stuff!

My motto since I was a wee lad is reuse, reduce, and recycle whenever possible. That goes double when I'm dealing with harsh chemicals. The more I can reuse it, the less I have to throw away. A good example is the method I use to make my paint thinner last a bit longer.

To clean my paint and varnish brushes, I pour the thinner into an old mayonnaise jar, and swish the brushes around until they're clean. Then, rather than dumping out the thinner, I grab my box of trusty paper coffee filters (which lives in my workshop) and another old mayonnaise jar (which I've labeled "recycled paint thinner"). I layer two filters, one on top of the other, and place them on top of the empty jar opening. But I don't pull them taut—I make them really 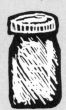 loose. Then I slowly pour the used thinner into the second jar through the paper filters.

Now, I use this recycled thin- ner only to clean my brushes; it's no good for thinning paint or varnish or stain, because there's always a little pigment left in it. But I'm always surprised at how long one tin of thinner lasts!

◆ THE MOODY BLUES

An added benefit to adding color to your walls is this: Scientists have found that color has an effect on our moods! So you can use paint to create a mood in a room. There are two types of color, those considered "warm" and those considered "cool". Here's a rundown…

Warm colors: include red, orange, and yellow (think of the colors of fire). They tend to be stimulating (some folks may even say stressful—think of sitting in a red room, for instance).

Cool colors: include blue, pur- ple, and green (think of the ocean). These tend to be more soothing than the warm colors.

How does this help you? Well, think about what happens in the room you're decorating and what kind of feeling you want to evoke. Do you want to encourage lively conversation in the dining room? Choose a shade of red, orange, or yellow. Want relaxing conversation in the den or living room? Then a shade of blue or green may be just the thing.

◆ BE A SHADY CHARACTER

How do you pick a color shade? Look around you, and start collecting "swatches" of the colors that appeal to you. A swatch can be a piece of clothing, a page from a magazine, a petal from a flower—anything that can show your paint dealer what you want. Of course, paint stores also have swatches, or paint chips, on cards that you can take home and see under the light conditions in the room you're going to paint.

A word of warning: Always look at the paint swatch or chips in the room you're going to paint, both with and without the lights on, so you can be sure of the true color.

Touch-Up Kit

Whenever you paint a room, put some of the leftover paint into a clean, reclosable baby food or mayonnaise jar. Not only will the paint keep better in the jar than in the original can, but now you'll have some paint readily available for touch-ups. Another plus— you won't have to pry open a messy, old paint can to see what's inside.

◆ GO LIGHT

Remember that if you do go the color route, choose carefully and (almost always) select a color that's a tad lighter than what you think you want. I can't tell you how many times I've come home with a can of paint, put it on the wall, and realized that it looked a whole lot darker on my walls than it did on that tiny paint chip. So my rule is to always err on the light side.

◆ A TEST FOR THE TIMID

If you get home with that can of sea-foam green paint and are too nervous to plunge right in and paint all the walls, pull the sofa out and paint a portion of the wall behind it. This way, you can get an idea of what the paint will look like in a good-sized area and, if you can't bear to go through with it, all you'll need is a can of primer and a quart of white paint to cover it up. No one will be the wiser.

◆ EASE INTO IT

If you just can't bring yourself to paint the walls, consider touching up just the trim and baseboard. This will let you introduce a little color into your room and help you get used to the idea before you go hog wild!

Hanging Pictures

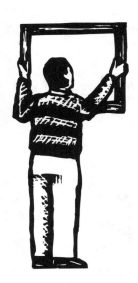

Sometimes all that your walls need are some decorations, either in the form of pictures or mirrors, to spruce things up. And don't be intimidated by the process; here's everything—and I mean *everything*—you need to know to do it right.

◆ IF YOU'VE GOT HANG-UPS

You just came home from the flea market with that beautiful "old-master" painting. Of course you want to hang it on the wall, but do you know how? And, just as importantly, do you know where to hang it on a wall? Here are some pointers on how to "install art" (as the professionals say).

☞ In rooms where you're seated most of the time, like the living room or dining area, pictures and mirrors look better if they're hung a little lower, because your line of sight is from a seated position.

☞ Conversely, hang a picture a little higher in halls and foyers, where folks are more likely to be standing.

☞ Wherever you decide to hang a picture, always do it with a helper. Hold it up so that your helper can see it, and ask him or her to hold it for you, *before* you start making holes in the wall.

☞ Have a pencil on hand, and use it to mark the wall at the top of the frame. This little bit of planning will save wear and tear on your walls.

◆ WHAT GOES UP SHOULDN'T COME DOWN

A picture hanger's worst enemy is guess what...gravity. Hanging a picture or mirror is all about supporting weight securely. (Did you know that in many cases the frame can make up most of the weight of a picture? That's what you actually need to support.) This can involve two main variables: the weight of the object and the type of wall it's going on. So be sure to use hardware that can handle the weight of the framed picture and is suitable for your type of wall material.

◆ IT'S WHAT'S ON BACK THAT COUNTS

You'll have a chance to admire your picture (or yourself in the mirror) after it's on the wall. But before you go to hang it, take a look at the back. There should be some kind of hanging device back there, either screw-eyes or some other kind of hardware that wire or picture hooks can attach to. If there isn't anything, go to the hardware store, and ask for a recommendation on what size screw-eyes and wire to use. Be sure to mention how heavy you think the object is.

> *Pictures get hung, but people get hanged.*

To insert those screw-eyes, place them in the frame, about one quarter of the entire height down from the top of the frame. In other words, if the frame is 12 inches from top to bottom, insert the screw-eyes 3 inches down from the top of the frame. To make things a little easier, rub some wax or soap on the screw to lubricate it and to keep the wood from splitting. This is especially helpful on old frames.

Use your awl (see "Jerry's Basic Tool Kit: Part I" on page 4) to start a hole in the wood, then turn the screw-eye in. Once you've started the screw-eye in the hole, finish screwing it in with your awl. Put the point of the awl through the hole, and then turn it, just like a handle.

◆ THAT'S A WRAP

To attach picture wire to screw-eyes, thread it through the hole of the screw-eye, and then wrap the end around the remaining wire several more times. Repeat for the other screw-eye. Allow a little slack in the wire—if it's too tight, you'll have difficulty putting it over the picture hooks. You should be able to pull the middle of the wire so that it reaches to within an inch to two from the top of the frame.

◆ TUG TEST

If there's already an old wire attached to the back of a picture or mirror, give it a good tug to test it. Better that it breaks now rather than once the picture or mirror is on the wall!

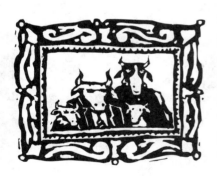

◆ HARDWARE HOLDING?

If your picture already has a wire, check the hardware that's holding it to the back of the frame. Does it look securely fastened? Tighten the screw or screw-eye if possible. You may need to remove the wire first and replace it later. If the hole in the wood looks too big, move the screw-eyes at both ends of the frame up or down about half an inch.

◆ A LIGHT WEIGHT

If the picture or mirror you're hanging weighs less than 75 pounds, it probably doesn't make a difference what kind of wall you hang it on—wallboard or plaster, painted or papered. As long as you measure carefully, when the time comes to move it, you won't have a major wall repair job to do.

◆ GET HOOKED

One standard-size picture hook (about ¾ inch long) uses one nail and is rated to hold 20 to 30 pounds. The next larger size uses two nails and is rated for 50 pounds. You can even get picture hooks with three nails rated for 75 and 100 pounds! So don't worry that the mirror you just bought is too heavy to hang. There are also picture hooks that use progressively larger nails to hold even heavier weights.

◆ TWO IS BETTER THAN ONE

No matter what size picture or mirror I'm hanging, I almost always use two picture hooks—especially if the picture will be hanging from picture wire. This isn't just because two hooks can support more weight than one, but because the picture will actually remain level longer on two hooks than on one. Hanging the picture or mirror on one hook allows the picture to rock like a pendulum; two hooks means it has less room to move.

Picture A-Weigh

Problem: You need to determine a picture's weight to decide what you'll use to hang it up with. But what if you don't have a scale to hop on? Just remember my practically foolproof picture-weighing system. (Now I'm a relatively fit guy, so you may have to adjust it to your own level of strength, but you'll get the idea.)

My solution: I give the frame a heft. If it's small enough to hold in one hand, then it probably weighs less than 10 pounds. If I can lift it easily, but it requires two hands, it weighs around 20 pounds. If I need to bend my knees, but I can still lift it without a strain, it's less than 50 pounds. If I need help, it weighs at least 100 pounds.

◆ LET'S GET ONE THING STRAIGHT

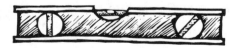

Here's how to make sure your picture or mirror will hang straight every time:

1. Hold the picture against the wall, and make a small pencil mark on the wall, at the very top center of the picture.

2. Next, look at the back of the frame: Remember, you want to use two picture hooks to keep it from rocking and rolling on the wall. If there's a wire on the back, measure an even distance along the wire between two points that begin and end a few inches in from the sides of the frame. Use a tape measure. For example, if the overall width of the frame is 18 inches, measure 12 inches across the wire, starting and ending 3 inches from the outside of the frame. This is how far apart the hooks should be on the wall.

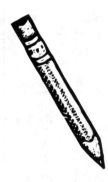

3. Now, with your fingers curled around the wire like little picture hooks, pull up on the selected points until the wire is the same distance from the top of the frame, at both points. Measure the distance from the top of the frame. (Let's pretend that it's 3 inches.) This is how far down from the top of the frame the hooks should go on the wall.

4. Go back to the wall and your original pencil mark. Measure down from this mark the same amount (our pretend 3 inches) as the wire was from the top of the frame. Mark that spot lightly with a pencil on the wall. Using that mark as a center point, indicate on the wall the distance between the two hooks you determined earlier. In our example, we used 12 inches. The 6 inch mark will be at the center point, with the 1 inch and 12 inch points at either sides. (This is why I like to use an even distance—it's easier to divide it in half.)

5. Next, measure down from the ceiling or up from the floor to determine the distance to your center point. Measure the two outside points to see whether they are the same. Nail the picture hooks into the wall so that the bottoms of the hooks are on your marks.

6. Now place the picture on the hooks, stand back, and admire your work.

◆ MEASURE UP

If the picture or mirror has no wire, but does have some kind of hanger on the back to which the hook attaches directly, don't

31 Ways to Hang Out

Of course you know that you can frame and hang a painting or mirror on the wall, but the choices don't end there. You're limited only by your imagination. To help you along, here's a list of 31 of my favorite "hangable" ideas:

1. Photographs

2. Old-time newspaper and magazine ads

3. Awards, certificates, and diplomas

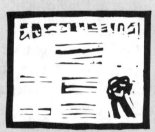

4. Picture postcards

5. Greeting cards

6. Calendar pictures

7. A stock certificate

8. An autographed jersey from a favorite sports hero

9. Maps and nautical charts

10. A menu from your first date or a favorite restaurant

11. Interesting stamps or an entire stamp collection

12. The board from an old board game

13. Your sports jersey from high school

14. Ribbons that you've won

15. A page from your high school yearbook

16. Your favorite record album cover

17. One of your old 45 or LP records

18. A lock of hair from each of your kids' first haircuts

19. A report card

20. Your cherished autograph collection

21. Old coins or other currency you've collected

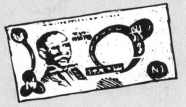

22. A favorite needlework project

23. A colorful scarf

24. Souvenirs from your vacation

25. Ticket stubs from a memorable theatrical or sporting event

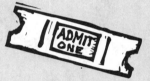

26. Your first paycheck stub

27. A picture downloaded from the Internet

28. Medals

29. Your mortgage (after it's paid)

30. A dust jacket from your favorite book

31. A special letter from a loved one or VIP

worry. Measure from the top of the frame to the top of that hanger. If there are two hangers, next measure the distance between the centers of the hangers. These are the two measurements that you need to transfer to the wall.

Be careful: This kind of hanging system requires slightly more accurate measurement to make sure the picture will be level. Since there's no wire, there's no margin for error.

◆ OOPS!

What if, after you see the picture up on the wall, you decide it needs to be raised or lowered a little? (Up a hair or down a drop, I believe, are the technical terms.) Do you have to pull the nails out of the wall and start over? Nope.

Simply remove the picture from the hooks, and unwrap the picture wire from one of the screw-eyes. Take up the slack in the wire, and you can raise the height of the picture. Add a little more slack in the wire, and you will lower it.

Whichever you do, do it in small increments, and don't forget to rewrap the wire securely around the screw-eye so that the wire doesn't slip and the picture doesn't fall off of the wall.

Antiques and Dust Collectors

I just love flea markets, tag sales, yard sales, garage sales—whatever you call them in your neck of the woods. I'm fond of junk and antique shops, too! There's nothing quite like finding a real, well, find. Over the years, I've collected some tips from friends and family that really help me out. I've gotten so many that I've decided to share the wealth. Here, then, are my golden rules for shopping the shows.

Tipsy Pictures

If the picture looks like it isn't level, slide the picture, wire and all, along the hooks until it's in the right place. As long as the hooks are level, the picture will be.

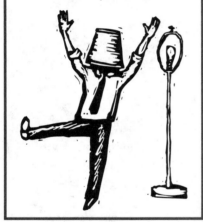

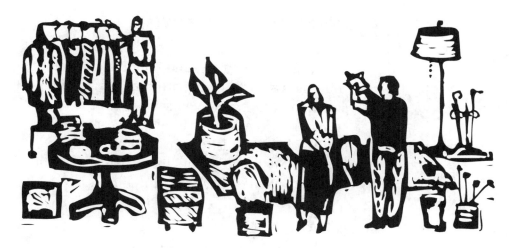

◆ EVERYTHING'S NEGOTIABLE

Especially at large, commercial flea markets and tag sales, be prepared to haggle. Once you get the hang of it, it's really kind of fun and exciting! Just make sure to decide the absolute maximum you're willing to pay for an item before you start to bargain. Remember, those guys are pros, and you may end up paying more than you bargained for!

◆ CASH AND CARRY

I don't understand how anyone can go to a flea market with a wallet full of credit cards and checks! Carrying cash, in small bills, is a terrific bargaining chip. Let's say there are two of you who want a vase. And let's say you're offering $50 in cash, and the other confident shopper is offering $60—in the form of a check. Who do you think will walk home with that vase?

◆ DRESS DOWN

It's better to look like a normal person rather than a snazzily dressed (and wealthy) antique buyer from the big city, especially if you're shopping in an upscale antique shop. A shop owner may be less willing to budge on a price for someone who looks like he or she can afford anything.

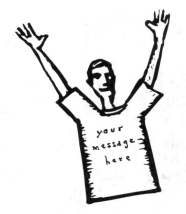

◆ IT PAYS TO ADVERTISE

A friend who goes to lots of big flea markets shared this tip with me, and I think it's brilliant. If you collect something in particular, say a china pattern or a toy, make yourself a T-shirt that says, "I collect Beanie Babies" or whatever it is you collect. Use big block letters that can be seen at a distance. My friend swears that when she wears her T-shirt, sellers flock to her in droves.

◆ NEITHER RAIN, NOR...

Rainy days might not be great for hitting the antique shops—they tend to be busy on rainy days, just as movie theaters and museums are. But those are terrific days to visit rain-or-shine outdoor sales. The crowds will be a lot thinner and the vendors will be a lot more eager to move their wares.

◆ RISE AND SHINE

The early bird gets the worm—and the best deals—at flea markets and outdoor sales. Daybreak isn't necessarily too early, but call ahead, or you just might find yourself sitting alone in an empty lot!

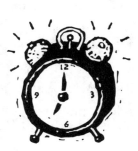

◆ THERE GOES THE NEIGHBORHOOD!

When you shop garage and yard sales, stick to the best neighborhoods. The goods you find there are likely to be of a superior quality.

◆ DO YOUR HOMEWORK

That Fiesta Ware you got for a song won't seem like such a bargain when you later find it on sale—and cheaper—at a discount store. If you're looking for collectibles, be sure to do your homework first so you don't get taken to the cleaners!

Refinishing for Fun

Furniture is the thing that I like to hunt for at flea markets. But it's not a priceless antique armoire I'm after. No, it's the diamond in the rough that I want: an old steamer trunk; a mahogany chest of drawers covered with black paint; a birch table buried under layers of dark stain. Of course, it takes a certain talent to see beyond the crusty old finish and envision the potential treasure beneath, but that's part of the fun! Refinishing furniture has become kind of a hobby of mine (and of lots of my friends). Here are some of the tips and tricks I've picked up along the way.

You Get What You Pay For

So, you've found a beautiful dresser or table or other piece of furniture at a tag sale, but it needs to be refinished. Great! Off to the hardware store you go to gather your supplies. Paint stripper, putty knives, sandpaper—hold on there. Now, if you're like me, this is when your frugal nature comes into play. You naturally reach for the least expensive sandpaper you can find. After all, what's the harm in buying cheap sandpaper?

Well, maybe you'll do no harm, but you may end up spending more in the long run. You see, the grit on inexpensive sandpaper is usually flint quartz, and it wears out very quickly. That means you'll have to change the paper more frequently, and that just makes the whole job go a lot more slowly.

My recommendation is that you spend a little more and get sandpaper that uses aluminum oxide, garnet, or silicon grit. If you're not sure, ask the fellow or gal behind the counter. You'll be glad you did!

◆ START SMALL

A word of wisdom: For your first refinishing project, I'd recommend choosing something simple, like an old wooden jewelry box or a trunk. Pieces of furniture that have intricate carving or turned legs may be a little discouraging for a beginner.

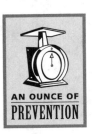

Keep 'Em Under Cover

When you're refinishing furniture, always be sure to wear gloves and safety glasses because even water-based strippers can be caustic.

◆ TAKE THREE

Refinishing furniture takes three steps:

1. Remove (or strip) off the old finish, whether it's paint or varnish.

2. Prepare the wood for the new finish by sanding it.

3. Apply a new stain and protective finish.

Now, I'm not going to walk you through the whole process step by step (that's a whole book!). But read on for some hints that will come in handy for each of those steps.

◆ TAKE IT OFF, TAKE IT *ALL* OFF!

Now, if you know me, you know that I sure like to do things the old-fashioned way, and that means using as few harsh chemicals as possible. We're lucky to have water-based paint strippers these days. Some take a little longer to work than the more caustic ones, but they're a whole lot safer. But that doesn't mean they're completely without risk, so please make sure to read and follow all of the directions on the container.

◆ GIVE IT THE OLD BRUSH OFF

It's true that, in general, you'll save money in the long run by purchasing good-quality tools and taking care of them. They'll last longer and give you better results than cheap tools. I learned that from Grandma Putt. However, when it comes to applying paint stripper, it's better to get yourself a cheap paintbrush. That's because once you've used it to apply stripper, it's not much good for any other job. So in this one case, the cheaper the better!

◆ LAY IT ON

One thing you need to keep in mind when you're applying paint stripper is that once it dries, it's useless. It needs to be wet to do its job. So if your piece is large, cover the surface with a generous helping of stripper—lay it on thick. If your piece is very large, work in sections.

◆ SWAB IT

Now if you've chosen a pretty simple piece for your first refinishing project, removing the finish should be fairly simple. But sometime down the road, you're probably going to have something a bit more intricate, and trying to get the paint stripper into all of those nooks and crannies (and back out again) can make you want to pull out all of the hair on your head! Here's the solution: Use a clean cotton swab to apply the paint stripper and an old, stiff toothbrush to remove it. Take it from me—both work like a charm!

◆ GIVE IT A REST

Once you've gotten all of the old finish off your piece of furniture, grab a clean rag and dampen it with paint thinner (again, keep those gloves on); then wipe the whole thing down. Here's the hard part: Once you get a good look at your clean, stripped-down piece of furniture, you're going to want to jump right to the next step. But take my word for it, patience is key here. Let your piece completely dry for a day or so; even longer if the weather is humid.

◆ KNOCK YOUR BLOCK OFF

Now that you've got your piece of furniture stripped down, it's time to start sanding. Use a sanding block, not your hands, for this job. You'll never be able to keep your hand level, you'll scratch the wood, and you'll end up with a cramp.

But don't run out to the hardware store for a sanding block. No, do what I do and make your own with a block of wood, like a scrap from a 2-by-4. Cover it with a piece of fabric like a left-over piece of felt and then wrap your sandpaper around it. It'll work just as well as a store-bought block—maybe even better.

◆ OH, THE IRONY

Sanding gets rid of most of the scratches on a piece of furniture that's not too beat up. This is true especially if you work in stages, starting with a coarse-grit paper, and gradually working your way down to a fine-grit paper. However, some dents and dings don't sand away.

If you encounter a particularly stubborn dent, try this old-time woodworkers' tip. Plug in your iron, and set it on high. Then get a couple of fabric scraps (cotton is best because it can take the most heat). Douse them with water, and place them on top of the dent. Now set your iron on top of the fabric, and press down. This will sometimes raise the grain again.

◆ GO WITH THE GRAIN

When you sand, always go with the grain of the wood; otherwise you risk scratching the piece and raising

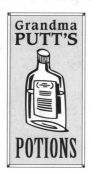

Ouch, A Scratch

Whenever I came home with a scraped knee, I knew what I was in for: some TLC from Grandma Putt. That was quickly followed by a trip to the medicine chest, where, after cleaning the wound, Grandma painted it with a little iodine.

Well, if your dark-colored wooden furniture gets scratched, you don't need to worry about germs. But you can camouflage that nick the same way that Grandma Putt took care of my knee. Use a cotton swab dipped in a little iodine. The purply-red stuff will hide the scratch in a jiffy. Just be sure to test it first in a hidden area, to make sure the color blends in nicely.

Make Your Own Tack Cloth

Now that you're an expert furniture refinisher, you probably know your way around the refinishing section of your local hardware store. And if you're like me, you're always looking for ways to spend less money or to make a tool or product yourself rather than paying for a ready-made one. Take tack cloth, for instance. It's the sticky cheesecloth that you rub over the piece of furniture you're refinishing after each sanding to remove the dust. You don't have to buy it—you can make it yourself.

Root through the kitchen drawers and get your hands on some leftover cheesecloth. Saturate it with linseed oil (okay, so you'll probably have to buy that from the hardware store). Squeeze out the excess, and store your tack cloth in a resealable plastic bag when you're finished with it.

the grain. Remember, your goal in sanding is to make the surface of the wood as smooth as silk (or a baby's bottom).

◆ ARE YOU AN OLD SOFTIE?

This is the fun part—now you're ready for the big, um, finish. If the piece you're refinishing is a soft wood, like pine, you'll have better luck with your stain if you first "seal" the wood. Now, you can buy a separate sealer or you can make your own by thinning some polyurethane with some paint thinner. Apply this sealer with a paintbrush and let it dry completely. Sand it very lightly when it's dry and give it a good going-over with your home-made tack cloth (see above).

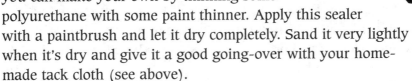

◆ THINK TWICE ABOUT STAINING

You know, you don't necessarily have to stain your wood. Some woods are beautiful without stain. Perhaps all yours needs is a coat of sealer. But how can you tell? Try this trick: Find an inconspicuous area on your piece of furniture and rub it with some paint thinner on a piece of cloth. That approximates how your wood would look with only a little sealer. Like it? Then all you need to do is apply your final finish. Not crazy about it? Then you ought to stain it.

◆ WHAT THE...

What the heck is stain, anyway? Well, it changes the color of the wood (makes pine resemble mahogany, for instance) and emphasizes the beauty of the grain. If you want the wood to look as natural as possible, use a light-colored stain. And please—just as with chemical strippers—it's very important to follow the manufacturer's instructions.

◆ POLY GO LIGHTLY

After you've applied your stain and have gotten the color you want, you'll need to apply some sort of protective finish. My recommendation is that if you're a beginner, use polyurethane. It's the easiest to work with.

◆ LEARN FROM MY MISTAKES

Once, not so long ago, I was refinishing a little cherry table I picked up at a yard sale. I took my time stripping and sanding and sealing it. But as this beautiful little table emerged, I started to get impatient. In my rush to admire my handiwork, I decided to take a shortcut, and hastily slathered on a thick layer of polyurethane.

Well, it never did dry the right way. And that eagerness completely undid all my hard work. And that's the final refinishing lesson I pass on to you: It's better to apply several thin coats of finish than one thick one. And after each coat dries well, go over it with some very fine sandpaper and then with your homemade tack cloth. Take your time, be patient, and your "new" piece should give you years of pleasure and enjoyment!

Surviving Household Emergencies

At one time or another, every one of us has experienced a power outage. There are some do's and don'ts you should know about when the lights go out to get through it with minimal distress. And if you've been fortunate enough to never experience a house fire, congratulations. But don't be too smug: It can happen to anyone at any time, so you must be prepared. Here's how to deal with these all-too-common household emergencies.

When the Power Fails

Some rain, a clap of thunder, a flash of lightning, and then, darkness. But what's this? The TV, radio, and all the lights are

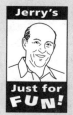

Jerry's Just for FUN!

Stormy Weather

What do Allen, Betsy, Fred, and Joan all have in common? No, they're not the Four Tops! They're hurricane names that have been retired. When a hurricane causes severe damage, its name may be retired. But it's not like when a baseball star's number gets retired—the reasons are a lot more ordinary than that. And it's not even a permanent retirement.

A hurricane name gets retired for 10 years to "facilitate historic references, legal actions, insurance claim activities, etc. and avoid public confusion with another storm of the same name." That's according to the National Hurricane Center.

But how are the names chosen in the first place? Well, way back in 1978, the World Meteorological Organization (that's a mouthful!) got together and came up with a list of 126 names—six years' worth, at 21 names per year. So the names on the list repeat after 126 hurricanes. When a name is retired, a representative from the country most damaged by that hurricane gets to nominate a new name. So now you know!

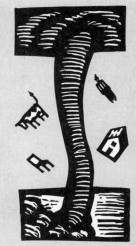

AN OUNCE OF PREVENTION

Be Prepared

That's the motto of the Boy Scouts, but it ought to be yours, too, and not just if you live in those parts of the country that experience tornadoes or hurricanes. Everyone, at some time or another, has had to deal with a power outage or a broken water main. But there's good news. You can minimize the unpleasantness for you and your family. All it takes is having a disaster kit and knowing how to use everything in it. Here's a rundown:

☑ Flashlight with extra batteries and extra bulbs. Just to be safe, check the bulbs and batteries every so often to make sure they work. I check mine at daylight saving time, the same time I check my smoke detector batteries.

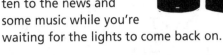

☑ Portable, battery-operated radio and extra batteries, so you can listen to the news and some music while you're waiting for the lights to come back on.

☑ Battery-operated weather radio. I like to listen to mine during a lightning storm or just for fun when I'm planning a picnic so that I'll know what the weather's going to be like.

☑ Emergency food and water. I have a couple of cans of tuna and salmon and other things that you can eat without having to heat them up.

☑ Non-electric can opener. Unless you're ready to open that can of tuna with your teeth!

☑ A first-aid kit and manual, as well as an extra bottle of any prescription medicines you take. See "A Well-Stocked First-Aid Kit" on page 141 for what needs to go inside it.

off, too. And where's the familiar hum of the refrigerator keeping all your goodies nice and cold? A power outage is probably the most common household emergency that you'll face. And to get through it takes more than a flashlight with a couple of burned-out batteries.

◆ NOW WHAT?

When the lights go out, the first thing you'll need is your well-supplied emergency power kit (see "Be Prepared" above). After that, whether you expect the power to be off for days (a hurricane? tornado? ice storm?) or just an hour or so, there are certain things you should do. Read on for more advice.

◆ TURN IT OFF

I know, I know, when the power goes out, all your appliances are already off! But think about what's going to happen when the power comes back on—each of those appliances will turn on at the same time. That can cause a surge, and knock the power out again! So what do you do? Go to each appliance and disconnect it or make sure the switch is in the "off" position.

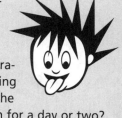

◆ WHICH ONES?

Which appliances should you turn off? Air conditioners, electric water heaters, freezers, furnaces, refrigerators, TVs, computers, and water pumps. So how will you know when the power comes back on? Leave one or two lamps turned on. When they come on, you'll know it's safe to plug in and turn on your other appliances.

◆ BUT I HAVE A ROAST IN THE FREEZER!

During a power outage, you'll probably be concerned with all that expensive food you have in the freezer. So you should keep checking it, right? Wrong! Every time you open the door, cold escapes.

The best way to conserve all that cooling power is to keep the fridge and freezer closed. If you keep your freezer door

Is It Safe to Eat?

Let's say the electricity in your neighborhood goes off. You already know to keep the freezer and refrigerator closed so that nothing goes bad, but what if the power doesn't come on for a day or two? Do you just throw away everything in the refrigerator, no matter what? What a waste that would be! But how do you know what's safe to eat and what isn't?

If the foods in your freezer still have ice crystals in them and are cooler than 40°F, it's perfectly fine to refreeze them. Some foods, such as fish, eggs, cheese, fruit, vegetables, and bread dough, while safe to refreeze, may lose some flavor. And no matter how short a time it's been warm, never refreeze ice cream.

If the foods in your refrigerator have been kept at a temperature lower than 40°F or if they've been held above 40°F for less than two hours, they will be fine to use. However, you should discard any food that's been held above 40°F for more than two hours.

closed, the food inside will stay frozen for up to 48 hours—if your freezer is fully loaded. In a half-full freezer, food will stay frozen up to 24 hours. So what are you waiting for? Load up that freezer!

Home Fire Safety

Here's one nobody wants to think about: fire. But I'm here to tell you that having a plan could save your life. So let's keep this short and sweet.

◆ HAVE A PLAN

You need to have a home fire-safety plan, even if it's just you and your spouse. Practice your plan from every room in your house. A good way to do this is with your eyes closed, feeling your way out. Learn to stay low to the ground, too, where there's more oxygen. Your plan should include a familiar place to meet after everyone gets out. This is especially important if you've got kids.

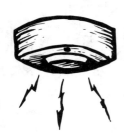

◆ THERE'S NO EXCUSE

You need to have at least one smoke detector in your home. At the very least. Why not one in every room? They're certainly cheap enough. And be sure to check the batteries at least once a year. A good way to remember this is to time your battery check for daylight saving time. When you turn your clocks back or ahead, replace your smoke detector batteries, too.

◆ DOWN AND OUT

Get yourself an approved escape ladder if your home has more than one story. And what good is it if you don't know how to use it? So practice using it! The first time you use it should *not* be during a fire.

CHAPTER 2

Spic and Span

I hate to clean! Now, maybe you're surprised to hear that from me, especially considering that I've written an entire chapter about the subject of cleaning. Well, that's the whole point. Everybody has to do *some* cleaning around the house, and since I dislike it so much, I decided to figure out the most efficient way to do it so that I could spend as little time as possible on it!

Lucky for me, I learned the ins and outs of it from Grandma Putt from the time I was a kid. She was an expert at cleaning, and a lot of what I know about it I learned from her, especially how to clean well without damaging the environment with harsh chemicals.

There was one important difference between Grandma Putt and me. You see, she loved to clean. Her house was always spotless, and she took great joy in tidying up a room, making her windows sparkle, and basking in the glow of the compliments she inevitably got from friends, family, and visitors about how neat her home was.

One thing about Grandma Putt's cleaning style was her cleaning credo: "Prevention is the best cure." She rarely spent a whole day cleaning; rather, she did a little bit every day. And almost every time she walked through a room, she did something to spruce it up. For instance, she'd pick up a book from a table and put it back on a shelf (she couldn't tolerate clutter), or she'd fluff the pillows on her sofa, or dust off the telephone as she walked by it.

Since I've learned so much about cleaning from Grandma Putt, I thought I'd pass what I know on to you so that you, too, can spend less time cleaning!

Cleaning Day to Day

Of course, I don't clean the same way every day that I do during spring cleaning (see "A Guide to Spring Cleaning" at right), but every day there are cleaning jobs to tackle. Here are some of my favorite methods and solutions for those daily chores.

Floors

We stand on them, we sit on them, we even put our furniture on them—what would we do without floors? And as long as we have floors, they need to be cleaned. How you go about doing that depends on what they're made of and what's covering them.

◆ GROOM YOUR BROOM

Grandma Putt had a trick for making a new natural-bristle broom last longer. Before she used the broom for the first time, she'd soak the bristles in hot salt water for half an hour; then she'd shake them out and let them dry thoroughly. She said it made the bristles tougher, and by golly, it did!

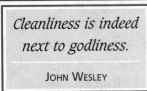

Cleanliness is indeed next to godliness.

JOHN WESLEY

◆ WALK OFF DIRT

Here's an old trick to cut down on cleaning carpets and floors, especially the areas near an entryway. Use walk-off mats before and after each entrance. For maximum effect, the mats should be at least four strides long. The idea is that you "walk off" the dirt from your shoes before you enter the room.

◆ RAG TIME

As much as I like to reuse old rags for cleaning, I sure can be fussy. I have my requirements. For me, the perfect cleaning

A Guide to Spring Cleaning

Like I said, Grandma Putt really looked forward to the month of April. Not only was that when robin red-breast returned, but Grandma's whole house also got a good going-over. Are you a little intimidated by the idea of cleaning your entire home, soup to nuts, top to bottom, all at once? Don't be. I'm here to give you a helping hand.

When it's time for spring cleaning in our house, I make a list of what needs to get done in each room and in what (general) order. That lets me keep track of what I've already finished, and what yet needs to be done—I'd hate like heck to miss something, or worse, do it twice (that means less time for napping!). Spring is also when I do all the bigger jobs that don't get done every week or every month during the rest of the year. My list looks something like this:

☑ Open all the windows and let in some fresh air.

☑ Remove books from shelves; dust and reorganize books and knickknacks.

☑ Reorganize drawers; get rid of any stuff I don't use anymore.

☑ Remove clutter; decide what's trash and what goes to the Salvation Army.

☑ Dust furniture—from top to bottom and underneath, too. If you use those dryer sheets they sell with built-in fabric softener, then you already have fantastic dusting cloths. After you use them in the dryer, store them in a box or drawer. Then whenever you dust, reach

for one. They pick up dust very well and it's always better to reuse something instead of just throwing it away.

☑ Dust entire rooms (on top of doors, around molding, and inside lamp shades, too).

☑ Wipe down and polish all woodwork.

☑ Vacuum rugs (don't forget to move the furniture!).

☑ Vacuum upholstered furniture; flip and fluff cushions.

☑ Wash all walls, windows, and any picture glass.

☑ Clean curtains.

☑ Wash floors and carpeting, if it's necessary.

Now, like I said, my zest for cleaning isn't as powerful as Grandma Putt's—she had all her spring cleaning done in about a week. So that I don't drive myself (and my family) crazy, I stretch out these chores over the course of a month, doing a room or two every weekend. That way, no one feels like a slave to cleaning, but the job still gets done. To make the atmosphere more fun, I like to put on some swing music. I tell you, nothing gets me ready for cleaning like Glen Miller's "In the Mood"!

How Much is Enough?

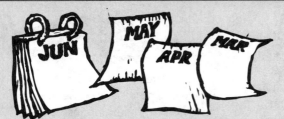

Do you know anyone who vacuums her home every single day? I sure do. Does *my* home get vacuumed every day? Not on your life! So how much vacuuming is enough to have a clean house? Although that decision is up to you, here are some general guidelines to help you decide when to do what household jobs.

DAILY OR WEEKLY

☑ Change kitty litter

☑ Clean bathroom and kitchen

☑ Clean mirrors

☑ Dust

☑ General tidying up

☑ Vacuum

WEEKLY

☑ Change bed linens

☑ Wipe down furniture

MONTHLY

☑ Thoroughly clean each room

☑ Wash/mop floors

☑ Wash windows

SEASONALLY (EVERY THREE MONTHS OR SO)

☑ Defrost refrigerator

☑ Wash and wax floors

ANNUALLY

☑ Shampoo carpets/rugs

☑ Spring Cleaning (see "A Guide to Spring Cleaning" on page 43)

cloth is made of cotton. Synthetic materials just aren't absorbent enough and, generally, can't be bleached. And while cotton is nice and soft, synthetics can be scratchy.

My favorite source for cleaning rags are terry cloth towels and bathrobes. Other good sources are sheets and pillowcases. Synthetic rags are great for disposable chores like wiping up paint spills, but for cleaning, dusting, and polishing, give me a nice, soft cotton cloth every time.

◆ A SQUARE DEAL

Whenever possible, I cut my cleaning cloths into 12-inch squares. And when I use them, I don't just ball them up in my hand—I fold them in half, and in half again, and in half one more time, leaving an exposed side that's 3-by-6 inches. This way, I can unfold the cloth as each side gets dirty, and I get 16 clean sides per cloth!

◆ STABLE SWABBING

One of the hazards of mopping the floor is that every so often someone, including the mopper, knocks into the bucket, spilling some or all of the cleaning solution out on the floor. If this happens to you more often than you'd like to admit, you may want to switch to my favorite kind of bucket—a square one.

I prefer square buckets to round ones because they're much harder to tip over. Other advantages to square buckets are that it's easier to pour out of them; a rectangular mop head will fit inside more readily; and if I need to clean higher up, like around the top of a window, the bucket will be more stable on a ladder platform.

◆ BRIGHT BUCKETS ARE BEST

Besides stability, another thing I look for in the perfect bucket is visibility. Go for a brightly colored one, and no one will accidentally knock it over because they couldn't see it, or slip on a wet floor because they didn't know you were mopping!

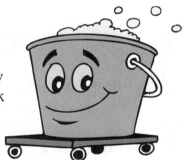

◆ LINOLEUM 101

Back in Grandma's (and Great-Grandma's) day, folks used linoleum to cover just about every floor in the house. In fact, many of the wooden floors that people today spend so much time and effort sanding and refinishing were never meant to be seen in the first place—they were always covered with at least one layer of linoleum.

True linoleum was made of ground-up cork and wood dust, mixed with pigments and a binding agent such as linseed oil, all attached to a canvas or felt backing, and cut into sheets and squares. You see very little linoleum today; it's been mostly

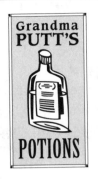

Floor, Sweet Floor

Grandma Putt used a secret formula to freshen the linoleum floor in her kitchen, and the secret was in her kitchen cupboard. Once a month, she'd mix a half-cup of apple cider vinegar into a gallon of warm water, and mop the floor with the solution. This stuff cut right through the grease—and left the room smelling sweet, too.

replaced by more durable and less expensive vinyl floor covering.

If you do have genuine linoleum, you need to give it special treatment on cleaning day. Linoleum is damaged by very hot water and strong detergents like ammonia. They cause the binding materials to dissolve. So when cleaning linoleum floors, use lukewarm water instead, and don't let it sit on the floor too long before mopping it up.

◆ SOAP AND STONE DON'T MIX

While good old-fashioned soap is good enough for just about any cleaning problem, once in a while you come across something like a stone floor, where ordinary soap just won't do. It's not that it won't clean the floor, but soap will leave a residue that won't wash away easily, and the floor will look kind of dull.

To clean stone floors, I like to use a mild detergent, like dishwashing detergent, mixed in hot water. About a teaspoon to a gallon is all you need to do the trick. Mop the floor once with this solution, and once with clear water.

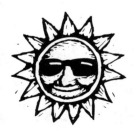

◆ SPONGE ON THE SHINE

To revive the natural shine on your stone floor, apply a little lemon oil (available at the hardware store) to the floor with a sponge or applicator mop. Wipe off the excess oil with an old towel, and buff to a nice shine.

◆ GO EASY ON THE VINYL

The key to maintaining a vinyl floor is to clean it quickly and frequently. While vinyl floor covering is pretty low maintenance, it's not maintenance free. All it requires is regular sweeping and damp mopping with a mild detergent, as well as a monthly application of a self-stripping, water-based sealer when the floor starts to look dull.

If you don't sweep regularly, the dirt and dust that builds up underfoot will quickly erode the factory finish on the flooring, which in turn makes it harder to get it clean with light mopping. The same thing happens if you use a strong detergent or very hot water. And once a vinyl floor has lost its factory finish, it's hard to keep it looking good.

◆ WOODEN YOU KNOW IT

If your finished wood floor has lost its luster, try this fantastic formula for perking up the shine. In an old pump-spray bottle, mix a solution of vegetable oil and white vinegar in equal amounts; about a pint of each, thoroughly mixed, should cover two 11-by-14-foot floors. Apply a thin mist to the floor, and rub it in well using cotton rags or a wax applicator you can get from the hardware store. Remove the excess with clean cotton rags, and buff to a shine.

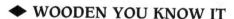

◆ GET BUFFED

Don't have a buffer for your wood floors? My favorite method these days is wrapping an old cotton towel around the bottom of a dry mop, and using that to buff my floors. When I was younger, I'd put on a few pairs of old cotton socks, and "skate" up and down the lengths of the floor boards, with the grain. A word of warning, however, if you try this method—watch out for splinters!

Keep Your Cleaners Clean

You wouldn't paint your walls with an old, paint-encrusted brush or roller, would you? Just the same, we often use an old mop or dirty broom to "clean" our homes with. Here are a few ways to keep those tools of the cleaning trade in tip-top shape.

Give it the clean sweep. Brooms don't just push the dirt around, they pick some up, too. And if yours isn't cleaned every so often, it'll deposit the dust someplace else in your home. To help keep your old broom sweeping clean, swish the tips of the bristles in a bucket of warm water mixed with a tablespoon or two of detergent, then shake it out as you would a paintbrush. Hang the broom up so that the bristles aren't touching the floor, and let it thoroughly dry.

Buck(et) the trend. Once you're done using your bucket, it's important to empty it out and clean it with a little disinfectant such as bleach, rubbing alcohol, or a pine oil cleaner made from 20 to 30 percent natural pine oil—but never, ever use a combination of those solutions. Damp, dirty buckets are breeding grounds for bacteria, which then get spread around your home, making it dirtier than when you started. Talk about one step forward and two steps back!

Cloth to perfect. Found a good cleaning rag that is just the right size and texture? You'll get more use out of it if you throw it in the laundry after a week's worth of cleaning. And don't forget to fully dry it in the clothes dryer so that it will be at its absorbent best.

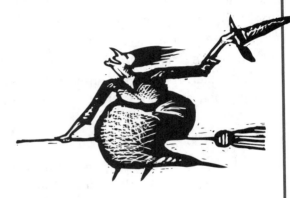

Dusty rides again. I remember one of my earliest chores as a young boy was to shake out the dust mop. If you're not lucky enough to live in a place where you can give your dust mop a good shaking in the great outdoors without disturbing the neighbors, give your dust mop head a going-over with the vacuum. When your mop gets especially grungy, wash it in the washing machine with a small amount of bleach and detergent. Once it's dry, treat it with a commercial product like Endust, or lightly mist it with a homemade solution made of two parts white vinegar and one part vegetable oil. Allow the mop head time to absorb the oil solution before using it, or instead of collecting dust, you'll be spreading oil!

Love those mop tops. Not the Beatles—we're talking about non-sponge mop heads here. At the very least, make sure to rinse and ring out the mop when you're done. Just because you were mopping with disinfectant cleaner doesn't mean that the mop is disinfected. For a more thorough cleaning, put the mop head inside an old pillowcase or mesh bag, and wash it in your clothes washer without bleach. A good-quality mop head will last a long time if it's cleaned regularly this way. Always hang the mop head out to dry so that the air can circulate through the string or fabric strips.

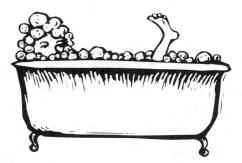

Soak it in. Rinse and ring out the head of a sponge mop in warm water with a little detergent mixed in after every use. Don't use hot water or bleach, or you'll break the sponge in half over time. Cleaning the head completely is especially important if your sponge mop does double duty as a floor wax applica-tor. Once that stuff dries on the mop, it's a lot harder to remove it, and the waxy buildup interferes with the sponge's ability to absorb.

Suck it up. Of course, you know that the vacuum bag needs to be changed regularly. But that's not all you need to do to keep the clean machine clean. When it comes time to change the bag, take a minute or two to check the beater bar (with the vacuum unplugged, of course) to make sure that nothing's caught in it. Then, run an old comb through the bristles to remove accumulated string and/or hair. If you've been doing some heavy-duty cleaning with the vacuum cleaner's attachments, clean those as well. Soak the attachments in a bucket of warm water mixed with a little detergent. Shake out the brush attachments, and make sure they're totally dry before you use them again or store them.

Running wet and dry. After using a wet/dry vacuum to clean up a particularly bad mess like the one left by a toilet that overflowed, run a bucketful of warm water and disinfectant detergent through the machine. Empty the reservoir, and give it a few moments to air out before storing it away.

Carpets and Rugs

When some folks hear the words cleaning and carpet in the same sentence, it conjures up the image in their minds of sweeping dirt *under* the carpet! But carpets themselves need cleaning every so often, too. Whether it's a quick vacuuming before the guests arrive, or taking care of a spill after they leave, you need to know what to do and when to do it.

Before you try any kind of cleaning solution on your rug or carpeting, *always* test the formula on an inconspicuous area, such as a dark corner or under the sofa, before you set to work. This little piece of advice will save you much heartache in the long run.

◆ OIL'S WELL THAT ENDS WELL

If your bottle of oil turned into a gusher and spilled on the rug, you need something to absorb it quickly before it has a chance to sink in and permanently stain. Sprinkle some baking soda or cornstarch on the stain to absorb the greasy mess. Let it dry, and then vacuum up the residue.

◆ A CLOSE SHAVE

If you drop your dinner on the dining room carpet, it's nice to have a man around...as long as he uses shaving cream. Borrow some from his toiletry bag and spray just enough of the foamy stuff on the area to cover the stain. Let it soak in for a few minutes, and then blot it up with a sponge dampened in cold water or seltzer. Shaving cream works especially well on food spills.

◆ YOU DON'T NEED TO BE A GUM SHOE

You can get gum out of a carpet by freezing it with an ice cube. Once the gum is hard, it'll be easier to remove by scraping it out with a putty knife or hard plastic spatula. You may need to reapply the ice every so often to keep the gum hard while you're working on it.

◆ SALT 'N' SOOT

Here's an old-time cure for taking soot and ash stains out of a hearth rug: rub salt and a little all-purpose household soap into the stain, and then rinse it clean with water.

◆ WOOF...OOPS

Even the perfect pet can make a mistake. Here's the expert's way to clean pet poop (but not urine) from carpeting. First, remove as much of the solids as you possibly can. Then wash the soiled area with a mild detergent solution (½ teaspoon of mild dishwashing detergent to 1 cup of water). Wash it again with a mild ammonia solution (½ teaspoon of ammonia to 1 cup of water). Wash the area a third time with equal parts white vinegar and water. (Test this treatment first because the vinegar might bleach some carpet dyes.) Flush the spot with warm water, and blot with a clean cloth or paper towels.

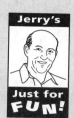

Don't Try This at Home

In 1898, H. Cecil Booth, the future inventor of the vacuum cleaner, was inspired by an exhibition of a "dust removing" machine that blew air into a carpet in order to remove the dust. Recognizing soon afterwards that there was probably a better way to accomplish the task, he tested his theory of sucking the dirt out by putting his mouth on the back of a plush chair in a restaurant, and inhaling as hard as he could. I don't suppose there was a line of women waiting to kiss him afterwards, do you?

◆ IN CASE OF A CAT-TASTROPHE

Don't use ammonia to clean pet urine, especially if the carpet was "sprayed" by a male cat marking his territory. The lingering ammonia scent (and I guarantee you that kitty will still be able to notice it, long after you think it's gone) will resemble the urine odor, telling him it's OK to have another go at that spot. And that's the last thing you want!

Instead, use a detergent that lists enzymes in its list of ingredients. Once the stain has been cleaned, spray the area with a commercial product like Nature's Miracle (available at most pet stores) that's specifically designed to neutralize the odor.

Upholstery

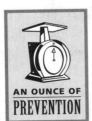

Here are some ways to keep Aunt Mabel's 75-year-old antique sofa (and your brand-new club chair) looking beautiful.

◆ UN-ZIP AT YOUR PERIL

If you're like me, you probably think the zippers on the backs of sofa cushions are so you can take the upholstery off the foam padding and clean it in the washer. Well, I found out the hard way that they're not!

If you launder sofa and chair cushion covers in a washing machine, you're only asking for trouble. The zippers and the rest of the fabric dry differently, and that may cause wrinkles. If you get a stain on your sofa or seat cushion, spot-treat the stain, and if that doesn't work, let your fingers do the walking and call in the professionals.

Antimacassars Revisited?

AN OUNCE OF PREVENTION

If you find that the top of your sofa gets soiled because of mousse, gels, sprays, and heaven knows what else people put in their hair these days, borrow an idea from the 1850s. Drape a matching fabric over the back (and arms) of your favorite sofa or chair. When it gets dirty, just wash it with the rest of the laundry. Grandma knew this handy item as an antimacassar, so-named because it protected her sofa from Macassar, a popular hair pomade way back when.

◆ RUB 'EM OUT

Got a smudge on the upholstery? Take a trip to the art-supply store. A rubber eraser, either the soft white rubber or the crumbly, gum kind (but not the pink kind—it'll leave a pink smear) will erase some stains like pencil marks and fingerprints from light-colored fabrics.

◆ SLICK STAIN FIGHTERS

Before a grease or oil stain has a chance to really soak into your upholstery, apply a poultice to soak it out. A poultice is an absorbent material that, when applied to a fresh

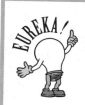

Mayonnaise Rub

You know those white rings left on the furniture by a hot mug or wet dish? Well, you can make them disappear with a little bit of mayo. Put a dab of mayonnaise on a cloth and work it into the ring, then immediately remove the excess. That'll do the trick!

stain, draws out the oil so that it can be brushed away, stain and all. Here are some of my all-time favorites:

Cornmeal. If the upholstery is light colored, use a light-colored absorbent material like cornmeal. Put enough on to cover the stain, and let it sit for a half-hour or so. After that, vacuum or brush the cornmeal away. You may need to dab the remaining stain with a little mild detergent solution.

Cornstarch and talcum powder. These finer-textured absorbents work as well as cornmeal at removing stains, but can be harder to remove from some upholstery. After you've let it sit on the stain for at least a half-hour, use your vacuum with the upholstery brush attachment to get it all up.

Fuller's earth. If the upholstery is dark colored, take a trip to your local pharmacy or hardware store, and buy some Fuller's earth. This is a natural clay product that is used in the manufacturing of fabrics. Apply it in the same way as the cornmeal. If you can't find Fuller's earth, try plain, unscented clay (not clumping) cat litter, ground to a rough powder.

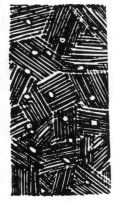

Walls

Don't climb them; clean them! It's easy if you know how. My number one tip? Don't wash your walls until the rest of the room has been dusted and vacuumed. That'll keep the flying dust from clinging to your nice, clean walls.

◆ LOOK MA, TWO HANDS!

For the cleanest walls in the west—not to mention the north, south, and east—try my two-hand, two-bucket system. Most walls, whether they're painted or covered with wallpaper, can be cleaned with this method. Before you begin, make sure to dust the walls. Here's what you'll need:

- ✔ 2 buckets
- ✔ 1 large clean sponge
- ✔ Mild dish detergent
- ✔ A few large clean cotton rags or towels
- ✔ A stepladder

1. Squeeze 2 teaspoons of detergent (a couple of squirts) into one of the buckets. Fill it ¾ full with warm water. Leave the other bucket empty.

2. Hold the sponge in one hand. Hold one of the cotton rags in your other hand, or tuck it into your back pocket or belt. Dip the face of the sponge (but not the whole sponge) in the sudsy water. Don't soak the sponge or the water will roll down the wall and your arm.

3. Starting at a top corner of the wall, work in an area as large as you can reach without straining—about three or four square feet—and wipe down the wall. Squeeze out the sponge into the empty bucket, and rewipe the same area on the wall. Then wipe down the same area one more time with the cotton rag or towel.

4. Move on to the next area, repeating step 3. If the cloth gets too wet or soiled, switch to another one. After a few tries, you'll get into a rhythm, and the entire wall will go quickly.

◆ CRAYON? SPRAY OFF

Did your little artist get carried away on your vinyl wall covering? Spray a little silicone-based lubricant on a rag, and use it to wipe away crayon marks.

◆ POWERFUL POWDER FOR DELICATE CLEANING

Painted walls and some wallpapers may be too delicate for some strong cleaners. If that's the case, make a paste of baking powder and water, erring toward the dry side. Apply this gentle cleaner with a clean sponge to remove smudges and stains like food splatters and handprints.

Just the Stuff for Scuffs

If the back of your chair leaves a scuff on the wall, here's a couple of tricks you can try to remove the mark:

☞ Scrub the mark with toothpaste (not the gel kind.) It'll work even better if you use an old, clean toothbrush.

☞ Erase it out. A rubber eraser, either the soft white rubber or the crumbly, gum kind, will erase most scuffs without hurting the paint or paper. Don't try this with the pink kind, or any other colored eraser because it may leave a new stain on the wall. You can pick up a good eraser at any stationery or art-supply store.

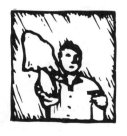

Windows

On a clear day, you can see forever. But through a dirty window, you can't even see across the street! Get a better view with these tips.

◆ SQUEEGEE: THE OLD PRO'S WAY

The most thorough way, by far, to clean a window is with a squeegee. This tool with the funny-sounding name is a T-shaped bar with a sponge on one side and a rubber blade on the other. It's often attached to a wooden handle, or can be screwed onto a broomstick for those extra-high areas. You can buy one at any good hardware or janitorial supply store.

Many folks today avoid squeegees because they think they're too messy to use or require special skill. But if you follow these instructions, your windows will be cleaner than ever. (Besides the squeegee, you'll need a bucket and a damp rag.)

1. Mix up a batch of your favorite window-cleaning solution, or put a couple of squirts of mild dish detergent in a gallon of hot water.

2. Dip the sponge side of the squeegee into the solution, just enough to wet the sponge. Wet the entire surface of the window, and then wipe it again with the sponge to dislodge any stubborn, stuck-on dirt. Wipe around the edge of the window one more time to get any dirt you pushed to the sides. Now it's time to put the the rubber blade into action to remove the water and dirt.

3. First, wipe the blade with the damp cloth to lubricate it so it'll glide along the window's surface. Begin at the top of the window, and draw the blade horizontally across the glass, applying light, even pressure. Wipe the blade with the rag, and go back to the top. This time draw the blade down vertically, starting in the dry area. Wipe the blade again. Work from one side to the next, overlapping the strokes, and wiping the blade in between. Finish by wiping the bottom of the sill with the damp cloth.

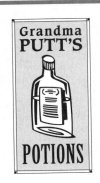

Window Wash

When it was time to wash windows, Grandma Putt mixed up a batch of cleaner made from a quart of warm water combined with ½ cup of white vinegar and 2 tablespoons of fresh or bottled lemon juice. It worked like a charm every time!

4. For large picture windows, split the job in two sections, cleaning the upper half first.

◆ IT MAY SOUND CORNY, BUT...

If there's a smoker in the house or you prepare a lot of fried foods in the kitchen, your windows probably need a little extra effort, and you can't rely on detergent alone to get them clean. Mix some cornstarch in with the ammonia and water to clean especially grimy windows. The cornstarch acts as a mild abrasive. Rinse with clear water.

◆ EXTRA, EXTRA!

My Grandma Putt knew what she was doing when she used crumbled-up newspapers to clean her windows. She knew it gave them a sparkle, but she probably didn't really know why. Well, here's why: By crunching up the paper, you create lots of edges to scrape the dirt off, and newsprint is pretty absorbent, too, so it does a good job of removing whatever cleaning solution you choose to apply. Best of all, newsprint is lint-free.

◆ NOW WHERE'S THAT STREAK?

Wipe windows up and down on one side of the glass, and left to right on the other in order to see streaks and missed spots. Then you'll know which side you need to redo.

◆ IT'S THE AUTO-MATIC CHOICE

If you insist on using a commercial product to clean your windows, consider using windshield washer fluid. It's available at any auto supply store, is sold in large quantities, is inexpensive, and you can pour it into an old spray bottle for easier application. You can't beat that!

◆ GIVE YOUR WINDOWSILL A RUBDOWN

Windowsills can get really grimy from all of the fingerprints and dirt that blows in from outside when the windows are open. Sometimes using detergent and water isn't enough to keep them clean. Try cleaning the sill with a cloth dipped in rubbing alcohol before you use the detergent. The alcohol should dissolve the dirt enough for the detergent to get down and do its thing.

In the Kitchen

With all the cooking that goes on in my favorite room of the house, the kitchen sure does get grimy. And it's not just the countertops that get yucky. Check inside the refrigerator, and you're bound to find some sticky puddle of something or other on the bottom shelf, or some leftover smelly food that looks like a science experiment gone awry. Here's how to take on those jobs and more.

Cleaning Your Appliances

Harsh chemicals to clean your appliances? Not on your life! Here are some of my (and Grandma Putt's) favorite earth-friendly methods.

◆ BAKING SODA TO THE RESCUE!

Here's a word you've heard a lot from me (well, really two words): baking soda. It's the all-time cleaning miracle substance. For appliances like your refrigerator or your stovetop, dampen a sponge with hot water, and sprinkle some baking soda on the sponge or right onto the appliance. Baking soda is a terrific, non-abrasive cleanser that will remove grease and grime of all sorts. And best of all, it doesn't harm the environment one iota.

◆ SPIT 'N' VINEGAR

Well, maybe not the spit, but the vinegar sure works well. If you're out of baking soda and you want to wipe the grime off your appliances, mix up a solution of hot water and vinegar; about 2 tablespoons of vinegar to 3 cups of hot water ought to do the trick. (I generally don't measure these things!) Dunk your sponge in that solution and wipe down the kitchen—it'll sparkle like new!

◆ A SALTY SOLUTION

You know when you make a cheesy casserole or a bubbly apple pie (say, that sounds good right about now!) in your oven and the filling drips all over the inside? Well, don't you dare reach for that caustic oven cleaner. It's not good for you or good ol' Mother Earth. Instead, do what I do—reach for the salt to get those baked-on nasties out of your oven.

First, I try not to even get those gooey problems started. Before anything goes into the oven, I line the racks with some aluminum foil. Then, if there's a leak, I just change the foil.

If some stuff does find its way to the inside of my oven, I attack it before it has a chance to harden. While the oven is still hot, I get out my trusty old saltshaker, and pour some on the spill. Then I just let the oven cool off; when it's cold, I take a rubber spatula or a scouring pad to it and the stain crumbles right off.

If the stain has already cooled and hardened, first I yell at whoever didn't put foil on the rack (it doesn't do much good, but it really makes me feel better). Then I dampen the stain with some water,

That's Good Coffee!

There's nothing better than a fresh cup of coffee. But if your cup's starting to taste stale or bitter, it's time to give the coffeemaker a good cleaning. Here's how to do it:

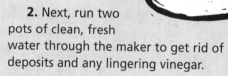

1. Fill the pot with a solution of one part white vinegar to one part water, and run that through the coffeemaker.

2. Next, run two pots of clean, fresh water through the maker to get rid of deposits and any lingering vinegar.

3. Do this every month or so, and you'll always be treated to deeelicious coffee!

add the salt, and scrub like crazy. Salt is a terrific, but gentle, scouring agent.

◆ INSIDE THE FRIDGE

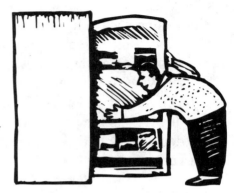

Uh oh, what's growing on in there? Now, I hate waste, so there usually aren't any left-overs in my refrigerator, but that doesn't mean mine does-n't need to be cleaned. Once a month or so, I fill a small bucket with hot water, add a half cup of vinegar, and give the inside a good going-over. The vinegar cleans and freshens it right up.

Then I get a plastic bowl, fill it with some baking soda, and put that in the back to absorb odors—but you knew that old trick, right? Don't forget to replace it every two months or so.

◆ IS YOUR STAINLESS NOT STAINLESS?

Is your toaster stainless steel? How about your breadbox? (Well, I still have a breadbox; I don't know about you!) How about your sink? Its fixtures? Here's my secret for keeping stainless from streaking and to remove stains: club soda! Yep, instead of drinking it, I pour some on a sponge, and rub it all over my stainless steel appliances. Then I buff them dry with a clean rag. They shine like new! To keep them shiny, finish up with a little car polish.

Of course, white vinegar works, too. I keep a little plastic spray bottle of it under the sink. Then when I've finished with the dishes, I spray it in the sink to shine it up.

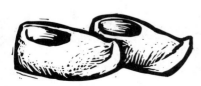

◆ DO A CLOG DANCE

Remember Grandma Putt's favorite cleaning adage: Prevention is the best cure. My kitchen sink almost never gets clogged and that's because every morning after I make my cup of tea, I pour the rest of the boiling water right down the drain. The hot water safely dissolves any oil or grease buildup in the drain, which prevents most clogs.

Also, I keep a drain basket in my sink at all times. Of course, that keeps anything but water from going down my drain. When I do get a clog, I try everything I can think of before using caustic drain cleaners. My favorite method is to pour about ⅔ of a cup of baking soda right into the drain. I follow that with about the same amount of white vinegar, and then I cover the drain with a bowl or a plate. While that mixture is doing its thing, I put a kettle of water on to boil. Once the water is boiling, I uncover the drain and pour the water down. The bubbling action of the vinegar and baking soda dissolves many clogs, and the boiling water usually gets the rest of the gunk down there.

One word of warning: *Never, never, never* use this method after you've used a commercial drain cleaner!

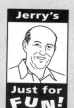

Good Help Was Hard to Find

In 1886, Josephine Cochrane, the wife of an Illinois politician—and a clever, wealthy woman— got tired of the fumble-fingered household help breaking her expensive dishes after formal dinners. "If no one else is going to invent a dish-washing machine, I'll do it myself," she declared. And she did, winning awards at the 1893 Chicago World's Fair for her invention. Unfortunately for her, the average housewife of the late 1890s and early 1900s did not regard dishwashing with the same disdain as did the socialite. So the idea of an automatic dishwasher wouldn't become popular until the 1950s.

Cleaning Pots and Pans

Looking for a way to shine up that copper pot? Or a surefire method for seasoning your cast-iron skillet? Well, you've come to the right place! Heck, I even have a way to shine up silverware.

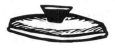
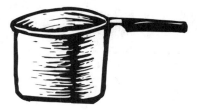

◆ 'TIS THE SEASON

Cast iron is my all-time favorite cooking medium. A cast-iron pan will last forever if you treat it right, and you can get the

Honest, I Meant Well

When I first went to stay with my Grandma Putt, I wanted to make a good impression. So I was always on the lookout for ways to be a "good boy". One day, I was in the kitchen looking for a snack when I noticed a big, old cast-iron skillet. It was absolutely filthy (I thought), blackened with years of use. I thought I'd found a perfect way to impress Grandma, so I set about scrubbing that skillet clean with a steel pad and lots and lots of soap.

Little did I know that "filthy" black skillet was a wedding gift to my Grandma many decades before, and it had taken her all that time to get the skillet seasoned so well. Who knew that I was undoing decades of work?

Well, Grandma Putt certainly did; you should have seen the look on her face when I marched out to the garden to show off my handiwork. When I think back on it now, she probably wanted to clobber me, but she didn't. All she did was take the time to very patiently explain what seasoning cast iron was all about. Then we went back into the kitchen, and re-oiled and baked that old skillet. All I can say is that it's a darn good thing that I was so cute!

pan good and hot without worrying about damaging it. And did you know that when you cook in cast iron, you're getting some of your daily dose of iron? That's right, some of the iron actually gets into the food and makes your meal better for you.

Before you can cook with a new cast-iron pan, though, you'll need to season it. That's a way of treating the pan to give it a non-stick surface and to keep it from rusting. Here's what to do:

1. First, wash and dry the pan in warm soapy water. Dry it very well. (I do that by putting the pan on the stovetop on low heat for a couple of minutes.) You really need to make sure the pan's absolutely, positively dry.

2. Next, I preheat my oven to 300°F and, using a paper towel, I coat the inside of the skillet with peanut oil. Then I pop it into the oven for a whole hour. When the hour's up, I take the pan out of the oven and wipe off any excess oil. *Caution:* It'll be hot, so wear an oven mitt.

3. After you cook in a seasoned cast-iron pan, never scrub it with scouring powder or a metal scouring pad. The best way to clean it out is with some hot water, then wipe it dry. I dry mine on the stovetop just to make sure.

Your pan will turn black over time, but that's good! That's what keeps food from sticking, so don't get the crazies and scrub it clean. If you get some stubborn cooked-on food in the pan, add a little water and put the pan on the stovetop. Bring the water to a boil, and use a plastic (not a metal!) spatula to remove the food.

◆ YOU DIRTY COPPER, YOU!

Copper is the best material for pots and pans because it conducts heat so well. Of course, it's also the most expensive and requires lots of care, so not many of us have copper cookware. More common are pots and pans that have a thin coating of copper on the bottom. It's also common for that copper to get really dingy and tarnished. Here's how Grandma Putt kept her copper clean.

She'd mix up some lemon juice and cream of tartar to make a thick paste. Then she rubbed it onto the copper with her fingers, and let it sit for about 10 minutes. When she wiped the paste off and washed the bottom, it shone like crazy. A quick buff with a rag added the final, finishing touch.

◆ SHINE ON

Grandma Putt had a great potion for cleaning the inside of discolored aluminum pots. She'd mix up a solution of one tablespoon of vinegar and one quart of water, and pour it into the pot. Then she'd heat the concoction for a few minutes on a low flame. Before you knew it, the pot was as shiny as new.

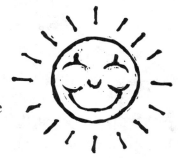

◆ SILVER ME TIMBERS!

One of the luxuries I enjoyed when I was growing up was real silverware, and even today, I still love to eat with it. It's so nice and heavy, and feels so good in your hands. Silver makes every meal feel special!

What's not luxurious about silverware is having to keep it

Don't Keep It Bottled Up

If you have a long-necked bottle with shoulders that you need to clean, don't drive yourself crazy looking for a bottle brush. Here's how to tackle this challenging cleaning problem with no muss and no fuss. All you'll need is a scrubby pad and a metal clothes hanger. Put some water and a little soap into the bottle, and then stuff the scrubby pad inside, too. Then bend the top of the hanger so it's straight, and use it to push the pad around the bottom and the shoulder to get the bottle clean. You can even put a little salt or uncooked rice into the bottle to act as a mild scouring agent.

polished. But it doesn't have to be too much of a job. Grandma Putt always wore cotton gloves when she polished her silver; I later figured out that if I wore rubber gloves, the silver tarnished more quickly. And she never used silver polish. You guessed it— she used baking soda. In a bowl, she'd put about a cup of baking soda, and then added enough water to make a thin paste. Then we'd set up an assembly line: I'd rub the silver with the paste, rinse it off, and pass it to Grandma, who'd buff it with a soft cotton cloth.

I loved silver-polishing day because that was one of the times that we'd spend the afternoon together talking and having fun.

In the Bathroom

We may not spend as much time in the bathroom as in the kitchen or bedroom, but by gum, the time we do spend there is quality time. So why not make that room as clean as the rest of your house? Here are some ideas to help you cope with the tough cleaning jobs you'll find in the bathroom.

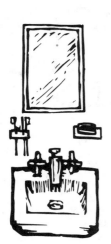

Cleaning Sinks and Tubs

Before you buy a truckload of bathroom cleaners, check out these tried-and-true homemade formulas for keeping sinks and tubs sparkling clean.

◆ JUST BLEACHY

The ring that shows the high water mark in your tub and sink can sure be tough to get rid of, even with a lot of added elbow grease. If scrubbing doesn't seem to work, try soaking. Soak white rags, such as old sheets, or paper towels in household bleach and lay them on the ring. Let them sit for one-half to one hour, then rinse to your heart's content. The rags keep the bleach in place on the stain, instead of letting it all run down the drain.

◆ START FROM SCRATCH

If your store-bought scratchless scrub powder doesn't quite do the trick on tough stains, give it a boost with something from the medicine chest. Make a paste out of the cleanser and some fresh hydrogen peroxide (make sure the date on the bottle is recent). Add a pinch of cream of tartar to it. Leave this poultice on the stain for a half-hour, then scrub it off with a brush or kitchen pad. *Caution:* Do this only with non-chlorine scrubbing powders. Combining chlorine with any other chemical can be dangerous.

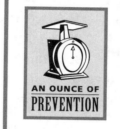

A Word to the Wise

Never, never, **NEVER** mix household ammonia with bleach. It creates very toxic fumes. So never ever do it. End of sermon.

AN OUNCE OF **PREVENTION**

◆ SHOWER SPRAY DE-MIST-IFIED

You've probably seen, and maybe even tried, those spray products that advertise "Never scrub your shower again." They actually work pretty well at controlling soap residue buildup and mildew. They work especially well if you start with a clean shower. But I have a formula for an after-shower spray made up of ingredients you already own. About the only thing you'll need to buy is a spray bottle, if you don't already have one.

In the spray bottle, mix 3 cups of water, ½ cup of rubbing alcohol, and 1 tablespoon of liquid laundry detergent, preferably one that lists enzymes in the ingredients. The last person out of the shower or bath each day sprays a mist of this concoction on all the wet surfaces—including the vinyl shower curtain liner. I won't promise that you'll never have to scrub again, but follow up once a month by wiping down the walls, and you should never see mold or mildew again.

> "Company" merges into family when clean towels are not kept in the bathroom every morning.
>
> WILLIAM ALLEN WHITE

◆ GREAT GROUT

They say that when in Rome, do as the Romans do. I say, when in the bathroom, use something from the bathroom to clean that ugly, stained grout. That's my roundabout way of telling you to save those old toothbrushes—they're the perfect-sized tool for this scrubbing job.

When it's time to clean stained grout, you could also use a little whitening toothpaste, but that could get expensive. Instead, make your own whitening paste by combining hydrogen peroxide with baking soda to make your own "scrubbing bubbles." This concoction works pretty well on your teeth, too; just remember to use a different toothbrush!

Cleaning Toilets

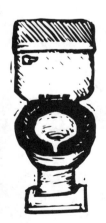

Toilets—we sure do appreciate having them around, but when it comes time for cleaning, we'd all rather be someplace else! But somebody's got to do it, and if cleaning the toilet is your job, take heart and heed my advice. I'll get you through it in no time at all!

◆ LESS TOIL TO CLEAN THE TOILET

Cleaning a toilet just sounds like a nasty job, but there's really not much to it, if you know what you're doing. First, you need the proper tool. Toilet bowl brushes are not all alike. I prefer one that has a ball-shaped head. Here's why.

When you pour cleaner into the bowl (I prefer household

bleach, but any disinfectant cleaner will do), it diluted in the water, so you need to use a lot more of it to do a thorough job. With the round brush, you can push the head down into the throat of the bowl several times, causing the

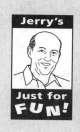
water level to go down. Now pour away, and you're cleaning at full strength. If you use bleach, make sure you remove any in-tank cleaners before you start because they may react with the bleach and release toxic fumes.

Give the inside of the bowl a scrub with the toilet brush, especially under the rim where the water enters. Use a little bleach on a cloth to wipe the seat and outside of the bowl. Do this once a week, and you'll never need to scrub hard again.

In the Laundry Room

My Grandma Putt started out doing laundry with a washboard and a hard cake of soap. Next came the wringer-type washing machine that many of us remember seeing down in our grandparent's basement or the corner of the kitchen. When you think about what a real chore laundry was way back then, it makes doing laundry today seem like a snap. But there are still some tips and tricks to make laundry chores go even faster. So the next time you head for the laundry room—whether it's to wash, dry, or iron—take these tips along with you.

If the Shoe Fits, Clean It!

One way to make your shoes last a whole heck of a lot longer is to take care of them, and part of taking care of them is keeping them clean and polished. You see, polish doesn't just make your shoes look good, it also protects them from the elements. Here's a rundown of some of the items you probably already have at home that will keep your shoes looking their best:

Art Gum Eraser. You can literally erase stains on suede with that eraser in your child's art kit. Follow up with a light rub of an emery board to bring the nap back up.

Beeswax. Rub some softened beeswax into your leather shoes (or other leather goods such as purses) to protect the leather and make it shine.

Lemon Juice. Apply a little on a soft clean cloth, rub it onto dark-colored leather shoes, and then buff lightly.

Olive oil. Rub a little olive oil onto your leather shoes to moisturize them and shine the leather.

Petroleum jelly. It does for your patent leather shoes what it does for your lips: makes them shiny and keeps them from cracking!

Wash Day

You sort by color and fabric content, you use the right detergent for the job, why you even make sure you have plenty of high-priced stain removers on hand. Well, you still may not be doing all you can to lighten your laundry load. Read on for some solid advice.

◆ SOFTER *AND* CHEAPER

Replace those expensive dryer sheets with a clean rag or sponge that has a teaspoon of liquid softener on it. Throw one in the dryer with each load.

◆ HOW SWEET IT IS

Here's a natural way to sweeten and freshen any load of laundry. Add half a cup of baking soda to the wash cycle and the same amount of white vinegar to the rinse cycle; use more if you have hard water.

◆ A SMOOTH MOVE TO TREAT GRASS STAINS

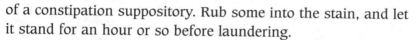

If you're like me and you do a lot of work in and around the garden, then a common wash-day problem is grass stains on the knees of your jeans. Well, I've got a great way to get rid of those tough stains, and I keep it in the medicine chest. It's called glycerin, and you may have heard of it; it's the main ingredient in many skin-softening lotions. It's also sold in pharmacies in the form of a constipation suppository. Rub some into the stain, and let it stand for an hour or so before laundering.

If you're using hand lotion, be sure it's pure glycerin; other ingredients might make the stain worse. The suppositories are 100 percent pure stuff. When you're finished treating the stain, make sure you rub some glycerin into your hands to soften your garden-tough skin.

◆ NEVER MIND THE BEEF, WHERE'S THE STAIN?

To get rid of organic, protein-based stains like milk, egg, and blood, make a paste of meat tenderizer mixed with a few drops of water. Work it into the stain, and then launder as usual. Tenderizers contain enzymes that break down proteins. If it works on a tough piece of meat, it'll work on a tough stain, too!

◆ BUBBLE AWAY STAINS

Grandma Putt always had perfect teeth, so I'm not sure where she learned this trick, but she used those effervescent denture-cleaning tablets to remove food stains from washable cloth items like aprons, napkins, and tablecloths. I guess she figured that if they could remove blueberry pie stains from false teeth, they would work like the dickens on her aprons, too. And do you know what? She was right!

To use the tablets, put the stained fabric in a container that's large enough to hold the stained portion, fill it with warm water, and drop in two of the cleaning tablets. Leave the material in the solution for the suggested time on the package, and wash it with the rest of the laundry. The stain will be gone.

◆ DON'T LET THAT STAIN SLIP IN

Did that pizza slice accidentally drip all over your lap? To stop a greasy accident from becoming a permanent stain, you need to act fast. Go into the kitchen for some baking soda, cornmeal, or cornstarch. All three are absorbents, so pick the one that's the handiest. Then sprinkle it over the stain. When it dries up, brush it off, and most of the oil will go along with it. As soon as you have the chance, launder as usual.

◆ RUST RELIEF

If you bleach a white garment and it comes out with what look like rust stains, it could be because the chlorine bleach caused iron in the water to leach out. This is a common problem in places where the water has a high mineral content—or in houses with rusty pipes. If you can't use household bleach to get your whites white, try this solution. Pretreat the rust stains with equal parts of lemon juice and water. Wash the garment again, this time without the bleach, and the stains should disappear.

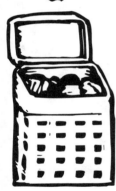

◆ THE RING CYCLE

If your dress shirts and blouses are looking kind of shabby due to the dreaded ring-around-the-collar, here are some ways to un-ring them:

☞ Rub some white blackboard chalk into the collar stain before you wash it. The chalk will absorb the oil that caused the stain.

☞ Don't know any teachers? Another way to tackle col-

Out, Out Darned Spot!

Many stains can be removed from clothing rather easily with common household products. Here are my favorite spot-busters:

Blood. Hit the stain immediately with some cold water or club soda; never use warm or hot water, which will only set the stain.

Chocolate. Well, I don't know how you managed to miss your mouth! No, don't try to do what my grandson, Zach, did and lick it off; rather, soak the garment in club soda before you wash it.

Ink. My favorite way to get rid of ink stains on clothing is to spray the spot with hair spray, and then launder the item as usual. I've always had great luck with this method. Another method is to blot the stain with rubbing alcohol.

Perspiration. Sponge the stain with a solution made up of 1 cup of water and 1 tablespoon of either white vinegar or lemon juice, and then launder the item as usual.

Soda. Soak a soda stain immediately with white vinegar, and then launder as usual.

Stains that aren't oily. For most any non-oily stain, you can use a mixture of a teaspoon of white vinegar and a teaspoon of liquid detergent mixed into 2 cups of warm water. Use a brush or sponge to apply the mixture to the stain, and then launder the garment as usual.

lar ring is to pretreat the stain with shampoo. After all, shampoos are detergents that are designed to dissolve oils.

☞ Fresh out of shampoo, or just a little thin on top? Still another way to get rid of collar stains is to pretreat the stain with an absorbent material like cornstarch or talcum powder. Rub it in and launder as usual.

◆ CLOTHESPIN CARE

Don't soil that freshly laundered shirt by pinning it to the clothesline with dirty old clothespins. Soak your wooden clothespins in a bucket of warm water with half a cup of bleach and a tablespoon of laundry detergent for about 10 minutes. Pin them up on the clothesline to dry in the sun. Not only will this get the clothespins clean, but it'll also kill the mildew that often develops on them.

◆ DRY(ER) CLEANER

Did your budding artist leave her crayons in a pocket, only to have them melt inside the clothes dryer? No problem! To get the crayon off, spray the inside of the dryer with a silicone-based lubricant like WD-40. Run the machine for 10 minutes on high. When the time's up, wipe out the drum while it's still warm with a clean, dry cloth.

Ironing Know-How

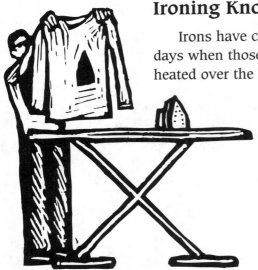

Irons have certainly come a long way from the days when those old anvil-type heavyweights were heated over the fire, and then used as quickly as possible before they cooled off. But there are still a few things we can learn from those good old days.

◆ STARCH FROM SCRATCH

You don't need to buy a can of spray sizing to have crisply starched shirts when you iron. Grandma Putt used to starch Grandpa's dress shirts with a homemade formula. She just mixed about a teaspoon of cornstarch into a cup of water, and poured it into a bottle with some small holes in the stopper to sprinkle the solution over the area she was ironing. You can use a spray bottle—just shake the bottle every so often to keep the starch from settling to the bottom. The more you spray on, the more heavily starched your shirt will be.

◆ SPUTTER BUSTERS

Hard water can leave mineral deposits that clog vents in a steam iron, causing it to sputter and possibly stain whatever you're ironing. To prevent this annoying problem, pour equal amounts of distilled, bottled, or otherwise filtered water and vinegar into your iron's reservoir. Heat up the iron, and let it steam and spray until it's empty. Good-bye sputters!

Another way to remove mineral deposits and built-up starch from the steam vents is to clean out the holes with a toothpick while the iron is turned off and unplugged. It's quick and easy.

◆ SALTY SOLUTION

If you like to iron with lots of starch, you may find that it begins to build up and burn on the sole plate, especially on an older iron that doesn't have a nonstick coating. In Grandma Putt's day, if her iron had starch building up on it, she'd pass the salt. You can, too. Turn on your iron to a medium setting. While the iron is warming, place a paper towel on the ironing board, and sprinkle table salt on it. When the iron is hot, pass it over the salt in a circular motion. This will gently scrub the bottom clean. When the iron cools down, wipe off any residue with a clean, damp cloth.

> ## Nonstick? No Problem
>
> Even if your iron does have a non-stick coating, burned starch can still build up. You can fix this by rubbing the sole plate (with the iron unplugged, of course) with a scrubber made for non-stick cookware. This will be gentle enough to tackle the starch without harming the coating.

Getting Rid of Odors

Whew! What the heck is that? Sometimes I wish we humans weren't equipped with such sensitive noses—there's so much to smell! I know, I know, many things

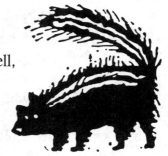

smell terrific: baking bread, freshly mown grass, a bouquet of flowers, a roaring fire in the hearth, babies (well, sometimes). But just think about all the stinky smells that can crop up around your home: mildew, mustiness, spoiled food, dirty socks, old garbage, cigar and cigarette smoke, a dead mouse in the heating vent...well, you get my point. Some odors you'll do just about anything to get rid of, and that's what these next couple of pages are dedicated to.

> *They're a poor lot, the men, all of 'em, and dirty, too—but the thing is, darlin', to get one that cleans easy.*
>
> GILBERT EMERY

Now, I know that you know that I'm not going to recommend commercial air fresheners, but it's not only because they're not natural. They're not good for you, either. Some just end up coating the inside of your nose with an oily film that diminishes your sense of smell! Yuck! That's not my style—nor was it Grandma Putt's. Here are some good old-fashioned ways to help your home come out smelling like a rose.

A Breath of Fresh Air

Sometimes, it's not that the air in your home smells bad, it's just that you'd like it to smell a little fresher, right? For those times, I have a lot of suggestions—read on, my friends.

◆ LET THE OUTSIDE AIR IN

My all-time favorite way to freshen a room is to throw open the windows and get a little fresh air circulating. I've been known to do this even in the dead of winter, which doesn't always make me immediately popular with the family. But they always thank me when I close the windows again and the air is fresh and crisp—and warmer.

◆ PUT THE KETTLE ON

To add a little fragrance to the air, put a large pot of water on the stove to boil, and add some cinnamon sticks and cloves to it. Let it simmer until the water's nearly gone. Then you can either put the whole shebang away, or just add more water and keep on boiling it. I especially like to do this in the winter when the air is dry. Not only do the cinnamon and cloves make the air smell good, but the simmering water also adds some much-needed humidity to the room.

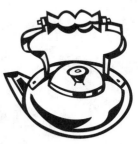

◆ EAU DE SCENT

My Grandma Putt had an old trick to perfume the air in her house: she'd dab a little perfumed oil on a cotton ball, and stuff it into the heating vent. When the heat came up, it would scent the whole room. Now that was a little too "girlie" for me, but she seemed to like it in her bedroom. She also liked to set little bowls of vanilla extract around the room, though some of you might find that to be an awful expensive way to do things.

◆ CHRISTMAS YEAR-ROUND

Setting potpourri out in a room is a lovely way to freshen the air. When the holidays are over, I love to save the pine needles from our Christmas tree, and set them out in bowls around the house. Every couple of months, I give the needles a stir, and the fragrance is refreshed. When the needles are completely dried out, I simply toss them in the fireplace.

To collect the needles from your tree, lay a large bed sheet or sheets of newspaper on the floor, and start the tree "shakin' all over." If the tree's dried out, you can collect most of them this way. Otherwise, you'll have to run your hands over the branches. Make sure you wear gloves, or you'll end up covered with sap!

Sweet-Smelling Surfaces

Sometimes it's not the air that's odiferous—it's your hands, or containers, or upholstery that holds on to bad scents. Try some of these sweet-smelling suggestions.

◆ ENOUGH WITH THE GARLIC!

Ah, the fragrance of sautéing garlic on the stovetop. *Argh*, the odor of raw garlic on your hands! Isn't that just the pitts? And no matter how much soap you use, the smell really lingers. Well, no wonder—you're using soap! The most effective way I have found to get rid of garlic or onion odor is to rub a piece of stainless steel on your hands while you run them under warm water. You can use any type of utensil, or even rub your hands on a stainless steel bowl.

Another cure: Grandma Putt always rinsed her hands with fresh lemon juice after she cut up onions or garlic. It works, but watch out—it sure does sting if you have even a tiny cut!

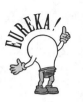

Perk Up Your Closets

Sometimes, when my closets get to smelling a bit musty, I grind up some coffee beans very fine; I pour the ground coffee onto a plate and put it on the top shelf of the closet for a day or two. The closet always ends up smelling better than when I started!

◆ CAN'T CONTAIN IT

Don't you just hate it when a food container absorbs the odor of the food that was last stored in it? How can you put a leftover piece of chocolate cake in a plastic container that once held onions? (On second thought, how can you possibly even *have* a leftover piece of chocolate

How'd You *Expect* Garbage to Smell?

I know, garbage cans aren't supposed to smell good, but that doesn't mean they have to smell bad! If you empty your can frequently, it shouldn't build up too much of an odor. To help prevent odors, I sprinkle the bottom of my trash can with baking soda (borax will do, too) before I put in the plastic liner. It absorbs most bad odors, and I can use it as a scouring powder when I wash the can out.

cake to begin with?) Anyway, here's how to keep food-storage containers smelling sweet: Fill the container with baking soda, and put the lid on. Let the container sit overnight or until the odor is gone. Then pour the baking soda down your drain to deodorize it.

◆ MUST BE A LITTLE DAMP

You've just found an old trunk in the attic, and it's full of books. But boy oh boy, does it ever smell musty. Here's how to get rid of that odor. First, get everything outside in the fresh air and sunlight if at all possible. Then put a few charcoal briquettes (not the kind doused with lighter fluid), some clay cat litter (but not the clumping kind), or baking soda inside the trunk, and close it up. Keep changing the charcoal, litter, or baking soda every few days until it's absorbed all the musty odor.

For those books (or anything else that smells musty), put them inside a paper bag for a few days with the charcoal, litter, or baking soda.

◆ YOU *MUST* TRY THIS

Basement carpeting can also get to smelling a little musty at times. So can any other carpeted area where there's a lot of moisture. Carpets also pick up odors from pets. You can deodorize the carpet by sprinkling some baking soda on it. Let it stand for about half an hour, then vacuum it up. It'll help freshen up your vacuum cleaner, too.

◆ URINE FOR TROUBLE

It doesn't matter if it was baby or puppy or kitty who committed the offense, there's no mistaking the unforgettable odor of urine. And there's no mistaking it for something pleasant. To get rid of the odor, dampen the spot and sprinkle it generously with borax, and then let the whole thing dry. When it's dry, vacuum the area well and the odor should be gone. If it does linger, repeat as necessary.

CHAPTER 3

Getting Organized

I know only a few folks whose lives are utterly and completely organized. Their garages are organized. Their bills are organized. Their closets are organized. Heck, even the junk in their attic is organized!

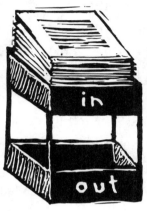

But what about the rest of us? How can those of us whose belongings aren't cataloged by size, shape, and color clear out the clutter and live ordered lives? Well, some of the answers are right in this chapter.

To me, coming up with a household organizational plan is a lot like coming up with a household budget. Think about it. When you create a budget, you take into account how much money (space) you have, what your expenses (items that need to be stored) are, and how they do (or don't) balance. The same is true with organizing.

The first step is finding out how much stuff you have. That means climbing into the attic and going through that old trunk; cleaning off those dusty, musty boxes in the basement; and sorting through your dresser drawers and closets.

The second step is to assess your storage space—basement, attic, bookshelves, closets, nooks, and crannies. If your storage budget is balanced, that is, you have a place for everything, then your job is easier. But if you have a space debt—less space than stuff—then you have some decisions to make. Do you get rid of stuff? Find more storage? Make better use of the storage space you have?

Are you confused now? Don't worry. I've got some great ideas to get you on the path to organizational bliss. Read on, my friends.

Now Where Did I Put That?

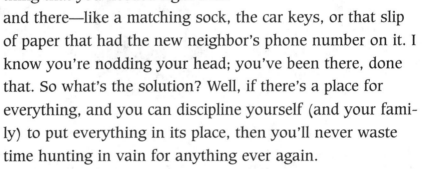

If you're like me, then there have been plenty of times in your life when you've lost precious moments (heck, actually a lot of time) looking high and low for something that you needed right then and there—like a matching sock, the car keys, or that slip of paper that had the new neighbor's phone number on it. I know you're nodding your head; you've been there, done that. So what's the solution? Well, if there's a place for everything, and you can discipline yourself (and your family) to put everything in its place, then you'll never waste time hunting in vain for anything ever again.

Sound too good to be true? Trust me, it isn't.

Eliminating Closet Chaos

Remember the old radio show where every week one of the characters would open a closet and—slam, bam, crash—piles and piles of junk came cascading down on him? If that image hits a little too close to home, you're not alone. Many of us just cram stuff into our closets the way we might, say, sweep dirt under the rug. But fear not, there are a few simple and fairly painless steps you can take to get that closet clutter under control.

> *Don't agonize.*
> *Organize.*
>
> FLORYNCE KENNEDY

◆ MAKE AN ASSESSMENT

First things first. How can you possibly get organized if you don't know what the heck you're organizing? The very first thing you need to do is to get into your closet and look at

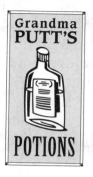

The Simple Cedar Solution

Back in Grandma Putt's day, the long-term storage of clothes was serious business. A good wool sweater, for instance, had to last many a winter season. Not only was it taken care of when it was worn, but it got special treatment when it was packed away for the summer so that the moths wouldn't get to it. After it was cleaned, it went into a cedar chest.

Grandma herself knew this well. But there was one time when she decided to make use of some space in the barn to store some clothes. Problem was, she didn't have another cedar chest to use. Her solution was brilliant. Grandma Putt knew how to turn any kind of box into a cedar chest. All she did was add some cedar chips!

Any clothes that she put into storage were safe from moths and silverfish. (You can do it, too. Just use the cedar shavings sold in pet stores as small animal bedding material—they'll be near the hamster toys.)

Grandma Putt kept the shavings corralled in an old, clean sock. If you do the same, find one that doesn't have too big a hole in it. Fill it with the shavings, and knot it at the top. An old stocking works even better. Place one or two of these sachets in any box that goes into storage and where there's a danger of infestation. They're even great in short-term storage areas like dresser drawers and closets.

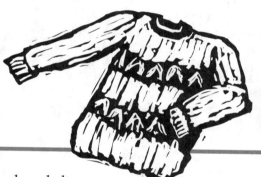

every single shirt, blouse, pair of trousers, shoe, belt, scarf, suit, and dress you have. Sound time-consuming? It may be, but look at it this way: By investing a few hours today in this task (and the ones that follow), you'll save yourself even more time—and a lot of frustration—later on down the road.

◆ PILE IT ON

Here's how I go about cleaning out my clothes closets. Twice a year, in spring and fall, I go through all of the clothing I have, then put each item into one of three categories: Keep, Give Away (or sell), and Throw Away. When I do this, I have one ironclad rule: If I haven't worn or used a particular item in three years it goes—*no ifs, ands, or buts about it!*

◆ ROTATE YOUR INVENTORY

Ever notice that in the dead of winter, it's hard to find a bag of charcoal or a beach chair at the local discount store? That's because when the warm weather rolls around, stores roll out their warm-weather wares. Makes sense, doesn't it?

Well, if you find yourself digging through parkas, mittens, and hats when you're looking for your bathing suit, I'd recommend that you try the same technique. When March or April rolls around, clean out all of your winter clothes, and transfer them to storage. At the same time, take your spring and summer gear out of storage, and put it in your drawers and on shelves where it's readily at hand.

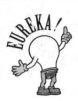

Take It to the Cleaners

Did you know that some dry-cleaning establishments store winter clothing? All it may cost is having your clothing cleaned there, although some establishments will charge a fee. If you don't have a lot of storage space at home, this may be just what you need to store bulky items like comforters and heavy winter coats.

◆ CLEAN 'EM UP

I'll say it again: Clean all your winter clothing before you transfer it to storage. Why is that so important? You've heard about moths eating wool, right? Well, technically, it's not the moths that do the damage; and they don't actually eat the wool. See, the moths lay their eggs on the wool, and when those eggs hatch, the little larva eat the *dirt* on the wool. If there's no dirt on the clothing, you won't have to worry as much about moths. End of lesson.

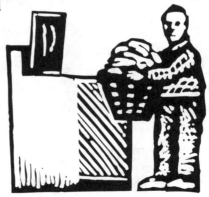

◆ BREAKING UP IS HARD TO DO

One of the things that I have trouble with is keeping all of my clothing items separate, but it's one of the best ways to stay organized. For instance, if you keep your tops, pants, sweaters, socks, and underwear in separate drawers, you stay a lot more organized than if you cram all of those items together.

Of course, if space is tight, you'll need to get creative. For example, all items don't need to go in drawers. I keep my socks in a medium-sized wicker basket that I found at a yard sale. Underwear goes in a flat tray that slides under my dresser and out of sight. Wire bins on wheels that you can roll into your closet are great for holding a variety of clothing items, and they're available at most home centers.

◆ REPEATING RODS

Take a look inside of your closet. Does it have only one rod? Well then, you're wasting lots of valuable space. Here's a nifty idea to try. Drape anything long, like trousers, over hangers. Then install a second closet rod about 40 inches up from the floor of your closet. Voilá—you've just doubled your hanging space!

This is an especially good idea in kids' closets, since children's clothes tend to be short anyway. (And maybe, just maybe, if your kids can reach the lower rods, they'll hang up their clothes!)

◆ DOING DOUBLE DUTY

I once met a man who worked with a theater group. Now that's a subject about which I know exactly nothing, so I asked him lots and lots of questions. Somehow, the topic of costumes came up; he told me that some costume rental companies charge by the hangerful. In other words, they let customers pile as many costumes on a single hanger as they can, then charge for one hangerful of clothing.

That gave me an idea. If a hanger is sturdy enough and the garment can take it, I hang more than one item on it. For

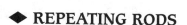

Give It Away

Local schools and theater companies are often desperate for clothing donations for their costume departments. So the next time you're ready to get rid of some old clothes, give those organizations a call. And don't forget to take the tax deduction!

instance, I usually hang two or three dress shirts from one hanger. The shirts don't take up any more space that way, and I'm able to hang three times as many shirts in my closet!

Kitchen Cleanup

It's the most popular room in the house and with all that traffic, it just may be the most unorganized, too. Many folks' kitchens are constantly cluttered with everything from today's mail to last Sunday's newspaper, as well as bills, school papers, and the like. Sound familiar? Lucky for you, I can let you in on my secrets for corralling that kitchen clutter.

◆ TOSS 'EM

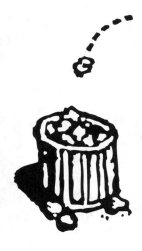

My rule about getting rid of items you haven't used in awhile applies in the kitchen, too, but I'm a little more lax here. I do feel that as soon as you get rid of the ice cream maker, you'll have a hankering for homemade ice cream. Of course, that doesn't mean you're off the hook—you still need to go through everything and give it a good, hard look. After all, do you really need three can openers? Six chipped saucers? Remember that if you can't use it, someone else almost certainly can.

You should also throw out old food. For instance, spices lose their pungency after six months or so (unless they're stored in airtight containers in the refrigerator), so get rid of those fennel seeds from 1972! And the next time you do buy spices that you don't use frequently, buy the smallest size. It may seem like an expensive option, but it's cheaper than buying in quantity, and having to throw it all out at the end of the year.

◆ HANG 'EM HIGH

Pots and pans are big and clunky, and they take up lots of space in your kitchen cupboards. The answer? Hang them from the ceiling! Kitchen shops and home centers are full of inexpensive hanging systems, but you can make your own rectangular or square system with some copper tubing and elbow joints. Hang it from the ceiling, add some sturdy hooks, and you're in business!

◆ BEHIND THE CUPBOARD DOOR

Talk about wasted space! Take a look at every cupboard door in your kitchen. Could the inside of the door accommodate some kind of storage rack without bumping into something inside the cupboard? Storage racks are inexpensive and well worth it, too, especially since they can almost double your kitchen storage space.

Jerry's Quick-Start Program

Did you ever notice that when you go on a diet, losing a couple of pounds quickly revs up your motivation? Well, if you're trying to get your home and your life organized, it can be a little overwhelming. And so, to rev up your motivation, I'm suggesting that you take 15 minutes a day for the next four days and tackle these four items. Getting them quickly organized will give you a boost of confidence!

Batteries. I don't know many people who don't have some old batteries lying around. Why the heck is that? Well, gather them all up, grab your battery-operated radio, and have a seat. Now go through every single battery and find out, once and for all, if it has power left for you to listen to the baseball game. Dead batteries should be properly disposed of (check with your local recy-

cling agency). The rest go into a box that's kept somewhere handy.

The underwear drawer. Open it up and pull out a pair. Then just ask yourself, "Would my mother be ashamed to see me in these?"

Pens and pencils. Look around your house. How many stubby little pencils and pens do you have that don't write? Now's the time to finally get them out of your life. If it writes, keep it; if it doesn't, get rid of it!

The sock drawer. Once and for all, get rid of those old, holey socks. Cotton ones are good to use as dusting rags and they make dandy shoe-shine rags, but don't keep every one or you'll end up with more socks than you'll know what to do with.

Junk Drawer Dilemma

You may not believe this, based on everything I've told you about my Grandma Putt, but even she had junk drawer!

She knew that it was better to have all those little knickknacks corralled in one place than to have them scattered helter-skelter all over her house. And believe it or not, the junk drawer really helped us to locate things, too. Since everything else that had a place was in that place (Grandma made sure of that), anything that didn't have a place would naturally find a home in the junk drawer.

Of course, periodically she'd go through the drawer and clean it out. Some items that accumulated there were transferred to a more logical storage area. Most of the other junk got thrown away—it was junk, after all.

Now I know most of you have junk drawers, too. But you may be wondering, when is it time to go through the junk drawer and get rid of useless items? Well, the obvious answer is when it's too full to pry open. But before you get to that point, try this: Keep a small pad of paper and a pencil near the drawer. Every time something gets put in, jot it down on the pad. When the top sheet is full, it's time start cleaning out the drawer.

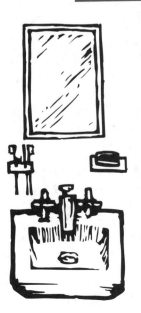

Clearing Out the Bathroom

It's usually the teeniest room in your home, but it may also be one of the busiest. And just think of all the stuff you need to organize in there: shampoo, lotion, shaving cream, razors, makeup, hair dryers, cleaning concoctions, towels, toilet paper, cotton swabs, and more. Here's some help.

◆ LOOK UP ABOVE

Just as ceiling racks can help you free up space in the kitchen, small metal hanging baskets can help free up space in the bathroom. Use them for everything from cleaners to face cloths to toiletries.

◆ BUILD UP, NOT OUT

What's on the wall behind your toilet? Nothing? Shame on you! Either build or buy some inexpensive shelving and make use of that space.

◆ RACK 'EM UP

When you're looking to save space in a small bathroom, consider installing towel racks that can be collapsed against the wall when they're not being used.

◆ LOOK OUT BELOW

If you have a free-standing sink, you can create extra storage space. Place a fabric skirt around the sink, and you can use the space under the sink to store cleaners and other supplies.

Foxy Boxes

Think shoe boxes are too ugly to use as storage containers? Try this: Cover them with scraps of fabric to match your room's décor, and use them to store everything from toiletries and recipes to sewing notions and yes, even shoes!

Picture-Perfect Playroom

Somewhere out there are kids who are neat as pins and who are naturally organized. They like to have all of their toys in a particular spot and in a particular order, and they don't mind putting their things away when they're finished using them.

The following is for all of the other families out there with little ones who need a tad more encouragement when it's time to straighten up the playroom, or any other room for that matter. I'm hopeful that the following advice will make the job seem a little less like a chore.

◆ MUSICAL CLEANUP

Make a game out of cleanup time. One way to do it is to play a favorite record or song. Like musical chairs, by the time a song ends, something has to be accomplished, such as putting a toy away in its proper place.

◆ BEAT THE CLOCK

Another way to play the cleanup game is to use a timer instead of music to play beat the clock. But just like in the game show, make sure there's always a payoff when the kids "win."

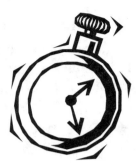

◆ HELLO DOWN THERE

Give your kids a fighting chance when it comes time to put their toys and clothes away. Make sure that shelves, hooks for clothing, toy boxes, and drawers that your child is responsible for are within easy reach. If they're too high or are just hard to get to, take a wild guess who'll end up putting things away!

◆ A HIGHER CAUSE

Having low shelves and hooks doesn't mean having wasted storage space higher up. Think of the area closer to the ceiling as deep storage. Put seasonal items like summer outfits or winter bedding up there.

> *Order is a lovely thing.*
>
> ANNA HEMPSTEAD BRANCH

◆ THIS TOY BOX BELONGS TO...

Kids love things that are exclusively theirs, like favorite toys. And that will go for storage places, too. To help give a child a sense of ownership over those storage spaces, let him or her decorate the bins with favorite colors or some other identifying theme, such as stickers or pictures of favorite cartoon characters.

◆ PLAY THE NAME GAME

Another way to help kids keep their stuff organized is to tape a picture or write the name (if it's appropriate for their age) of the items to be stored on the outside of the box. Even the youngest of kids can match the item to the picture, and figure out where everything goes.

Secrets of My (Organizational) Success

Here are my tips that will help you to get a grip on household clutter.

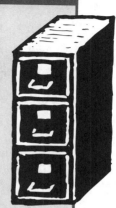

☑ **A place for everything, and everything in its place.** When every single item you own has a place to live, you'll know where it is when you need it, and it won't be in the way when you don't.

☑ **Reduce, reuse, recycle.** Don't forget these three Rs of organizing.

☑ **When in doubt, throw it out.** If you can't think of a good use for it, then there probably isn't one.

☑ **KISS (Keep It Simple, Silly).** File and store things in a logical way, and it will be easier to find them later and to maintain your system.

☑ **Deep storage, not permanent storage.** When you do store items, put them away with the goal of being able to retrieve them easily later on.

☑ **Label storage containers.** It's faster to read a list than to rummage through (and re-pack) a carefully packed box.

☑ **Do something. Anything.** If you feel completely overwhelmed by the prospect of getting organized, start small. Very small. For example, put this book back on the shelf when you're done reading it. After all, as a wise man once said, "A journey of a thousand miles begins with a single step."

☑ **Do it now, while you're thinking about it.** Can't get your coat in the closet without a struggle? Pull out the one most likely to go to the Salvation Army while you can see the need to.

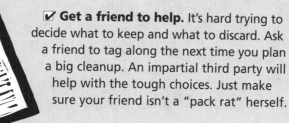

☑ **Get a friend to help.** It's hard trying to decide what to keep and what to discard. Ask a friend to tag along the next time you plan a big cleanup. An impartial third party will help with the tough choices. Just make sure your friend isn't a "pack rat" herself.

Work Smarter

In the home office, workshop, or craft room, if you're not organized, there ain't much work getting done! Read on for my tips on clearing out the clutter and getting down to business.

Cuttin' Clutter in the Home Office

Even if you leave home and commute to an office every day, you still have a home office. It's anywhere you pay your bills, do your taxes, or make out Christmas cards. Here are some tips to help you keep your work area organized.

Don't Throw That Away!

Before you head to the local office-supply or home store looking for organizers, take a look around—you may already have just what you're looking for. Some everyday household items can be used as office organizers. Check out these ideas:

✔ Pencils, pens, and markers can be stored on your desk in an old mug or a vase; even a small flowerpot will do the trick.

✔ You can keep small office supplies such as push pins, thumbtacks, and paper clips organized in drawers by storing them in old ice cube trays. They're stackable, too!

✔ Cast-iron doorstops or old-fashioned irons make terrific bookends!

◆ WHERE, OH WHERE, CAN MY HOME OFFICE BE?

I'm lucky in that I have a whole extra room in my house that I use as my home office. But I know that not everyone does. Here are some other spots in your home to consider using.

☞ Do you have kids who are in school all day? Well, if they're tolerant of having you in their bedroom or playroom (and they can be trusted not to snoop or mess up your files), set up shop in there. Who knows? Maybe there's even a half-empty dresser that you can use as storage.

☞ You may be able to convert part of your own bedroom or living room into office space. Separate it from the rest of the room with a piece of furniture, a decorative screen, or even some large plants.

☞ A space doesn't have to be large to be a home office. Corner desks are pretty darn easy to come by these days. And how about a stair landing? Yours may be large enough to accommodate a small desk and a bit of storage.

☞ One of my favorite places for a home office is underneath a stairway. Add a small desk, and you'll have the coziest office nook in town!

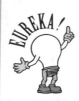

Desk Set

Do you have a home office area with a desk? Take a look at the area under the desk where your legs usually go. You just might have enough space there for a little storage. I've got a plastic storage bin, about the size of two shoe boxes, under my desk for storing extra pads of paper and other small office supplies. The best part is that it makes a dandy footrest!

◆ TAME THE PAPER MONSTER

Just about all of us have to save receipts and other bits of paper for tax time or budgeting. Here's the patented Jerry Baker method:

I have a couple of credit cards that I pay by phone. The company has a system in which I call in a payment, then it just transfers the money out of my checking account. The thing is, those two credit card companies still enclose envelopes with my bill. But rather than throwing away the envelopes, I put them to good use as storage for my receipts. Each envelope is labeled: gas receipts, grocery store receipts, dry cleaning receipts, etc. That way, when it comes time to do my budget and taxes, my receipts are already organized for me! The best part is, I didn't spend a dime on one of those fancy organizers that the office-supply store sells.

◆ A CLOSET CAREER

If you're lucky enough to have a spare closet, then you just may have the solution to your home office problem. Remove the door or doors and use that space! You may have to get clever, using vertical wall storage, but devising ways to make it work can be half the fun.

◆ OFFICE ON THE GO

If all else fails and you simply can't eke out enough space for a home office, don't worry—you can make a portable office. All you need is an old (clean) tackle box or tool kit, where you can stow all your office supplies, from a small stapler and tape to paper clips and bills. Best of all, it's small enough to tuck away when you're not using it.

◆ DO IT NOW!

Since I do a lot of work out of my home office, I own several filing cabinets. As long as I stay on top of filing everything, my desk stays pretty clean. Here's a lesson I learned years ago that helps me stay on top of the filing.

When something crosses my desk—a bill, paperwork, a phone message—I take care of it right away. Now, that doesn't mean I always stop what I'm doing to answer a message or pay a bill. What it does mean, though, is that rather than letting the phone message sit on my desk, I make a note in my agenda book to return the call, and then I either file or throw away the note. When a bill comes in, I note (again in my agenda) the date it needs to be paid, then I file it in my "Bills to Pay" file.

Everything that could land on my desk has a home in my filing cabinet, and if something needs to be done to it, I note it in my agenda book. My desk is almost always clear because I file everything. And I rarely forget to complete tasks because they're all noted in my agenda book. This method works like a charm!

◆ FILE IT

Almost everything I own has a file. I have a file for paid utility bills, paid credit card bills, home improvement ideas, vacation ideas, taxes, and car information. But the smartest file I ever came up with is the one called "Warranties and Equipment Information."

Do you know where the instruction booklet for your five-year-old iron is? I know where mine is. I also know how to order a replacement blade for my blender and whether the warranty has expired for my vacuum cleaner. It's a simple solution, and it's saved me all sorts of time and money.

Head to the Store

When I have a sticky organizing problem, I head to the store. No, not to spend my hard-earned cash on fancy organizing systems, but rather to see how they organize. Hardware, stationery, kitchen, and fabric stores are great places to check out. After all, those places have to display and store many of the same items that we do.

◆ READ ALL ABOUT IT

Magazines are probably one of the most common items piled up in your home. You mean to read each copy, but you don't get to it and so it lays there for a couple of months (or more). Here's how I handled my magazine, um, issues.

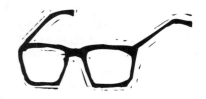

The first thing I did was make a list of all of my subscriptions. Then I took that list to the library. Any magazine on my list that the library carried got a checkmark; those were the magazines I would cancel. Why pay for what I can read for free? That left me with just three subscriptions.

Now, on the last day of the month, like clockwork, I sit down and look at my three magazines. If there's an article I want to read, I read it then and there or make notes about it. I don't clip anything unless I'm absolutely sure I'll use it. If I do clip it, I file it right away, but this is *very* important: I meticulously and ruthlessly clean out my files every six months. That means there are no clippings from 1968 clogging my files.

In no more than 2½ hours, I've finished with all three magazines, and they're ready to go out with the recyclables.

◆ THANK YOU FOR SHARING

Do you have friends who share the same interests and read the same magazines that you do? If so, consider sharing magazine subscriptions. Not only is it a terrific money-saver, but it saves clutter, too. (This is a great idea for catalogs, too.) Decide among friends who will receive which magazines, then call the various publishers' toll-free numbers and make the subscription arrangements. When the magazines arrive at each member's house, the member keeps them for a week or so, then swaps them among the other members. By the end of the month, everyone should have seen every magazine, but only has one or two to dispose of.

◆ READ FREE

These days, almost everybody has access to the Internet, either at home or at a local library. And many magazines and catalog companies make their information and wares available on-line at no charge. Does that give you an idea?

Sad, But True

Here's a tale of truly tragic irony. Brothers Homer and Langley Collyer weren't much for organizing. Neither liked to throw anything away and, consequently, junk piled up in their New York apartment for years. Among those items were 14 grand pianos and several tons—yes, tons—of old newspapers.

Here's the tragic part: The brothers died when, one day in 1947, Langley tripped and was crushed by bundles of newspapers and other items. Homer, who was paralyzed and unable to get help, starved to death days later.

◆ BUT THEY CAME WITH A BOX!

I once bought raffle tickets for a friend and was at his house to pick up his check. He opened up his checkbook and realized that he was out of checks. When he reached for the box of checks, I had one of those slap-yourself-on-the-forehead moments. For years, I bought small accordion files to store my canceled checks. What a waste of money, when I could just put them in the original check box, behind the new ones!

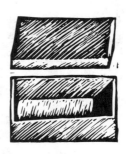

Organizing the Workshop and Craft Room

You can't do good work if your workbench is buried. And how crafty can you be behind all the clutter? Here are a few tips to keep your work spaces in working order.

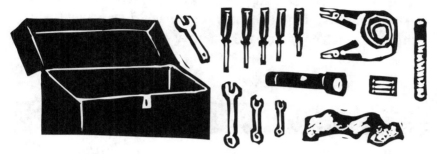

◆ PARTS PLACE

Whenever I have a project that involves keeping track of lots of small parts, I break out an old muffin tin. I have one that I keep on hand for these occasions. The compartments are terrific for separating nuts, bolts, screws, and what-have-you, and I can readily see what I have without kicking them all over the place.

◆ EGGS-ACTLY WHAT YOU NEED

Another great, but temporary, organizer is an egg carton. Just be sure to clean it off first.

◆ THE TWINE'S FINE

You can keep a ball of twine from getting tangled by storing it in a clean plastic container, like the kind that yogurt comes in. Poke a hole in the cover, and feed the end of the twine through. Drop the rest of the ball into the container, and replace the lid. If you want to be able to just yank at the twine, put a heavy weight, like a stone, in the bottom of the container before you insert the ball of twine.

Don't Be Shelf-Ish

Do you never get around to putting things back on their shelves? Well, maybe it's not you, but the shelves! The optimum height for shelves that hold things you use frequently is between your hips and your shoulders. That way, you won't have to bend or grab a chair to put things away. Of course, shelves for items that you don't need frequently can go higher or lower.

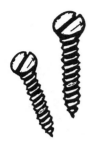

◆ ALL SCREWED UP

On the wall behind my workbench is a shelf that I put up at eye level. Under that shelf, I keep a few baby food jars. The lids are attached to the underside of the shelf with a single screw through the middle, so that the glass jar will screw up into the cap, hanging from the underside of the shelf. I can open them with one hand. Those jars make a great place to keep nails, screws, and other small spare parts.

Storage Solutions

If you've got a large attic, a basement, and/or a garage, consider yourself lucky—you've got even more opportunity for storage. Now don't let the wide-open spaces scare you. I've got some surefire ways to make the most of these super storage areas.

Organizing the Attic

The good thing about living in a house with an attic is that you have a great place to store items like that spare cot, the holiday decorations, and all of those out-of-season clothes. That's terrific, because they don't end up in the back of the closet, under the bed, or just underfoot. The bad part is that this wealth of storage space can get away from you, becoming the final resting place of old grammar-school text-books, board games with missing pieces, and table tennis sets with only one paddle. Here are some ideas to consider when packing things off to the attic.

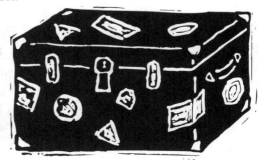

◆ TEMPERATURE COUNTS

Although the attic is a great place to store items that you don't
need readily at hand, remember that not all items can withstand an extended stay up there. This is because most attics
are unfinished spaces in which the temperature can fluctuate
widely—over the course of a day as well as a year.

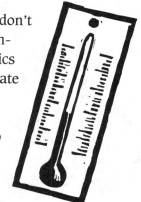

If your attic isn't temperature controlled, don't store
items such as vinyl records, photographs, audio and video
tapes, computer discs, or musical instruments up there.
None of these can withstand the extreme temperature
changes that often occur.

◆ A ROOM FOR ALL SEASONS

Unless your roof leaks, the attic is a great place to store things
that need to stay dry, and that can tolerate extreme hot or cold,
like seasonal clothes and furniture as
well as sports equipment.

◆ TURN YOUR ATTIC INTO A CLOSET

A winter coat is mighty welcome when
the weather turns nasty, but it sure
seems to take up a lot of room when
summer comes. Here's one way to keep
those bulky items organized during
their off season. Install a closet pole
from the rafters near the entrance to the
attic, and you'll have a great place to
hang winter coats and snowsuits, as
well as the kids' team uniforms and any
other items of clothing that are worn
during a particular season.

The easiest way to hang the pole is
by screwing it directly to the exposed
rafters. Make sure to install it high

Read 'em and Bequeath

If there's one category of "stuff"
that can be found in most folks' attics,
basements, and garages, it's books.
Boy, do they ever take up a *lot* of
room, but folks hate to throw them
away. I agree. Don't throw books
away. *Give them away!*

Periodically go through your
books, and choose ones that just
aren't keepers. Then divide them
among a few piles. For instance, one
pile can be for the library, another for
the grammar school, yet another for a
local nursing home, or your friend
Bob. Chances are you've got a few
books that any of those people or
organizations would be happy to
have, and you can bet that they'll be
grateful to get them.

enough so that a long coat won't touch the floor, but not so high that it's impractical to use.

◆ SHED A LITTLE LIGHT ON THE SUBJECT

If you use your attic for storage, there needs to be enough light up there so you can see well. A flashlight is the simplest solution, but it may be hard to rummage through a box with one hand while holding the flashlight with the other.

If your flashlight has a place to attach a lanyard, here's a real neat solution: Screw some cup hooks into the rafters, spaced throughout the attic. Hang the flashlight by the string over the area where you need light.

No way to tie a string to the flashlight? Another way to let there be light is to install inexpensive battery-operated closet lights. These handy items are sold at most hardware and home-improvement stores.

◆ SUPPORT THE HEAVYWEIGHTS

Unless your attic has a finished floor, remember that the "floor" of your attic is actually the ceiling of your living room, dining room, and so on. Storing heavy items such as furniture or boxes of books can turn into a real headache if they come crashing through into the living space below.

So before storing large items in the attic, lay some inexpensive lumber, such as pine boards or old shelves, across the ceiling joists, and place the heavy items on them.

◆ YOU'LL LIKE IT

One way to organize items in the attic (or anywhere else for that matter) is the "like goes with like" method. For instance, you can designate a storage box for each of your children or one just for financial records. Keep it simple. Write a short description on the outside of the container, and you'll never search through the wrong box to locate a stored item again.

◆ DON'T STUFF YOUR STUFF

If you follow the "like with like" system (see above), remember that it's OK to have a half-empty container. In other words, don't feel that you need to stuff everything full to make efficient use of your space. A half-empty container will fill up eventually. And isn't it good to know that when the time comes to put something else away, it has someplace to go?

◆ THE LAYERED LOOK

You know those traditional Russian dolls that open up to reveal another doll and then another and another inside? Use this same principle when storing items in the attic. For instance, that pair of winter boots will fit nicely inside your empty suitcase. Tape a small list on the outside of the larger package to help you remember what's stored inside of it.

◆ HARD HAT AREA

There's an area in my attic where the ceiling's just a little too low for me to stand up to my full height. And the results of my forgetting that have ranged from a big ol' bump to a nasty cut from an exposed roofing nail. If you spend as much time as I do rooting around in your attic and have suffered a knocked noggin, try my solution.

Right inside the entrance to my attic, I keep an old yellow construction hard hat hanging on a nail. I bought it at a yard

---

Take a Picture, It Lasts Longer

Running out of room to keep those keepsakes? Don't agonize over their loss—if you own a camera. Take photographs of all of those things, whether they're old sports jerseys, kids' band uniforms, whatever it is that you've been hoarding away in the back of the closet. Save those pictures in albums marked "Athletic Endeavors" or "High School Days." The pictures will take up less room than the genuine articles, and they will give you almost as much pleasure as the real thing.

sale. If you can't find one yourself, and don't want to purchase a new one, improvise. A souvenir batting helmet or even a small sauce pot will work well. Put it on every time you enter your attic, and your head will thank you time and again.

Organizing the Basement

Got some room down below to put things away? Before you do, take a look at the next few tips.

Don't Get Boxed In

One way to waste limited storage space is to save every cardboard box that new purchases come in. Me? I save a box for about a month only, just in case the product is defective and might need to be returned. After that, if I can't reuse the box for something else, it gets put into the recycling bin.

The exception to my rule would be if you're planning to move or know in advance that you'll need boxes for some project in the near future. In that case, the best thing to do is carefully unfold each box, and store it flat until needed.

◆ CUPBOARDS AREN'T JUST FOR CUPS

If you're remodeling your kitchen and decide to change the cabinets, don't throw them away—reuse them in your basement. Old kitchen cupboards are a great place to store tools and workshop items. They make terrific long-term storage for laundry or garden supplies, too.

◆ STAIRWAY TO STORAGE

If there are open stairs leading to your basement, you have a great place for all kinds of storage. Place a small chest of drawers under the stairs or build some shelves to fit. You may be surprised at how much you can fit in this hidden nook.

◆ STUDLY STORAGE

If the walls of your basement are unfinished, take advantage of the exposed studs and turn them into an organizing opportunity. Build small shelves in the space between the studs using scrap wood from the lumberyard.

◆ SKI-DO...

Need a place to store your skis? Mount two shelf brackets on the wall, about three feet apart, high up near the ceiling. Lay your skis and poles across them. They'll be out of the way, but easy to retrieve when the snow begins to fall.

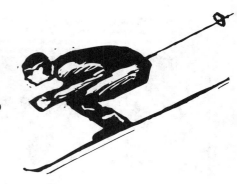

This is is a great way to store canoe and kayak paddles as well!

◆ JUST HANGING AROUND

Lots of items can be stored hanging against a wall. In fact, one of my all-time favorite inexpensive gizmos is a wire hanger. I especially like the kind used by dry cleaners, you know, the ones that are part wire and part cardboard tube. First remove the tube and save it for later (it makes a great paint stirrer, among other things). Then bend the wire into a sturdy hook for things like boots, a plastic sled, empty backpacks, or just about anything else light enough to hang on the wall.

Organizing the Garage

Another one of those places around the home that can be a storage blessing (or a curse) is the garage. I think one of the reasons a good parking space is hard to find is because people have their garages filled with everything but their cars!

Just as with the attic, items in the garage may need to be protected from fluctuations in temperature and temperature extremes. Here are a few more rules to keep in mind while you decide where else to park the car.

◆ THEY DON'T CALL IT A GARAGE SALE FOR NOTHING

A great way to clear some space and maybe make a few dollars in the process is to hold a garage sale. Even if you don't sell anything, the simple act of organizing for the sale will motivate

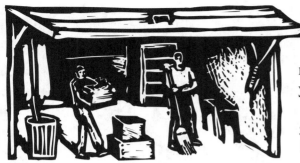

you to straighten up in the first place. And what do you do with the stuff that's left over? Well, if nobody else wants it, doesn't that tell you something?

If you decide to hold on to your goodies when the sale is over, at least it will all be in neat little groups!

◆ DON'T BUILD A HOUSE OF CARDS

I'm not a big fan of stacking boxes because it makes it hard getting to the one on the bottom. But sometimes it's unavoidable. So if you're going to stack, do it right. For instance, always try to use boxes of similar size in one stack; that way, they won't wobble. If that method isn't an option, stack pyramid style with the larger boxes on the bottom.

◆ MAKE MINE PLASTIC

If you store books or other paper goods in the garage, one thing you need to be wary of is moisture. For this reason, whenever I need to store items in the garage, I skip cardboard boxes. I prefer to use those inexpensive plastic boxes with lids that are sold in household stores and five-and-dimes. These containers are air- and moisture-tight. Another benefit of using the plastic bins is that they're easier to get stuff in and out of, and they don't fall apart over time.

Lend a Hand

Everyone knows that a surefire way to cut down on clutter is to make a donation to the local thrift store. But if you're like most folks, you collect a big pile of stuff and place it near the front or back door, where it sits, and sits, and sits, waiting to be taken to the Salvation Army. Now you have a new organizing problem: what to do with that big pile of stuff in front of the door. A molehill like that can turn into a mountain before you know it, causing even more work to truck it all out of the house.

Instead of trying to do all your sorting and donating in one fell swoop, change your approach to the whole matter. Starting tomorrow, and once a week from now on, make a sweep of the house with an eye toward finding just one item each time to donate to the local thrift store. If you think of it as doing a weekly good deed, you'll find that you're more likely to get rid of your junk. And when you do it in small batches, it doesn't seem so overwhelming.

Cash In

One way to motivate yourself to clear the clutter from your life is to make a little money from it. How? Have a yard sale. But wait—don't use the vague notion of a yard sale someday in the future as an excuse to hold on to junk you don't need.

Right now, grab your calendar, and pick a date for your sale. To attract a bigger crowd, get your neighbors involved, and make it a block-wide or neighborhood-wide sale.

Between today and the day of your sale, you're going to label three large boxes or set aside three areas in your basement for the items that you're going to sell. As you clean and organize your home, each item you choose to sell will go into one of three labled boxes or areas: keep, throw away, or sell.

Be sure to clean all of the "sell" items well (clean items sell more readily than old, ratty ones) and put a price tag on them, before putting them in their appropriate area. By the time your sale comes around, you'll be all set!

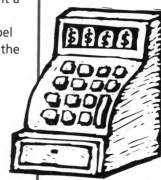

◆ ALL THAT GLITTERS MAY BE...

Silverfish. These little critters love damp areas, and they feed on organic matter such as paper. So storing books and magazines as well as fabrics like cotton and wool in a damp garage can be like ringing the dinner bell for these critters. So be sure to put anything that could potentially become infested in sealed plastic bags, or wrap them tightly in plastic. While you're at it, include a small amount of mothballs or moth flakes around the packaging for added insurance.

◆ NATURALLY BETTER

A safer alternative to toxic naphthalene mothballs or flakes is to use cedar wood chips or dried lavender flowers. They'll keep pests away—and they sure smell a whole lot better!

◆ SHELF HELP

A shelf on the back wall of the garage is a perfect storage place, and it's easy as pie to install. Just remember to measure the height of you car's hood (or trunk, if you back in) first. And don't forget to include the hood ornament in your measurements!

◆ HAMMOCK TIME

If you're a busy person (and who the heck isn't these days!), you may not have much time for hanging around in a hammock, but don't let that stop you from buying one. A hammock is a great place to store things that only get used occasionally like spare life vests or the extra cushions for the chaise lounge. Hang your hammock from the ceiling of the garage, and make sure that it doesn't hang too low when it is full. After all, you'll need enough room to drive the car under it.

If you're really clever, you can rig up the ends to a clothes-line pulley and a cleat to raise and lower it when you need something from it. It doesn't get any easier than that!

CHAPTER 4

What's Cooking?

Hey, good lookin'! Whacha got cookin'? Hope you've got something cookin' up for me!

I don't know anybody who doesn't like to eat. I certainly do. And I like to cook, too. Surprised? Don't be—after all, I learned from the master, Grandma Putt. What exactly did I learn from her? Well, some of the ideas that Grandma Putt cooked by included the notion that waste was as bad in the kitchen as it was in the garden and the rest of the house; that you should use fresh ingredients whenever possible; and you should make the most of less-expensive ingredients.

Grandma Putt believed that eating was a joyful experience and that no matter what we were munching on—a steak, corn on the cob, or even pizza (not that she ever had much of that)—we should be grateful and thankful for it.

But her cooking know-how went well beyond generalities. She was full of hundreds of practical hints and tips. I've included loads of them here, in addition to a bunch of clever ideas I've picked up from friends through my travels over the years. For instance, did you know that you can fix a too-salty stew by adding potatoes to it? Or that you can peel fresh ginger with a spoon? Or that cooking in a cast-iron pan adds up to 100 milligrams of iron to the food? Or that you can dehydrate fruits and vegetables or make your own jerky at home? It's all as easy as pie!

Read on and enjoy some more pearls of my and Grandma Putt's wit, wisdom, and experience.

Preparing Foods

A good meal (or even a good snack, for that matter!) always starts with good food preparation. It doesn't do any cook a bit of good to spend time finding the freshest produce or the tastiest meats, only to mess things up in the kitchen! So, if you're unsure about how to marinate meats or zest a lemon, take a look at these tips.

Chicken and Meats

Many of my meals during the week have meat or chicken in them. Since I spend so much time making these dishes, I've come up with lots of tips for shopping and preparing them. And, of course, lots of those tips came right from good ol' Grandma Putt herself. Thanks, Grandma!

◆ MARINATING WITH EASE

I'm no vegetarian—I love a good piece of meat every once in awhile. But I'm a save-a-tarian, too. That means I like to save money whenever possible. When I do prepare meat, I purchase the less-expensive cuts.

Take London broil, for instance. It can be a pretty cheap cut of meat—and it can be a pretty tough cut of meat, too. But mine is always tender and tasty because I marinate it in a salad dressing mixture for a whole day or two, which tenderizes and flavors the meat. Then I cook it to medium rare, which keeps it from getting too tough.

To make marinating the meat easier, I pour the marinade into a plastic bag, put the meat inside, squeeze out all of the air, and then close it securely. This way, I don't have to flip the meat because the marinade completely covers it.

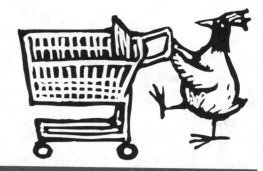

◆ ONE WAY TO SKIN A CHICKEN

I think the saddest day of my life was when I found out that most of the fat in chicken was in the skin. But I took it like a man, and now I always remove the skin from chicken before I prepare it. (I never buy skinless chicken—it's more expensive.) Of course, getting the skin off is a whole other issue. It's slippery and icky and can be a pain in the neck to remove. That is, unless you use my surefire method.

I grab a clean kitchen towel (mine's terry cloth), and put it over my hand. It lets me get a good grip on the chicken skin, and it yanks right off. Works every time! (Just remember to keep that towel separate from the rest of your laundry, and to use bleach when you wash it to kill any bacteria.)

◆ THE BIG CHILL

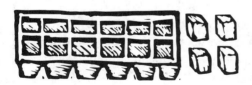

As good as it tastes, the fat in your chicken stock is just no good for you, either. Here's a trick that Grandma Putt taught me to remove the fat when she didn't have time to let the stock chill. Grab a clean piece of kitchen cheesecloth (a paper towel will work, too) about 12 inches by 12 inches square, and put it on your countertop. Grab a big handful of ice cubes, and dump them in the center of the cloth. Gather up all four corners of the cloth, forming a sack, and tie them together or hold them tight. Now take

How Much *Is* Enough???

OK, so you're having a small family gathering, 12 of your nearest and dearest. But wait. How much pot roast will you need? How much zucchini, and how much pie? Here's a quick and easy way the pros use to figure it out:

If you're serving meat, figure on about a half pound for each person (so for 12 people, you'll need a 6-pound roast). If you know that these folks are big eaters, make that three-quarters of a pound.

For side dishes, figure on a cup to a cup and a half of each per person. That means a cup of green beans, a cup of salad, and a cup of rice or mashed potatoes for each person. (By the by, 1 pound of white potatoes is the same as 2–5 medium potatoes or 2–3 cups cooked and mashed.)

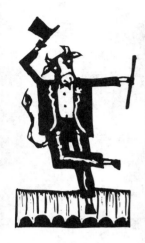

Homemade Beef Jerky

I once heard that one man's reason for fishing was to have an excuse for having a drink in the afternoon. Well, I'm not much of a drinker, but when I was a lad, fishing was the perfect excuse to eat some beef jerky. Grandma Putt made some every so often and gave it to me to take along as a snack; to this day, her recipe still can't be beat. To make about a half pound of the best beef jerky in town, you need:

2 pounds of flank steak
²/₃ cup of low-salt or regular soy sauce
²/₃ cup of Worcestershire sauce
4 to 5 cloves of garlic, crushed or finely chopped
1 small onion, finely chopped, or 1 teaspoon of onion flakes
2 teaspoons of seasoned salt (optional)
Additional spices like crushed red pepper, to your liking

1. Slice the flank steak along the grain of the meat into very thin slices about an inch wide. If the meat is slightly frozen, it's easier to slice.

2. Combine the remaining ingredients and marinate the meat overnight, or at least eight hours, in the refrigerator. (I put it all in a one-gallon, reclosable plastic bag. Turn the bag once or twice during the process to make sure that all of the pieces get covered.)

3. Remove the meat from the marinade, lay it out on paper towels to soak up the excess, and pat the slices dry.

4. Place the meat in a dehydrator or on a rack in the oven, as far from the heating element as possible. Lay the meat in a single layer to ensure good air circulation. Place aluminum foil or a cookie sheet under the oven racks to catch the drippings.

5. Set the oven temperature to 140°F for the first eight to 10 hours, or until the meat is ²/₃ dry. After that, lower the temperature to 130°F until the meat is fully dry. Leave the oven door slightly open during the drying time.

6. Occasionally pat the jerky with paper towels to remove excess moisture. You'll know the jerky is done when a cooled piece bends like a green stick, but won't snap like a dry twig. There should be no moist spots. Store the finished jerky in an air-tight container. It'll keep for several months.

that bag of ice, and drag it through your stock. The fat will harden and stick to it.

If you don't want to fuss with the cheesecloth, just dump some ice cubes into your stock. The fat will harden and collect on the ice cubes. Use a slotted spoon or a strainer to remove the cubes before they melt too much.

Fruits and Vegetables

You know what they say—an apple a day keeps the doctor away! That goes for all of the other fruits and vegetables out there. Eat plenty of those, and you're sure to be healthy. Here are some of the preparation tips I've picked up along the way.

◆ FOR THE LOVE OF BROCCOLI!

I love broccoli (unlike one of our past presidents). And it's good for you, too, because it's loaded with vitamin A, vitamin C, and folacin.

I'm always surprised when I have broccoli at a friend's house and they serve all florets, and no stalks. What a waste! (I can just imagine Grandma Putt frowning down from above.) After all, the stalks are just as delicious and healthy as the rest of the vegetable. I know, I know, the florets and the stalks cook at different rates, so that when the florets are a delicious crisp-tender, the stalks are still hard and inedible. Once again, Grandma Putt comes to the rescue with one of her ingenious, but commonsense, solutions.

When she prepared broccoli, she first cut off the florets. Then she flipped the whole broccoli upside down and split the stalk to about halfway up (just like you'd split a piece of firewood). That way, when she steamed or boiled it, the stalks came out just as tender and tasty as the florets.

◆ PEEL OUT (AND OFF)

Peeling tomatoes, peaches, and other thin-skinned fruits and vegetables can be easy, if you know about blanching (or dunking food into boiling water for a short time). Cut an X in the bottom of the fruit or vegetable, and then dunk it into boiling water (15 to 30 seconds for a tomato and about a minute for a peach). As soon as you remove the fruit or vegetable from the water, plunge it into ice-cold water (called shocking—that stops the cooking). Now the skin will peel right off.

◆ RAPID RIPENING

I'm one of those people who likes his bananas ripe—I mean really ripe, almost completely brown. Unfortunately, though, when I go to the fruit stand to buy bananas, most are on the green side. But that doesn't mean I have to wait weeks to eat my bananas. I just grab an apple, and put it in the bag with the bananas. Apples give off ethylene, a gas that causes bananas (and other fruit) to ripen. Bananas give off the gas, too, so if I have a riper banana around (instead of an apple), I put that in the bag with the unripe bananas to speed up the ripening process. But an apple is my first choice because apples give off more of the gas than bananas.

Grandma's Words of Wisdom

When you cook cauliflower, don't use a cast-iron or aluminum pot. A chemical reaction between the cauliflower and these metals will make the vegetable turn colors like yellow-brown or blue-green. Not very appetizing!

But do use cast-iron for your other cooking. When you do, the food absorbs some of the iron, which will boost its nutritional value!

◆ THE ZEST OF LIFE

Did you ever have a recipe that called for lemon zest? That's the yellow part of the lemon rind (not the white, bitter pith underneath). It contains a flavorful oil that gives, well, zest, to all kinds of foods. These days, they sell all sorts of fancy contraptions to scrape the zest off. You're not going to buy one and risk the wrath of Grandma Putt, are you? Grandma Putt removed zest from lemons (and limes and oranges) with her trusty vegetable peeler, being careful to remove only the yellow part of the fruit. Then, if it needed chopping, she'd do that with her chef's knife.

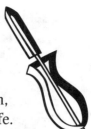

Storing Foods

Now that you've filled the pantry with flour and sugar, and loaded up on lots of other must-haves for your kitchen, how do you keep everything from going bad? Try some of Grandma Putt's suggestions. They work for me.

Into the Fridge

Some foods do best in the refrigerator or freezer. Here's what you need to know.

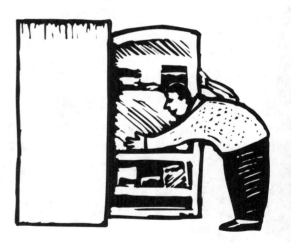

◆ DON'T FEED THE BUGS

I don't like to find mealybugs in my flour, so I store my flour in the freezer, sealed well in a plastic freezer bag. It will keep for months and months there. But I always let it come to room temperature before I use it.

◆ WHAT A CHEESY IDEA!

I love cheese—all kinds of cheese. What I don't love is when I spend my hard-earned money on a wedge of cheese, and then find that the sides are all hard after a few days in the refrigerator. The answer? Butter! Before I wrap the cheese and put it in the refrigerator, I coat the sides with a little fresh butter. It seals in the moisture, and keeps the cheese from drying out.

Eggs-actly How Fresh?

Granted, fresh eggs do keep for a long time in the refrigerator—four to five weeks, in fact. So how can you be sure that they're still fresh?

A fresh egg that is broken will stay intact. If the yolk breaks right away, no matter how gently you broke it, it's not fresh. Another way to check is to put an unbroken raw egg in a bowl of cool salted water. If it floats, toss it. If it sinks, it's okay to use.

Keep in mind that fresher eggs (a week or less old) are best for all uses, but they are better for frying and poaching. Older eggs don't work so well for those kinds of preparation, but are fine for baking, hard-boiling, and scrambling.

Old-Fashioned Additions

Long before refrigeration, housewives struggled with ways to keep foods fresh. Here are some tried-and-true methods that are still good rules for today's cooks.

◆ JOHNNY APPLE SPUD

Buying potatoes one at a time is a waste of money. But you know what happens when you buy a whole 5-pound bag. That's right, they start to sprout and bud. The solution is not to go back to wasting your money. The answer (as usual) comes from Grandma Putt: Put an apple in the bag with your potatoes. For some reason, that keeps them from budding!

◆ IS THERE ANYTHING APPLES CAN'T DO?

An apple a day keeps the doctor away. But that's not all it can do. A slice of apple—any old kind will do, so choose the least expensive—will soften hard brown sugar. Place the slice in the bag with the sugar, and in about a day, the sugar will be ready to use. This is a preventive measure, too. Store the slice in the brown sugar, seal it tight, and you'll never have hard sugar again.

If you don't have an apple around, but you do have a microwave, put the hardened sugar in a microwave-safe plastic bag, and put the whole shebang in the oven. Microwave on HIGH for about 30 seconds, and then check the sugar. If it's still hard, keep microwaving it at 15-second intervals until it's soft.

If you don't want to use a plastic bag, put the sugar in a bowl, and put it in the microwave oven along with a cup of water in a microwave-safe mug. Microwave as above until the sugar is soft.

Be Grate-ful

When the brown sugar is hard and you need just a spoonful or two for your oatmeal, simply grate the sugar on your box grater.

◆ SALT RICES TO THE OCCASION

I remember the first time I noticed that there were always a few grains of rice in Grandma Putt's salt shakers. To me, it was the strangest thing in the whole world! But, as always, she had a perfectly reasonable—and clever—explanation. The rice absorbed any moisture in the shaker and kept the salt from clumping! Now if you come to my house, you'll always see rice in my shakers.

◆ TAKE AN ICY DIP

Help! My parsley's wilted! Here's how to perk it up again: Snip off about an inch or so of the stem ends, and put the whole bunch into a big bowl of ice water. In no time, your parsley will be ready for anything!

A Cook's Tour of Tips

From using up leftovers to grilling, Grandma Putt always had the best suggestions, and I still follow them today. At the end of this section you'll also find a slew of miscellaneous tips—in my opinion, they were just too good to leave out, and I think you'll agree.

Using Up Leftovers

Waste not, want not, that was my Grandma Putt's motto, and it's mine now, too.

◆ WHAT A GRATE IDEA!

Leftover bakery bread? I never throw it away, no siree. I leave it in a paper bag until it's as hard as a rock, then I grate it on my box grater for delicious homemade bread crumbs. Then, for every two cups of bread crumbs, I add a teaspoon of garlic powder, a pinch each of dried oregano and basil, and a half teaspoon of white pepper. Just before I use it, I add a tablespoon of Parmesan cheese. Dee-lish!

◆ BE FRUITFUL

I admit it, sometimes I buy canned fruit, like peaches, when they're out of season. Here's a tip I picked up along the way to make use of the leftover liquids that they're packed in. (Remember: Waste not, want not!) Put the liquid in a saucepan, heat it up, and thicken it with some cornstarch. A little of this juice on a piece of pound cake makes a delicious glaze.

◆ FREEZE!

So just what do you do when you have a little itty bit of leftover chicken, beef, or vegetable stock? You certainly don't throw it away. Grab a clean ice cube tray, and pour the leftover stock into that. When the cubes are frozen, transfer them to heavy-duty freezer bags. Then, anytime you want to add flavor to vegetables, sauces, or soups, you can simply add a few stock cubes.

Kitchen Substitutions

Just because you don't have unsweetened chocolate squares on hand doesn't mean you can't whip up a batch of brownies. Here's a handy list of substitutions you can refer to when you run out of an ingredient you need:

IF YOU DON'T HAVE	YOU CAN USE
3 ounces of semisweet chocolate	1/3 cup of unsweetened cocoa powder plus 2 tablespoons of granulated sugar plus 2 tablespoons of butter
1 ounce of unsweetened chocolate	3 tablespoons of unsweetened cocoa powder plus 1 tablespoon of butter or margarine
1 cup of corn syrup	1/2 cup of water and 3/4 cup of granulated sugar
1 tablespoon of tomato paste	1 tablespoon of catsup
1 teaspoon of baking powder	1/4 teaspoon of baking soda plus 1/2 teaspoon of cream of tartar
1 cup of sour cream	1 cup of cottage cheese blended with 1/3 cup plus 1 tablespoon of buttermilk
1 cup of self-rising flour	1 cup of all-purpose flour plus 1 1/2 tablespoons of baking powder and 1/4 teaspoon of salt
1 cup of buttermilk	1 cup of milk mixed with 1 tablespoon of vinegar (let stand for five minutes at room temperature before using)
1 tablespoon of prepared mustard	1 teaspoon of dry mustard plus 1 tablespoon of cider vinegar
1 cup of bread crumbs	3/4 cup of cracker crumbs
1 cup of cream or half-and-half	7/8 cup of whole milk plus 1 1/2 tablespoons of unsalted butter
1 whole egg	2 egg yolks plus 1 tablespoon of cold water

◆ KEEP ON CUBING

Leftover stock isn't the only food you can freeze in ice cube trays. Here are some others: egg whites, pesto (without the cheese), tomato sauce, and tomato paste.

Can't-Fail Grilling and Barbecuing

There's something about cooking over a wood fire that can't be matched by any oven or stove indoors. If you follow my advice, you'll be a master barbecuer in no time at all.

◆ BARBECUE OR GRILL?

Most folks use the terms interchangeably, but they're really two different ways of cooking. Barbecuing is slow cooking over low heat, often to impart the flavor of the wood being cooked over. Barbecue sauce is used to keep the food from drying out during the process.

Grilling, on the other hand, is what most folks do in their backyard. With this method, you cook more quickly over high heat to sear the outside of the food. Barbecue sauce generally shouldn't be used until the end of the process, or else it will burn.

Except where specifically mentioned, the following tips apply to either style of cooking.

◆ A CLEAN START

I can't think of a less appetizing idea then eating the last cookout's food along with tonight's barbecue. The way to avoid this is to start with a clean grill. To get your grill nice and clean, start your fire early. Get it good and hot so that it'll burn off any residue from the last time you cooked. Then use a wire brush or a balled-up piece of aluminum foil to scrape off what's left.

◆ LIGHT MY FIRE

Here's my foolproof method for starting a fire for a barbecue. I use a charcoal chimney that I made from an large, old coffee can. To make yours, remove the bottom of a can so you have a metal tube, and use the pointed end of a bottle opener to punch holes all around the side at one end for plenty of ventilation. Now you're ready to get glowing.

1. Place the chimney in the center of the barbecue, with the punched-hole end down. Put some dry, wadded-up newspaper at the bottom, and pour your charcoal into the can.

2. Wet the charcoal sparingly with lighter fluid after it's in the chimney, and put the can of lighter fluid away. Never add lighter fluid to burning coals.

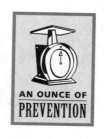

I Wooden Use These

Don't cook with soft woods like cedar, fir, pine, or spruce. The sap from these woods will make your food taste like it was basted with turpentine. Especially avoid plywood, pressure-treated wood, and any other kind of processed lumber. These can contain glue and other poisonous chemicals.

AN OUNCE OF PREVENTION

3. Light the paper through one of the holes at the bottom of the can, and in about 15 minutes, the charcoal will be ready to go.

4. Slowly lift the chimney with a pair of pliers, letting the glowing coals spill out of the bottom. Spread them out evenly with an old garden trowel. If you plan to barbecue and add some wood chips for flavor, now's the time.

5. Allow another 10 to 15 minutes for the petroleum vapors from the fluid to burn off before you start to cook. By then the charcoal should have a coating of gray ash. If it does, you're ready to barbecue.

◆ MAKE A FLAVORFUL FIRE

Adding wood chips to a barbecue is an excellent way to subtly flavor food. Some kinds of wood traditionally used for barbecuing and smoking are alder, apple, apricot, ash, butternut, cherry, hickory, maple, mesquite, oak, peach, pear, pecan, sassafras, and sweet birch. Each imparts a different flavor. Many are available in gourmet food stores as chips, but stop by a local orchard to see if it has any (untreated) wood to spare from pruned trees.

> *Tell me what you eat:*
> *I will tell you*
> *what you are.*
>
> ANTHELME BRILLAT-SAVARIN

◆ SOAK 'EM

Keep in mind that dry wood chips need to be soaked in hot water for at least 30 minutes before you add them to the barbecue so that the wood smolders instead of just burning up. Drain the chips, and add a handful to the hot coals. If you find wood that is still green, you won't need to soak it—it'll already have enough moisture in it.

◆ WHEN THE GRILLING'S DONE

Always allow the coals to cool to the touch before you discard them. Then move them to a covered metal container—an empty bucket or small trash can works well. When the ashes are cold, they can be trashed, or placed in the garden or compost pile.

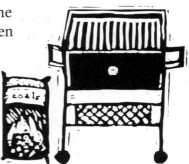

◆ NO LYE

Don't ever leave old ashes in the grill. While the ashes themselves are no problem, the trouble starts when they become wet. Water combines with the ashes and creates a corrosive compound (lye) capable of eating through the metal grill.

◆ AN OPEN-AND-SHUT CASE

When grilling, I always recommend keeping the lid up. The reason is that the cover tends to smother the fire and create soot.

The lid is, however, useful for controlling flare-ups. When you're barbecuing, you want to keep the heat low, so go ahead and lower the lid.

◆ HOLD THE SAUCE

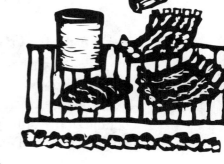

Most commercial barbecue sauces are made with sugar and tomatoes. Both of these ingredients burn easily, so use them when you're almost done grilling or when the charcoal is almost out. The temperature should be hot enough only to dry the liquid out of the sauce, not cook or burn it. Or you can use a barbecue sauce that contains no sugars or tomatoes, and thin it with water, apple juice, beer, or wine.

◆ A SPRITZ IN TIME

If you're slow-cooking meat on the grill and need to keep the meat from drying out, spritz it with plain water from a clean spray bottle.

◆ MAKE MINE MARINATED

Instead of using barbecue sauce, try your favorite oil-and-vinegar-based salad dressing as a marinade before you put your meat on the grill.

Miscellaneous Kitchen Tips

Here's a hodgepodge of tips and tricks that just don't seem to fit into any one category. These are some of my favorites.

◆ DON'T PAN THIS CLEVER IDEA

I'm not crazy about nonstick cookware. It's too delicate for the way I cook. I like to cook over high heat, and most of the non-stick pans can't take that kind of treatment. And I like to use my metal spatula—a real no-no with nonstick pans. My old standby is my seasoned cast-iron skillet. And food never sticks. My secret? I always heat the skillet well before I add the oil. Hot pan + cold oil = food that doesn't stick.

◆ WE ALL SCREAM FOR ICE CREAM!

What could be better on a sultry summer night than a delicious ice cream cone? But, uh oh, when that ice cream melts and drips out the bottom of the cone, you've got a sticky mess on your hands—literally. Here's a solution that works for me every time.

Before I load up the ice cream, I put a mini marshmallow or a chunk of leftover cake in the bottom of each cone. Then I scoop the ice cream into the cone. The cake or marshmallow catches the dripping ice cream—and makes for a delicious surprise treat when I get to the bottom of the cone!

Look, But Don't Eat!

Nasturtiums are beautiful, edible flowers that make for lovely garnishes on your food. But there are lots of other flowers that you can use, too. They include chive blossoms, daisies, geraniums, jasmine, lavender, marigolds, pansies, and violas. *Caution: NEVER eat flowers from a florist shop—they may have been sprayed with pesticides. Any flowers you plan to eat should come from a supermarket or gourmet shop, or from your own organic garden.*

◆ FREEZE AND SLICE

Some recipes call for you to slice food that's soft, like cheese, chocolate, or raw chicken or beef. Here's how to make that chore go a lot faster and easier: freeze it! If you place whatever it is you need to slice in the freezer just until it begins to harden slightly, slicing will be a breeze.

◆ FAT IS GOOD

Not for your pot belly, but fat's terrific for your pot—that is, it can keep your water from boiling over when you cook. So, next time you make spaghetti, oil the sides of your pot before you add the water, and I *guarantee* that the water won't boil over.

Flavored Oil

Here's a savory oil to use over salads and pasta.

2 cups of extra virgin olive oil
2 to 3 cloves of finely chopped garlic
½ dried chili pepper, crushed, or ¼ teaspoon crushed red pepper flakes (optional)
½ teaspoon of coarsely chopped parsley, dried or fresh
½ teaspoon of coarsely chopped basil, dried or fresh
½ teaspoon of coarsely chopped oregano, dried or fresh

1. Heat the oil over medium heat. Add the garlic, pepper, and herbs. Reduce the heat to low, and let steep for 1 hour. Keep the temperature around 170°F (use a candy thermometer to check) . Don't let the oil get too hot or it'll burn.

2. Remove the pan from the heat, and carefully strain the hot oil and herbs through a paper coffee filter into a Pyrex measuring cup or some other heat-resistant container. Let the oil cool to room temperature.

3. Strain the oil once more into clean storage bottles.

4. Refrigerate the oil and don't keep it hanging around any longer than three weeks.

◆ BETTER BUTTER

To soften cold butter in time to spread it on the rolls with dinner, I just put the butter dish on top of the stove while whatever I'm making cooks. Usually, the heat generated by food cooking on the stovetop or in the oven is just enough to soften the butter for spreading.

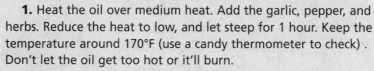

◆ SAY NUTS TO CABBAGE

Don't get me wrong: I love walking into the house and getting a whiff of something delicious. But when that something delicious is cabbage, the odor is anything but. When Grandma Putt boiled cabbage (and believe you me, she did it often back in those days), she would drop a whole, unshelled walnut into the water. I don't know why, but I never noticed an unpleasant odor again.

That makes me remember the jar of unshelled walnuts she kept in the kitchen cupboard—the walnuts for cabbage cookin'—not for nibbling. But one day Grandma was out of walnuts, so she threw in a big old slice of bread, and guess what? It worked just as well!

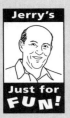

Old-Time Temperatures

Back in my Grandma Putt's day, folks didn't refer to temperatures when they talked about preparing something in the oven. Instead, they used phrases such as "Bake in a slow oven until done."

So just in case you're using a really old cookbook, here's how to translate that old-time phraseology:

Very slow oven: 250°F to 300°F

Slow oven: 300°F to 325°F

Moderate oven: 350°F to 375°F

Hot oven: 400°F to 425°F

Very hot oven: 450°F to 475°F

Extremely hot oven: 500°F to 525°F

◆ COFFEE FOR A CROWD

Need to make coffee for 50? Then you'll need a pound of ground coffee. A half pound of coffee will make enough for 25 people, and a quarter pound will make enough for 12.

Food Folklore

Here's a handful of fun food facts that won't necessarily make you a better cook, but I just couldn't resist including them here because they're so much fun. Enjoy!

◆ THE ORIGIN OF SOUP

The English word for soup comes from the Middle Ages. The term used then, "sop", referred to a slice of bread over which roast drippings were poured.

These days, we have an infinite variety of soups, both hot and cold, but around 6000 B.C., according to archeological discoveries, the main ingredient was hippopotamus bones.

◆ THE FIRST FAST FOOD

John Montagu (a.k.a., the Fourth Earl of Sandwich), an English lord and well-known gamesman in the 1700s, is credited with inventing the popular repast that shares his title: the sandwich. Legend has it that he had his cook place slices of beef between pieces of toast so he could play cards and eat at the same time.

◆ SAY WHAT?

In the West Indies, there is a variety of chili pepper called *bouda à Man Jacques* or Madame Jacques' bum (don't ask me why).

> *Friends of the present day are like melons—you must try fifty before you find a good one.*

◆ THE SKIN TEST

Folks used to believe that you could forecast the weather for the coming winter by the thickness of an onion's skin. The following is an old proverb: When the onion has three skins, winter will be very cold.

Surefire Baking

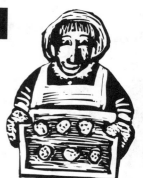

Nothing beats the aroma of something baking in the oven. Cookies, pies, cakes, you name it; if you make it, I'll eat it! Most of these tips are Grandma's—she sure knew how to bake a mean loaf of bread!

I Like to Loaf Around

You might not know it to look at me, but I've made a loaf or two of bread in my time. To me, kneading bread dough is like working the soil in my garden—I like to get my hands into it and enjoy the feeling of satisfaction when I see those beautiful loaves rise and brown in my oven.

If you've never tried baking bread, you ought to—it's very

therapeutic. For those of you who do make bread and are still in search of a perfect loaf, here are some pointers I picked up from Grandma Putt (and a few more that I've even learned myself along the way).

◆ SOME LIKE IT HOT; YEAST DOESN'T

The quickest way to a lousy loaf of bread is to kill the yeast right off the bat. Remember, yeast is a living organism (no, you can't see it move). It needs a little tender loving care, some warmth, and just a touch of sugar to spring to life, expand, and make your bread light and fluffy.

So what's that mean? Mostly that the water you mix with the yeast should be hot—but not too hot—no more than 115°F. Dip your fingers into the water; it should feel like a hot bath. It doesn't matter if the water you add is cooler (the yeast will rise more slowly, that's all), but if it's much hotter, it spells doom for the yeast. The easiest and most accurate way to make sure your water is the correct temperature is to use a thermometer. If you have a candy thermometer around, that'll work just fine.

Tried-and-True Techniques

Do you know how the pros separate eggs? Or the secret to really great whipped cream? Try these tricks, and you'll be a better baker in no time at all!

◆ NO MORE SEPARATION ANXIETY

If you've ever been frustrated trying to separate eggs without breaking the yolks, take a tip from Grandma Putt, and separate them in your hands. Make sure your hands are very, very clean, and then just break the egg into your palm. The yolk will stay put, while the white will run into your bowl. It's easier than using the shell halves (which never break evenly anyway) or any of those silly store-bought contraptions. To make the job even easier, make sure the eggs are cold when you separate them.

◆ YOU CAN'T BEAT THESE IDEAS

As I just said, eggs separate most easily when they're cold, but egg whites should be at room temperature before you whip them up. And make sure your bowl and beaters are clean, clean, clean. Any speck of leftover food or grease will keep the whites from beating up.

◆ GIVE CREAM THE COLD SHOULDER

When whipping cream, think *cold*. I mean really cold. The cream, the bowl, and the beaters should be ice cold for best results. I use a metal bowl, which seems to retain the cold better. I put my beaters inside that bowl and put them in the freezer for a while before I even attempt to whip cream.

◆ RAISIN' YOUR RAISINS

Tired of the raisins and nuts sinking to the bottom of your quick bread or muffins? Next time you bake, dust the raisins or nuts with some flour before you add them to the batter. The flour keeps them evenly distributed in the batter, and prevents them from sinking to the bottom in the final product.

Kitchen Reference Guide

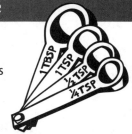

Here's a handy equivalents list for you to copy and hang on your refrigerator. Next time a recipe calls for a pound of brown sugar, you'll know exactly how many cups that translates to.

INGREDIENT EQUIVALENTS

THIS MEASURE	IS EQUAL TO THIS MEASURE
1 pound powdered sugar	4 cups
1 pound granulated sugar	2 cups
1 pound brown sugar	2¼ cups, firmly packed
1 pound all-purpose flour	3½ cups
1 pound cake flour	4 cups

◆ BISCUIT KNOW-HOW

My motto—if it's fattening, I love it! Take biscuits, for example. Put a basket of piping hot, fresh-from-the-oven biscuits in front of me, and I can polish them all off in a second. Must be the butter that makes them so good!

Now, some folks like biscuits with soft sides, and some like them slightly crunchy all around. (I'm a slightly crunchy type of guy). If you like them soft, place the biscuits very close together on the baking sheet, even touching ever so slightly. If crunchy is your thing, keep them farther apart, up to 2 inches away. That lets the heat in your oven circulate around the biscuits, getting them all nice and crunchy.

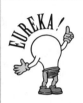

This Can Can

Save that tuna can! Wash it really, really well and remove the bottom, too. Then you can use it as a cookie or biscuit cutter or to shape perfectly round fried eggs.

Have Your Cake and Eat It, Too!

Grandma Putt never, ever used store-bought cake mix. She always made her own. And she was always coming up with clever ideas to make a cake look or taste better.

For instance, most folks know that you should butter and flour a pan before pouring in the batter. But Grandma Putt even went one better. When she was preparing a chocolate cake (my favorite, of course), she dusted the pan with unsweetened cocoa instead of flour. That did two things: It added a little bit of flavor, but it also eliminated that white flour residue on the sides of the cake. That was a real bonus when she was making a cake that she didn't want to frost.

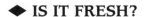

◆ IS IT FRESH?

Just how old is that baking powder of yours? Here's how to find out if it's still fresh. Add 1 teaspoon of the powder to $\frac{1}{3}$

cup of hot water. If it bubbles like mad, it's
still fresh. If not, toss it out.

And what about that baking soda? Well,
you can find out if that's still good by pouring
some vinegar or lemon juice into a cup or
bowl, and adding a teaspoon of baking soda
to it. If it bubbles like a science experiment,
it's fine. If it doesn't do much of anything,
you can toss it out (though it will still absorb
odors in your refrigerator).

Floss to the Rescue

Dental floss isn't
just for cleaning
teeth and cutting
cakes. You can use clean, unflavored floss to cut through soft
foods including cheese and
doughs (like when you're making sweet rolls). Simply wrap
the ends of a length of floss
around one finger of each
hand, hold it taut, and slice
through the food.

◆ BAKERS RECOMMEND FLOSSING!

Did you ever prepare one of those cake
recipes that directed you to cut a cake into
two or three layers? Then you know how
tricky it can be to keep those layers even.
Here's a neat trick I learned:

Let's say you want to split a single layer
cake into two halves. First, grab a bunch
of toothpicks, and stick them all around
the cake where you want to cut it. Those are
your cutting guides.

Now, you could grab your longest serrated
bread knife, and cut the cake at the toothpicks. Or
you could go into your bathroom and get an 18-inch-long piece
of clean, unflavored dental floss. Wrap the two ends around
your fingers, and then use it to slice through the cake, again
using the toothpicks as guides.

◆ DOILY DÉCOR

Here's a clever tip I learned that's terrific for decorating an
unfrosted cake: Place a clean paper doily on top of the cake,
and then dust it with some confectioners' sugar (for a chocolate
cake) or unsweetened cocoa (for a white cake). Carefully lift the
doily, and voilá! A beautifully decorated cake!

Drying Foods

When Mother Nature blesses you with a bountiful harvest, or if you just like to buy produce in bulk to save money, there's nothing worse than throwing away spoiled goods. But you don't have to if you use this old-fashioned way of preserving your fruits and vegetables for long-term storage: dehydration.

It's Drying Time Again

By slowly removing moisture from food with dry heat, and carefully packaging the food, you can enjoy the fruits of your labors for weeks—and sometimes months—after the food would normally have spoiled.

The process is easy and similar for most kinds of produce, but the amount of drying time required for each fruit or vegetable differs, depending on the variety. So see the individual instructions below.

◆ OUR FRIEND BLANCH

Before you dehydrate them, fruits and vegetables need to be pre-treated. This stops the organic process that allows foods to spoil. The easiest and most reliable method is steam-blanching.

Put several inches of water into a deep pot with a tight-fitting lid, like a spaghetti or lobster pot, and bring the water to a rolling boil. Set the cut fruit or vegetables in a wire basket or rack, in a layer no more than 2 inches deep, making sure it's high enough to be clear of the boiling water. Cover the pot, and let the food steam. About halfway through the recommended time (see "Food Drying Guidelines" on page 132), uncover and check to see that the pieces are all steaming uniformly; adjust accordingly, then finish steaming.

Once it's been blanched properly, the fruit or vegetable

will feel soft and wilted, but it will retain most of its color. Remove the food and spread it out on paper or fabric towels, and cover with the same to remove the extra moisture. Now it's ready to be dried.

◆ THE HEAT IS ON

It might have been good enough for our ancestors, who first discovered how to preserve foods by drying, but I don't recommend drying foods outdoors. Unless you live in an area that has low humidity and extended days of sunshine, it takes much longer—and you spend a lot of time chasing away flies and other pests that are looking for a free meal. For most folks, indoor drying, either with a store-bought dehydrator or your oven, is the only way to go.

◆ TABLE-TOP DRYING

First, let's talk about store-bought dehydrators, which you can find in health food stores and the houseware section of department stores. These range from the inexpensive kind (around $20) that

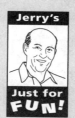

Jerry's Just for FUN!

You Say Tomato; They Said Poison!

Would you believe that some foods we commonly eat were once thought to be poisonous? Take, for instance, those botanical cousins— tomatoes and eggplants.

It wasn't until explorers returned from Mexico and Central America with the *tomatl*, compatriot of the tobacco and potato plants, that Europeans got a taste of this savory fruit. The people of Naples called it *pomodoro*, or golden apple. In Provence, it became known as *pomme d'amour*, or love apple.

The folks back then noticed that tomato plants kept ants and mosquitoes away, so they assumed that tomatoes must be poisonous. To make matters worse, the tomato also happens to belong to the same plant family, *Solonaceae*, as the Deadly Nightshade, a well-known poisonous plant. So tomatoes were grown as ornamentals, primarily for medicinal purposes. Fortunately, there were a few brave souls who dared to eat it, to the eternal thanks of pizza lovers everywhere!

It wasn't until the end of the 17th century that eating tomatoes caught on, and by the 1790s, there was a common saying in France, "It is the tomato (sauce) that makes good meat!"

Eggplants share a similar story. Once known as the raging apple, it was believed to cause epilepsy, fever, insanity, and uncontrollable lust. Today, the Italians still call it *melanzana*, a derivation of *mala insana*, or mad apple.

are basically fill 'em up, plug 'em in, and go, to more expensive models that are equipped with thermostats, timers, and fans to

Grandma Putt, Salt of the Earth

One day, Grandma Putt was making a big pot of chicken soup. Well, I was just dyin' to help. So I picked up the salt shaker with the intention of adding a few shakes of salt. Unbeknownst to me, Grandma had taken the top off earlier to add a teaspoon of salt to some other dish. But instead of screwing the top back on, she just gently set it back down on top of the shaker. So when I turned over the shaker, the top fell off, and several table-spoons of salt tumbled into the soup. I burst into tears and ran out of the kitchen!

Grandma came back into the room and figured out what had happened when she saw the shaker lid in the soup and heard me whimpering in the next room. She called me in and used my mistake as another one of her "teaching moments."

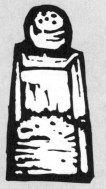

She grabbed a big potato, peeled it, and cut it into thick slices. Then she put it in the soup, saying that the potato would absorb the extra salt. About an hour later, she fished out the potato chunks and served the soup. It was as good as new!

better circulate the warm air. The simple ones work about as well as their more expensive cousins, but they may take a little longer and require more supervision.

Most dehydrators come with multiple stacking trays (additional trays are usually available from the manufacturer). Because food drying takes hours, the advantage to using a dehydrator is that it uses considerably less energy and is therefore less expensive to use than your oven. Since each individual model is different, follow the manufacturer's guidelines for use.

◆ SOMETHING'S IN THE OVEN

If you're not sure you're ready to purchase a new gadget for your kitchen, you can still use your oven to dehydrate foods. Here are a few suggestions if you do.

☞ Preheat the oven to 140°F or 60°C. If your oven doesn't go this low, set it for the lowest setting and leave the door open a crack. You may want to purchase an oven thermometer if you don't already have one, to keep an eye on the temperature.

☞ When you first put a tray in to dry, lower the temperature about 10 degrees (or open the oven door a little more) for the first hour, and lower it again for the last hour. Remember,

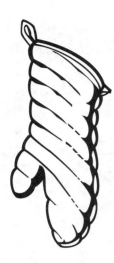

you want to *slowly* remove the moisture from the food to preserve it, not cook it.

☞ Place food on racks away from the heat source. If you have a gas oven, the heating element is usually at the bottom, so place the food on the upper racks. If you have an electric oven, the heating element may be at the top or the bottom, so place the food on the racks farthest from the element, and maybe place an empty cookie sheet on the empty rack to help deflect the direct heat.

◆ ROTATE YOUR TRAYS

Whether you use a dehydrator or your oven, you'll need to rotate the trays from top to bottom about every hour to ensure uniform drying. Don't neglect to do this, or you'll end up burning the foods closest to the heat source.

◆ SMALLER IS BETTER

Keep in mind that the more food you try to dehydrate at a time, the longer it'll take, so work in small batches for better results. And smaller is better when it comes to the size of the food, too. Cut or slice fruits and vegetables into smaller pieces for faster drying.

Storing and Using Dried Fruits and Vegetables

After you've spent your time and effort carefully slicing, blanching, and drying your foods, don't go and undo everything you've done by improperly storing your dried produce! I can't tell you how disappointing it is to find mold growing on your dried apples and pears just a few days after you've put them away. So heed my advice, and make your dried foods good to the very last bite.

Food Drying Guidelines

Here are some general guidelines for drying fruits and vegetables. For more detailed instructions, call your local county extension service, listed in the phone book, or look for a copy of *Putting Food By* by Janet Greene, Ruth Hertzberg, and Beatrice Vaughan (New York: Dutton, 1991). This book is the last word on the proper methods of preserving all kinds of foods.

FOOD TO DRY	WHAT TO DO
Apples, apricots, and pears	Peel, core, and remove all of the stones and seeds. Slice the fruit into ⅛-inch-thick pieces. Sprinkle them with a little lemon juice to keep the slices from turning brown.
	Steam blanch the slices for 5 minutes, and press out the extra moisture by placing them between paper towels and rolling with a rolling pin or pressing with a heavy pot or skillet.
	Place the fruit on a cookie sheet greased very lightly with vegetable oil (if using an oven) or in the tray of your dehydrator, in a single layer. The average total drying time will be about 6 hours. You'll know they're done when they feel leathery and there's no moisture when a piece is cut and squeezed.
Tomatoes	Halve and remove seeds, stem base, and the tough midrib. Spread them out on a platter cut side up, and salt to remove moisture (about 1 teaspoon of salt per pound of tomatoes). Stack them in layers, and press with a weighted plate for about 1 hour. Steam blanch the halves for 4 minutes.
	Place the tomatoes on a cookie sheet greased very lightly with vegetable oil (if you're using your oven) or in the tray of your dehydrator, in a single layer. The average total drying time will be 4 to 5 hours. Fully dried tomatoes are pliable, but not soft.
Green, red, or yellow bell peppers	Quarter the peppers, and remove the seeds and fleshy core. Steam blanch for 12 minutes, then place the slices on a cookie sheet greased very lightly with vegetable oil, if using an oven, or in the tray of your dehydrator, in a single layer. Start at as low a temperature as possible (120° F) for the first hour, gradually increasing the temperature to 140° F and reducing again when nearly dry. The fully dried peppers will be crisp and brittle.

◆ KEEP YOUR COOL

Once your dried food has cooled, place small amounts in air-tight plastic bags or containers. Store these in a cool, dry place where the temperature won't go above 60°F. Use one small batch at a time to avoid exposing the rest of your stash to moisture or parasites. The food should last indefinitely this way, but if it shows any sign of mold or dampness, get rid of it!

◆ PLUMP 'EM UP

I usually eat my dried fruits and vegetables out of hand, but once in a while, I yearn for a more juicy treat. That's when I reconstitute the dried fruit or vegetable (that's a fancy word for putting the water back in).

It's not hard—simply place the dried slices in a saucepan, and pour enough boiling water over them to just cover. Simmer, covered, for about 10 minutes. Add more water if it's quickly absorbed. Remove from the heat and let cool.

Drying Herbs

You can dry herbs without using any fancy equipment. The simplest way is to tie the stems together, and suspend them upside down in a small brown paper bag or in old clean panty hose in a warm, dry place, such as an attic. Cut a few small holes in the paper bag so moisture can escape. It will take about a week for the herbs to dry. Here's what else you need to know.

◆ REMEMBER THE SUN BLOCK

Don't dry herbs in direct sunlight, because the light will cause the color to fade, and the herbs will lose their aroma and flavor.

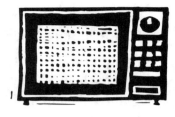

◆ ZAP!

Microwave ovens are great for drying small quantities of herbs and it takes just minutes. Here's how:

1. Place the herbs between sheets of paper towels.

2. "Cook" the herbs for 2 to 4 minutes on HIGH power, depending on the amount of herbs you're drying. Start with the least amount of time. Then, if the herbs need to dry a little more, do it a few seconds at a time so as not to burn them.

3. Let the herbs completely cool before storing them in a reclosable, airtight container.

Flavored Vinegars

Homemade infused vinegars add extra flavor to salads and are a lot less expensive than store-bought ones.

1. Place three or four sprigs of your choice of fresh herbs into a bottle (see some of my and Grandma Putt's favorite mixtures, at right, for suggestions). Then add the other ingredients, like fresh garlic, peppers, or fruit.

2. In a non-reactive (that is, not aluminum or copper) pan, heat 2 cups of vinegar to just boiling. Carefully pour the hot vinegar through a funnel into the bottle. Cover and let it stand in a cool, dark place for about two weeks. There's no need to refrigerate it.

3. Strain the mixture through a paper coffee filter into a glass measuring cup or pitcher. Discard the herbs or fruits, and pour the flavored vinegar into a clean bottle. Store at room temperature or refrigerate for up to three weeks.

Here are some of Grandma Putt's (and my) favorite combinations for flavoring vinegars, along with the kind of vinegar that I think works best:

Basil-Orange: Distilled white vinegar, the peel from one orange, and basil sprigs.

Chili Pepper-Cilantro: Distilled white vinegar, 1 to 4 chili peppers (depending on how hot you think you can stand it), and cilantro sprigs.

Dill-Peppercorn: Cider vinegar, 1 tablespoon of peppercorns, and 1 tablespoon of dill sprigs.

Garlic-Chive: Rice vinegar, 2 to 3 cloves of peeled and chopped garlic, and chives.

Lemon-Thyme: Distilled white vinegar, the peel from one lemon, and thyme sprigs.

Raspberry-Mint: Distilled white vinegar, 1½ cups of fresh raspberries, and mint sprigs.

Sage-Rosemary: Red wine vinegar, sage, and rosemary sprigs.

CHAPTER 5

Here's to Your Health

You know the old saying, "When you've got your health, you've got everything." Well, most of us don't even realize how smoothly all of our body parts are working until something goes wrong—you step on a bee in your bare feet and get stung (ouch!); you try to pick up a heavy box and wrench your back (umph!); you have a little too much of that delicious pepperoni pizza (urp!) and wind up with a nasty case of heartburn.

Well, in this chapter I'm going to let you in on a few of my secrets for good health as well as some of my favorite homemade and homegrown remedies for a whole bunch of aches and pains (all alphabetically arranged so you can find what you're looking for quite easily). One of my mottos is that prevention is the best cure, so I'll start by telling you about my favorite tonic for maintaining good health. (Hint: It comes out of your tap.) We'll finish up with a variety of formulas and ideas to help you keep looking your best: from smooth, clear skin, shiny, full-bodied hair, and sweet-smelling breath to feet that you'll be proud to show off.

But before we get started, there's a little fine print (isn't there always?). Even though all of my remedies, mixtures, and formulas are made from all-natural ingredients, you should test them on a small patch of your skin, just to be sure you're not allergic or sensitive to anything. And, of course, if you suspect something serious may be the underlying cause of any ailment, I want you to contact your doctor immediately.

My Prescriptions for Good Health

The best cure-all I know of is prevention—and prayer (please God, don't let me get sick!). In other words, the best way to cure illness is to not get sick in the first place! Now, I'm no doctor, but I'm a pretty healthy old bird (and so was my Grandma Putt), so I think I've learned a thing or two about staying well the natural way. See what you think.

Water, Water Everywhere

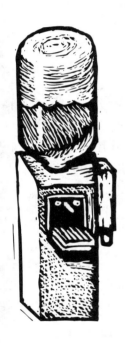

You probably remember from grammar school that your body is mostly made of water—according to experts who study such things, water makes up between 55 and 75 percent of your body weight. Water's the gasoline that makes your body go. It regulates your body's temperature, it carries away waste, and it circulates nutrients throughout your body. That liquid stuff is pretty important to your health, so read on for tips on how to get the most out of the water your body needs.

◆ 10 CUPS OR BUST

According to those in the know, you lose about 10 cups (yes, *10 cups!*) of water throughout the day through urination, breathing, and sweating. That's a heck of a lot of sweat! And all that water needs to be replaced—every day. Do you drink enough water to replace all that you lose? When you don't, you can suffer from all sorts of ailments. Headaches, for instance, are a prime example.

So the next time you get a headache, *before* you reach for the aspirin, ask yourself how much water you've had that day. For many of us, a headache is the first symptom of dehydration (even before thirst). Try drinking a glass or two of cold water (your body absorbs cool or cold liquids more readily than warm or hot ones) before you pop a pill.

◆ THE LIST GOES ON

In addition to headaches, dehyration can cause sluggishness, a lightheaded feeling, nausea, and even anxiety. (You thought you were nervous about that mortgage payment, when all along you just needed a glass of water!) So make sure you get enough water throughout the day. For many of us, that's at least eight 8-ounce glasses. Water comes in many forms, and the best can include herbal teas and juices, but *not* beverages with caffeine or alcohol. Of course, if you're active or the weather is hot, you're going to need a whole lot more.

> *He who enjoys good health is rich, though he knows it not.*
>
> ITALIAN PROVERB

◆ A SIMPLE TEST

Here's a surefire way to know if you're getting enough fluids throughout the day—and no laughing allowed! Take a look at your urine. If it's clear or very light in color, you're drinking enough. If it's dark, then head to the faucet; you need to drink a whole lot more.

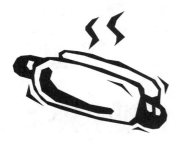

You Are What You Eat

Don't worry. I'm not going to lecture you about your diet. Well, maybe just a little. Here's how I make sure I eat all the food my body needs each and every day.

◆ HAVE A POSITIVE FOCUS

Rather than thinking about all those yummy foods I *shouldn't* be eating lots of (bacon, full-fat ice cream, and soda pop to name a few of my ex-favorites), I take a look at the food pyramid and concentrate on getting all the foods I *should* eat in a day. Here's how it works:

I get up in the morning knowing that I've got to eat six to 11 servings of breads and grains; two to four servings of fruit;

three to five servings of vegetables; two to three servings of meat, poultry, or fish; and two servings of milk products. That's a lot of food! Then, when I want a snack, I don't concentrate on what I can't have, but rather what I need to have. That way, I don't feel deprived. I fill up on healthful foods, and don't have enough room or appetite for the no-no's.

Jerry's Just for FUN!

Leech Me Alone!

In ancient times, bloodletting (by applying leeches to the area) was the preferred treatment for a whole host of ailments. Yikes!

◆ KEEP MOVING!

It's been a while since I've taken part in a pick-up basketball game, but I do exercise regularly. You've got to believe me, it makes such a difference in my life. My wife and my doctor are happier, and so am I.

Did you know that exercise can actually help you feel better when you're blue? And you don't need to become an exercise nut. All it takes is doing something (like brisk walking) for at least 20 minutes, three times a week. Now, I know you're busy, but most of us can manage that. You'll really be doing yourself a favor.

First Aid and Home Remedies

It's hard to go through life without needing a little first aid once in a while. You buy a new pair of shoes and get a blister. You nick yourself shaving. You get bitten half to death by mosquitoes. And what about those minor health concerns, like an upset stomach or an earache? The good news is that you can handle almost any minor mishap or malady using some all-natural remedies. Heck, Grandma Putt did it back in her day, and you can, too.

Abrasions

Abrasions, you say? Why, that's just medical jargon for cuts and scrapes. Here's how to treat 'em.

◆ CLEAN IT UP

The most important step you can take when you get a boo-boo is to make sure that it's clean—that'll keep it from getting infected, which can spell big trouble. So wash it well with soap and water. Then put a dab of antibiotic ointment on the spot, and cover it with a bandage strip.

◆ TURN UP THE HEAT

When I was just a small boy and I got a cut, my Grandma Putt would take me by the arm and walk me into the kitchen. After washing that cut really well, she'd sprinkle just a teensy bit of cayenne pepper onto it. No, she wasn't being mean. And no, it didn't sting—not too much, anyway. What it did do, she told me, was help stop the bleeding and close up the cut faster. Of course, don't try this on a huge cut—for one of those, you'll want to get right to the doctor.

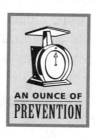

AN OUNCE OF PREVENTION

Natural, but Not Nice

Just because it's natural doesn't mean it's good for you. Herbs, and the oils and teas made from them, can be powerful medicine and can cause dramatic results—but sometimes not the results you were expecting.

So, be sure to test any remedy before you use it for the first time, especially if you don't know whether or not you're allergic to it or are sensitive in any way. Rub a small amount of the herb or oil on the back of your hand. You should know pretty quickly if you're allergic to it by your skin's reaction.

If you do get a reaction, immediately run your hand under a stream of cold water. And steer clear of that remedy from now on.

Aches and Pains

Is there anyone out there who doesn't suffer from aches and pains at one time or another? I know I sure do. Sometimes they're a real surprise, too. How many times have I mown my own lawn? Hundreds? Thousands? You'd think that these old muscles would be used to it by now. But every once in a while I wake up with an aching back.

Now, I'm not one to take a commercial painkiller at the drop of a hat. I'd almost always rather try to treat myself with some good old-fashioned, down-home remedies—and aching muscles are no exception. Read on for my advice.

Schedule a Spring Cleaning

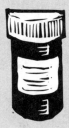

Is looking into your medicine cabinet like peering into the deep dark recesses of your past? If so, then it's time for a cleaning. Go through the cabinet, and *throw away* any old or unfinished prescriptions or other expired medicines.

You should do this at least once a year so that you don't end up taking old medicine. Expired medications probably won't hurt you, but they do lose their strength. A final word to the wise: If you have old antibiotics laying around, *get rid of them.* Antibiotics are prescribed to be taken from start to finish, so you shouldn't have any leftovers to begin with. A partial course of them won't cure anything and may actually end up making you feel worse.

◆ RICE IS NICE

The first thing I do for an ache or pain is to use a little RICE. No, I don't make myself a snack. RICE stands for: Rest, Ice, Compression, and Elevation.

First, when my muscles are tired out, I give them a *rest.* Next, I *ice* them up. Then I use a little *compression,* meaning that I wrap the injured body part with an elastic bandage. Finally, I *elevate* the achy limb. For instance, if my calves are tired, I soothe them with a cool compress, applying pressure, then I kick back and put my feet up.

◆ IT'S IN THE BAG

You know what I use to ice up my sore muscles? A bag of frozen peas or corn! Yep, that's right—I head for the freezer and pull out some bagged veggies. The bag molds nicely to the contours of my arm, leg, neck, shoulder, or whatever's bothering me. Then I wrap it with an elastic bandage to keep it in place.

I keep a couple of bags of vegetables in the freezer just for this purpose. When one starts to thaw, I simply reach for the other one! And while I'm resting my tired, aching body, I drink up a cup of strong comfrey tea—Grandma Putt's favorite remedy. She told me that it reduces swelling, just as the ice does.

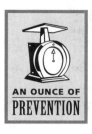

AN OUNCE OF
PREVENTION

A Well-Stocked First-Aid Kit

I'm a big stickler for safety. I check all my smoke detectors at least twice a year (at daylight saving time). I've installed several fire extinguishers around the house and workshop. And I keep a fresh, well-stocked first-aid kit in my workshop and one in the house.

I'm always surprised when I find out that a friend's or neighbor's first-aid kit consists of a few old Band-Aids and a crusty old bottle of iodine. If you're one of those folks, take this list with you the next time you head to the drugstore, and put together a useful kit. Keep the items together—in an old shoe box, a big re-sealable plastic bag, in fact, anything big enough to hold them. Then write "FIRST-AID" on the container. Make sure every-one in your family knows where it is. Now, for that list:

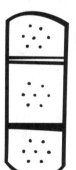

☑ **Bandages and gauze.** Several different sizes and shapes to dress different size cuts, scrapes, and minor injuries.

☑ **Alcohol or hydro-gen peroxide.** To clean wounds (after you've washed them with soap and water).

☑ **Antibiotic ointment.** Put this on cleaned, dried wounds to speed healing and prevent infection.

☑ **Aspirin or ibuprofen.** For pain and swelling.

☑ **Acetaminophen.** To reduce fever and pain.

☑ **Instant cold packs.** To reduce the swelling of muscle strains and pulls.

☑ **Elastic bandage.** To wrap sprains and strains.

☑ **Tweezers.** To remove splinters.

☑ **Cortisone cream.** To reduce itch-ing caused by everything from poison ivy to minor rashes.

☑ **A thermometer.**

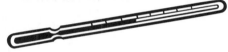

☑ **Miscellany:** Sharp scissors, swabs, tissues, and a first-aid manual.

You may notice that some of the items in your kit have expiration dates. That means you need to check your kit periodi-cally to make sure that the items in it are still fresh.

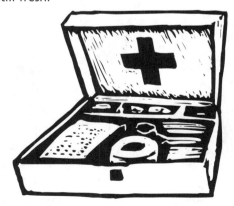

Acne

You don't have to be a teenager to suffer the ravages of acne. And don't believe those old wives' tales about chocolate and potato chips bringing on acne. It's actually caused by over-productive oil glands in your skin, not by anything you eat or drink. Read on for some time-tested tips for clearer skin.

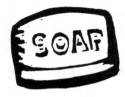

◆ GO EASY

Since acne is caused by overproductive oil glands, you may be tempted to wash the heck out of your skin. Well, in a word, don't. You'll just make the problem worse. Overwashing dries out your skin and irritates it. That makes it red. And that makes those old pimples more noticeable (and sore). Instead, use a very mild astringent, like witch hazel, to soothe irritated skin.

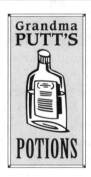

Grandma
PUTT'S

POTIONS

A Thyme-ly Tonic

Here's an old-time mild astringent that Grandma Putt first showed me how to make:

Go out to your garden, and grab a 4- or 5-inch-long sprig of fresh thyme. Put that in a pot with 2 cups of water and bring it to a boil. Take the pot off of the heat, and leave the thyme in the water for five to seven minutes to steep. When the mixture cools down, remove the thyme and throw it away. Then add a teaspoon of lemon juice to the liquid. Pour this concoction into a glass bottle with a top, and store it in the refrigerator.

Rinse your face with this refreshing mixture just before bedtime; you may be surprised to find the acne clearing up in a hurry.

Athlete's Foot

You don't have to be an athlete to get a case of athlete's foot. And you don't need to be a brain surgeon (or even a foot surgeon) to prevent it. Here's what you need to know.

◆ COOL THOSE HOT DOGS

Athlete's foot (not to mention blisters and foot odor) are usually caused by the combination of two things: moisture and heat. By rubbing a little baking powder on your clean feet before putting your shoes and socks on, you'll go a long way toward keeping your feet dry. That's because baking powder is very absorbent. It keeps your feet cool, too, because it reduces the friction between your foot and the shoe. Friction causes heat. Take away the moisture and the heat, and you take away the foot troubles they cause.

◆ MAKE A CORNSTARCH COOLER

If you're out of baking powder, dust your feet with a little cornstarch—right from the grocery store shelves, not from the drugstore—before you put your shoes on.

Then, before you go to bed at night, and after your shower, douse your feet with some white vinegar. That'll help kill the fungus.

◆ TAKE A CINNAMON SOAK

Another folk remedy for those itchy dogs is cinnamon. Steep 15 or 20 broken cinnamon sticks (you can buy them cheaply in bulk at some grocery stores) in about 8 cups of boiling water. Remove the pot from the heat, and let the mixture steep for about an hour. Put this "tea" in a bucket, and soak your feet in it for 15 minutes or so. When you're done, rinse your feet. They'll smell great— and the athlete's foot will be on its way out the door.

> *The sovereign invigorator of the body is exercise, and of all the exercises, walking is the best.*
>
> THOMAS JEFFERSON

Bad Breath

Do your friends grimace or look the other way when you talk to them? Uh-oh. Sounds like you may have a case of bad breath. If you're not brushing and flossing regularly, start there. Next, try some of these breath-freshening tips.

◆ CHEW ON THIS

Reach for that sprig of parsley. You know, the one the chef puts on your plate as a garnish? After you finish eating, pop it into your mouth and munch on it. Your mouth will feel refreshed, and your bad breath will be just a memory.

◆ HERBS AND SPICE ARE NICE

Some other remedies for halitosis (the scientific name for bad breath): chew on cloves (the ones you were going to put in your Easter ham) or drink some peppermint tea.

◆ DRINK BETWEEN MEALS

Not only can you decrease your chances of developing bad breath with good oral hygiene, but you can also do so by chewing your food well and drinking lots of water *between* meals. If you drink too much water (or anything else) *with* your meal, you'll dilute your gastric juices and make digestion more difficult. And that can cause, among other things, bad breath.

Baldness

I once met a guy at a party who was trying to sell what he claimed was a cure for baldness. He told me all about his new business, how his new tonic would give me a full head of hair in no time. I pretended to be interested, asking him lots of questions. The punch line was that he was as bald as a cue ball. He said he took his own cure, but that he simply liked to keep his head shaved. Hmmm. Sound kind of suspicious to you?

If the only thing I told you about in this entire book was a surefire cure for baldness, it would be a million seller. Unfortunately, as far as I know, there isn't a guaranteed way to stop hair loss. But there are some old-time methods to keep your scalp healthy, and a healthy scalp is less likely to lose hair.

◆ YOUR HAIR WILL (PEPPERMINT) STICK

Here's an old trick for improving the circulation in your scalp and helping your hair to stay put at the same time. Rinse your hair with peppermint or spearmint tea. If you're not growing these herbs in your kitchen garden or window box, you can use the kind you buy in the health food store.

I'm not saying you'll grow hair where there is none, but by improving the blood flow to your scalp, the hair that you do have will stay put because your scalp will be healthier.

◆ HAIR CAESAR

Make a mixture of a raw egg and olive oil, and apply it to your hair. Rinse it out with warm water. Do this every so often and keep that hair right where it belongs—on your head and not on your pillow.

◆ SAGE ADVICE

Some folks say that eating sage helps you grow hair, too. Pick some out of your garden and add it to the foods you eat (it's darn good in my spaghetti sauce).

Head for Tea

An old-time remedy for baldness is to shampoo with a tea made from the herb yarrow. This will supposedly open the pores on your scalp and encourage those reluctant hair follicles to grow. Brew some extra to drink, too; it's mighty good for you.

◆ SEE? WEED!

Wakame and hijiki are said to prevent balding. What are they? They're seaweeds that are common in Japanese cuisine, and they're readily available in health food stores. If you don't eat a lot of exotic foods, these may take some getting used to. But even if they don't keep your hair from falling out, they're very healthy because they're loaded with vitamins and minerals.

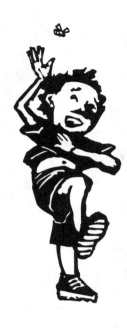

Bites and Stings

Remember when you were a kid and you spent most of your time in the summer barefoot? And remember all those bees you stepped on? Most of us don't have a problem with insect bites and stings. That's not to say that we like them, it's just that few of us have severe allergic reactions (like shortness of breath or a swollen tongue). If you know that you do experience severe reactions, you need to talk to your doctor about carrying something called an EpiPen—it's a prescription injection of epinephrine that you give yourself if you get stung. As for the rest of us, here are a couple of ways to take the sting out of a sting or relieve the itching of a bite (bee or otherwise) without scratching yourself silly.

◆ SCRAPE FIRST

Ouch! If you've been stung by a bee, the first thing you need to do is get that stinger out. But don't reach for the tweezers— instead, use your fingernail or a credit card to gently scrape out the stinger. Since it contains venom, squeezing the stinger may release even more venom under your skin.

Next, clean the area with soapy water, then relieve the pain with one of the remedies below.

◆ BAKING SODA SOOTHER

One of the easiest ways to soothe a bite or sting (first get that stinger out—see "Scrape First," above) is to mix up a thick paste from some lukewarm water and baking soda and apply it to the area. Applying vinegar helps with the stinging and itching, too, as long as you haven't already started scratching.

◆ CHILL OUT

Chill the pain of a bee sting with ice. Put ice cubes or crushed ice in a cloth or plastic bag and place it on the sting for 15 to 20 minutes. You'll say *ahhhh!*

◆ A DAB'LL DO YA

Ammonia works to soothe bites and stings, too. Seem drastic? Not really. The next time you're in the pharmacy and are tempted to buy one of those over-the-counter anti-itch sticks for mosquito bites, take a look at what's in it: good old-fashioned ammonia. Put just a little dab of household ammonia on a cotton ball or a cotton swab, and apply it to your bite before you've scratched it. But be forewarned: If your skin's broken at all from scratching, you'll be doing the "Ooo, Ow, Ooo, Ow, Ow, It Stings!" dance.

◆ MORE STING RELIEF

Here are a few more of my home remedies for bites and stings:

☞ Aloe vera works wonders. You can squeeze some juice fresh out of your houseplant, or buy gel at your local pharmacy or health food store.

☞ Grandma Putt always put a dab of honey on my stings when I was little—and I don't remember ever being itchy.

☞ I've also had good luck with making a paste of lemon juice and cornstarch, and applying that to the itchy area.

◆ BANANA BONANZA

One of my secret weapons in the war against bug bites is… bananas. Or, rather, the lack of bananas. You see, for some reason that I cannot explain, eating bananas attracts all sorts of biting and stinging pests. So I never, ever eat bananas when I know that I'll be spending a great deal of time outdoors.

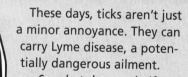

A Slick Tick Solution

These days, ticks aren't just a minor annoyance. They can carry Lyme disease, a potentially dangerous ailment.

So what do you do if you find a tick on your skin? Don't use that old trick of holding a lit cigarette near it. The tick may just burrow more deeply into your skin, and then you've got more problems than you started with.

If the tick is crawling on you, don't crush it in your fingers; you don't want tick innards (which carry disease) on you. Rather, flick it off your skin and smash it between two rocks—then wash your hands. If it's already bitten you, cover the tick with some oil—olive oil, motor oil, suntan oil, any kind will do. That'll loosen its grip on you. Then, carefully (with tweezers) remove the entire tick, and wash the bite area well.

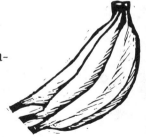

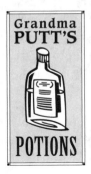

Aw Shoo!

My favorite way to stop the sting and itch of bites and stings is to not get bitten or stung in the first place! That means using some sort of insect repellent. But I really don't like to use store-bought repellents. They contain an ingredient commonly known as DEET—which is a poisonous insecticide. Now, you can buy non-DEET products, but they get pretty expensive. So I like to brew my own insect repellent, based on one my Grandma Putt made many years ago.

I head to the health food store and buy some pennyroyal tea. I make two or three cups of tea, then add a drop or two of eucalyptus oil. I pour the tea into a small spray bottle and apply it to my exposed skin whenever I go outside. Most times, it keeps those pesky bugs away like a charm.

Blisters

Those brand-new shoes sure look pretty, but after you've been walking around in them all day, you feel that little hot spot developing on your heel. Now, if you're smart, you'll take that shoe off and put on a bandage strip or some moleskin. But if you're human, you'll let it go until you've got a big old, juicy blister. So now what do you do? Read on.

◆ DRAIN IT

First, get yourself a needle and douse it well with (at least) 70 percent isopropyl rubbing alcohol. Then pass it through the blister and drain it. Don't remove the skin of the blister, though, because that's what's protecting the delicate skin underneath. Wash the blister well with soap and water; dry it, and give it a dab of antibiotic ointment. Now keep it covered with a Band-Aid until it toughens up.

◆ BREAK 'EM IN

We've all been guilty of it: We buy new shoes for a special occasion, then we put them away until the day we're going to wear them. This is a sure way to get a blister. No matter if you've bought new shoes for dancing the night away or for walking while on vacation, don't wait until the last minute to wear them! Instead, break them in a little at a time by wearing them around the house for an hour or so the first day or two, then for half a day, then all day. Now they're ready to reside on your feet for the long haul.

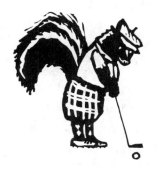

Body Odor

Something stinks! Is it you? We all get a little...well...gamey, sometimes, whether it's after a day of working out or just working in the yard. And if you don't like the idea of using a store-bought deodorant, try these terrific tips.

◆ POWDER POWER

Use some powder in place of deodorant. But don't buy talc or baby powder—it's so expensive. Instead, go to the grocery store, pick up a box of cornstarch for about $1.29, and dump it into that old powder bottle (you'll have to tug a bit to get the top off, but it can be done). Sprinkle it under your arms, on your feet, and anywhere else you'd use commercial powder. The cornstarch absorbs the moisture, and once you get rid of the moisture, guess what? You get rid of the odor!

◆ GO SOAK YOUR TOES

If it's your feet that are a bit, shall we say, odoriferous, try this cure: Brew up a couple of quarts of extra-strong black tea, and when it's cooled sufficiently, soak your feet in it for about 10 minutes. The tannins in the tea will dry out your feet long after the soak is done—and that reduces the odor.

Bruises

Ouch! You bumped into the edge of the bed again, and that means another nasty bruise on your shin. Say, here's an idea: Move the bed! But first, here's how to treat that bruise.

◆ TRY AN ICE-CYCLE

Put some ice on your bruise for 10 to 15 minutes, then take it off for the same amount of time. Repeat this on-and-off cycle for up to three times a day until the bruise fades away.

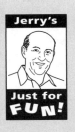

Healing with Witch Hazel

Jerry's Just for FUN!

Early Native Americans used witch hazel to treat every-thing from bites and bruises to muscle aches and pains.

◆ MULL OVER MULLEIN

To make a homemade ointment for bruises, steep some mullein flowers in a little warmed olive oil. Rub the oil onto the bruise once or twice a day; it will help it to heal faster.

Burns

A hot stove or a steaming iron—at one time or another, just about everyone's skin has made contact with one of their hot surfaces. Here's how to cool the burn, instead of feeling it.

◆ DRENCH IT

For minor burns, hold the burned area under cool or cold water for several minutes to reduce tissue damage. Apply aloe vera gel or cucumber juice to soothe the pain and reduce the swelling. Apply antibiotic ointment and keep the burned area covered.

◆ LEAVE BLISTERS ALONE

When a burn blisters, that's a good sign—the blister is a protective cover for the damaged skin, so leave it alone. If it should pop on its own, don't panic. Simply wash the area with mild soap and cool water, then apply antibiotic ointment and cover it up.

◆ HOLD THE BUTTER!

Never, never, NEVER put oil on a burn. The same goes for other oily substances like butter and lanolin. Oils trap in the heat and encourage further burning, so don't use them at all.

◆ KNOW WHEN TO GET HELP

If your burn was caused by contact with chemicals or electricity and your skin is charred and white, get to a doctor right away. In all likelihood, you've got a third-degree burn, which needs immediate medical attention. Don't think that if you're not in pain, it's a good sign. These burns usually are not painful because they destroy nerve endings.

Colds

It seems that every year we hear that scientists are getting closer to finding the cure for the common cold. Well, it hasn't happened yet, so here are some time-tested tips for helping yourself when a cold strikes.

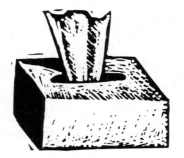

◆ SNIFF MINT

One way to reduce the sniffles associated with a cold is to sniff some peppermint oil. That will open up those stuffy sinuses, and it smells good, too.

◆ HOT STUFF!

My favorite way to clear my sinuses is to eat a big spoonful of horseradish, but you've got to like hot food if you're going to try this! If you're a real glutton for punishment, eat a spoonful of wasabi, a potent green horseradish paste that is traditionally served with Japanese foods like sushi. Your sinuses will be clear in no time at all—and so will your tear ducts and the sweat glands on your upper lip!

Jerry's Believe It or Not!

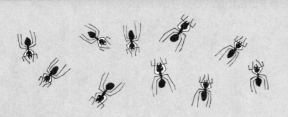

Just when we think we've cornered the market on amazing medical breakthroughs—transplants, miracle cures, etc.—we learn something about the abilities of ancient civilizations that simply amazes us.

Take, for instance, ancient Hindu surgeons. They were performing surgery thousands of years ago. Not only did those docs of yore perform operations on their patients' intestines, they devised a remarkable way to stitch up their work. What they did was to place large ants side by side along the cut. The ants chomped down and closed the wound. Then the doctors would cut the ants' bodies off, leaving their chomping heads on the cut to keep it closed. Then the doctor would close up the wound, leaving the heads, which would eventually disintegrate in the body.

Amazing, but don't try this at home!

◆ TRY A SWEET TREAT

If spicy foods aren't your idea of a soothing cure, put a tablespoon or two of honey into a cup of hot water and add a teaspoon of lemon juice. Keep drinking this throughout the day to soothe your throat. Better yet, boil the water and squeeze some fresh lemon into it, and then float the lemon slice in this homemade lemon-honey tea. The steam rising from the mug will help open up your stuffy sinuses as you sip.

Constipation

Well, no one likes to talk about these things, but let's face it, it does happen. When I was a kid, Grandma Putt was always asking me about my bathroom habits. When? How often? How much? It was awfully embarrassing for a little boy, I'll have you know, but it certainly did make me more aware of my own body and how it works.

◆ WATER HELPS

Now, constipation is nothing to be ashamed of, and there are lots of natural ways to deal with it and to keep it from happening again. First off, you should know that this condition could be yet another way your body is telling you that you're dehydrated, so make sure to drink lots and lots of water.

◆ GET FRESH

To keep constipation at bay, add lots of fresh fruits (rather than juice) and vegetables to your daily diet. Their fiber keeps things moving along quite nicely.

◆ GET GOING

Lack of exercise can also contribute to a lack of, um, movement. Starting your day with a brisk walk around the block or neighborhood is oftentimes enough to get you back on track.

Corns

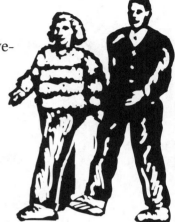

A corn is really nothing more than a callus on your foot—of course, knowing that doesn't make you feel any better, does it? Well, some of the following tips may help.

◆ STRONG BREW

Whenever Grandma Putt got a corn on her dogs (get it?), she would brew up 6 ounces of very strong chamomile tea. Then she'd apply it to the corn frequently throughout the day with a cotton ball. She'd do this for several days, and swore it worked like a charm.

◆ TRY A SALTY SOAK

You can relieve corn pain by soaking your feet in a mix of Epsom salts and warm water. Then dry your feet thoroughly, and cushion the corn with a non-medicated corn pad that you can buy at your local pharmacy.

Coughs

Yes, I know there are lots and lots of over-the-counter cough syrups and drops, but before you run out and spend a fortune on the stuff, give my old-fashioned tips a try.

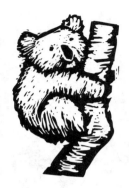

◆ MAKE LIKE A KOALA

Whenever I get a cough that's a real humdinger, I rub the out-side of my throat with a little eucalyptus oil. Not only does it help me get rid of mucus, but it also relaxes me, so that I can get some much needed rest.

◆ OR, MAKE LIKE A FISH

Of course, one of the all-time best remedies for a cough is to gargle with warm, salty water several times a day. Even "modern" medicine has caught on to this cure!

Dandruff

Here's a problem that's plagued man (and woman) for millennia—and you can be sure that there are plenty of old-time remedies available.

◆ TRY A RINSE

One of my favorite dandruff cures is to make a strong tea of yarrow and chaparral. After I wash my hair, I apply the tea, let it sit on my hair for a minute, and then rinse it out. Here are some other old-time tea cures:

Very vinegar. Mix 3 tablespoons of white vinegar with a cup of warm water. Rinse your hair with the mixture. It cuts through the residues left in your hair by shampoos and conditioners—residues that can irritate your scalp and cause flaking. If the odor of vinegar lingers, keep rinsing until it's gone.

Tea time. Make a tea of water, sage, and rosemary, then rinse your hair with it—it has a delightful fragrance and soothes scalp irritation.

Dermatitis

I'm one of those guys who never takes off his watch. It's not that I always need to know what time it is, it's simply a habit. That means it's on no matter what I'm doing: washing dishes (my wife loves that), working in the garden, washing the car, or cleaning up in the workshop.

One afternoon not too long ago, I realized that my wrist was as itchy as could be. At first I thought it was poison ivy, but a friend pointed out that the rash was confined to the area under and around my watch. I did a little research and discovered that what I had was called contact dermatitis. It's sort of an allergic reaction; mine was probably caused by a buildup of dirt or old soap around my watch. Here's my solution.

> *The best of healers is good cheer.*
>
> PINDAR

◆ SAY ALOE, AND GOODBYE

The first thing I did was to take that old watch off and give the band a good cleaning. Then I did the same for my wrist, scrubbing it with soap and water. After I dried it well, I put a little aloe vera juice on it (you guessed it, a Grandma Putt remedy). The itching stopped almost immediately, and by the next day, the rash was gone, too!

Diarrhea

Everyone suffers from diarrhea at some time or other—and usually it's caused by something we've eaten. Of course, as soon as you realize you have diarrhea, you want it to stop! But don't be too quick to reach for over-the-counter medicines. Try some of these home remedies instead.

◆ LET NATURE RUN ITS COURSE

Think of diarrhea (if you must think of it) as your body's way of getting rid of some kind of toxin—spoiled food, bacteria, etc. If you take an anti-diarrheal, you plug up your system, so to

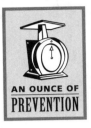

AN OUNCE OF
PREVENTION

St. Bernard Had It Wrong

Long ago, it must have been a welcome sight for skiers and stranded hikers in the Alps to see that big, friendly dog with the cask of brandy tucked under his chin. What better way to take out the chill than with a little nip, right? Wrong! Nowadays we know better.

If you're outside in cold weather and need to warm up, taking a drink isn't a good idea. Alcohol may be good for many things, but warming you up when you're cold isn't one of them.

The alcohol actually makes your blood rush to your skin's surface, causing it to flush and feel warm—but (and it's a big but) it reduces your body's core temperature, taking heat away from where your body needs it most. The liquor can also cloud your judgment, making you more relaxed and less vigilant about keeping bundled. You might even think that you're warmer than you actually are. The best thing to do to retain the heat your body is already producing is to put on another layer of dry, warm clothing.

So when that big rescue dog shows up, give him a big hug, and tell him to fetch...help, that is. Whatever you do, don't let him buy you a drink!

speak, and trap those toxins in your body. So the best cure is to let nature run its course, keep hydrated, and eat bland, easily digested foods like crackers, white rice, and bananas. Avoid alcohol and caffeine, which will further irritate your system.

◆ NOSH ON NUTMEG

When you have diarrhea, you can speed your recovery by eating a teaspoon of ground nutmeg three times a day. The nutmeg will help your body form a healthy stool.

◆ AN OLD, OLD CURE

Long ago, Europeans would boil unripened vanilla beans, strain them, and add them to sweetened brandy. They would drink this concoction to cure diarrhea and other bowel problems. I can't say if it worked, but it sure sounds tasty!

Dislocations

If you suffer dislocation of a joint (shoulders are the most common), don't try to reset it yourself. Get to your doctor or a local emergency room right away. Otherwise, you risk doing further, more permanent damage.

Dizziness

When I was a boy, a friend of mine and I had a who-could-hold-your-breath-the-longest contest. I won, which means that I passed out and woke up on the floor. I don't remember feeling dizzy before I passed out, but if I had, you can be sure that I would have followed Grandma Putt's advice.

◆ JUST A PINCH...

When you're feeling dizzy, pinch the skin between your eyebrows with your index finger and thumb. This has always worked like a charm for me.

◆ GET YOUR SUGAR UP

Now, dizziness can be a symptom of something as easily remedied as low blood sugar or dehydration. The cure is to drink some cold water with a little honey and salt mixed into it, and then get yourself a real meal and some water. But if you find yourself becoming dizzy for no obvious reason, you should be checked out by a doctor.

Dry Skin

My women friends seem to suffer more from dry skin than us guys, but no matter who's suffering, I always give the same advice. As soon as you get out of the shower, and definitely before you dry off, slather yourself with aloe vera gel or vitamin E oil. They will help trap moisture against your skin. Here are some other tricks I've picked up over the years.

◆ GREASE UP

A nurse told me this one: Put a little vegetable shortening on your hands and feet before bed, and then put on cotton gloves and socks and sleep with them on. The shortening moisturizes your skin as you sleep!

◆ YET ANOTHER REASON TO DRINK UP

I find that when I haven't been drinking enough water, my skin—and especially my lips—gets chapped. So in very dry weather, I make extra sure to drink plenty.

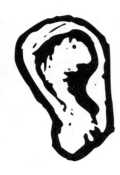

Earaches

I still remember the very first earache I ever had. I was in third grade, and I recall a pain deep in my ear that I couldn't even reach to massage it. And to this day, I still do what Grandma Putt did for me that day. I wrap a cold pack with a towel and hold it against my ear. The cold restricts the blood flow to the area, and that reduces the pain.

Eczema

If you have eczema, you may be tempted to use cortisone cream. After all, it certainly does stop the itching. Unfortunately, it has another side effect—it thins, and ultimately damages, your skin. Here are some of my better options.

◆ COD, THAT FEELS GOOD!

If you're looking for natural remedies for eczema, try using cod liver oil or aloe vera gel to ease the itching. I've also heard that some folks get relief by avoiding dairy products.

◆ GOOD OL' OATMEAL

Here's a time-honored remedy that helps with eczema and itching related to almost any kind of skin condition. First, get yourself some uncooked, plain oatmeal. Grind it in your blender or coffee grinder, and place the oatmeal powder in the center of a cotton handkerchief or washcloth. Gather up the corners of the cloth and tie them to make a pouch. Dip the oatmeal pouch in some warm water, and dab it onto the eczema. The oatmeal "juice" will soothe the itching and bring blessed relief.

Fever

We all know that you should drink plenty of fluids when you have a fever. But did you also know that parsley can help reset your body's thermostat? Read on, my friends.

◆ HIGH FEVER? HI, PARSLEY

Only an old-time country doctor may know that a tea made from parsley, taken often throughout the day, will help reduce a fever. Place a teaspoonful of dried parsley in a tea ball and steep it in a cup of hot water for about seven minutes. If you're going to drink plenty of fluids, the fluids you drink may as well be plenty good for you! And parsley tea is one of the best.

Headaches

One of mankind's most common pains in the "you-know-what" is, well, the headache. But before you try any remedy, drink a couple of big glasses of cool water. Your headache may simply be the result of dehydration. If that's not the culprit, I've got some other simple solutions to this age-old problem.

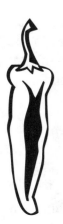

◆ SOME LIKE IT HOT

Go to the kitchen and break out the cayenne pepper. Massage it into your temples, forehead, neck, and shoulders. Like those commercial "hot" rubs, the pepper will increase the circulation in your skin and help relieve the headache.

If you accidentally get pepper in your eye, flush it with a few drops of milk. The same applies if the cayenne gets too hot on you skin. Wash it off with a cloth dipped in milk.

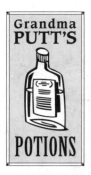

Grandma PUTT'S POTIONS

A Surefire Hangover Cure

When I was a young fella, my Grandma Putt always told me that the only sure way to avoid the consequences of overindulgence (that's what she said my Uncle Art did on Friday evenings) was not to overindulge. It wasn't until I was much older that I learned that even though she preached moderation, being the resourceful person that she was, she still had a formula for dealing with "the wrath of grapes."

First, forget that old wives' tale about "the hair of the dog that bit you." If you're like most folks, the morning after a festive occasion, you don't even want to go near the kennel, never mind sample the dog's hair! The last thing you need is another drink—of alcohol, that is. You should, however, drink plenty of water.

And then there was Grandma's secret ingredient. She would go to the wood stove, and remove a small piece of charcoal. I'm not talking about one of those commercially processed briquettes that folks use in their backyard barbecues, or mineral coal, but an actual charred bit of the seasoned hardwood she burned in her stove. She'd crush a piece the size of a small chestnut, and give it to me with a large glass of water. The charcoal didn't have any taste, but it was kind of dry.

Grandma Putt wasn't the first person to try this trick. In the 19th century, chimney sweeps swore by a glass of warm milk with a spoonful of soot mixed in. Nowadays, many of us don't have wood-burning stoves, but we can buy activated charcoal for medicinal use at the local pharmacy.

◆ **BE A SWINGER**

The ancient Chinese remedy *Li Shou* is another cure for headaches. It's a Chinese phrase meaning "hand swinging." It's really very simple: you just swing your arms back and forth for several minutes. Swinging relaxes your mind and directs blood flow away from your head to your hands. Reduced blood flow means reduced pain!

Hemorrhoids

Unfortunately, from time to time, hemorrhoids are something many folks are forced to deal with. What to do? Take a trip to the cabbage patch. An old farmers' cure for relieving the symptoms (and believe me they know a thing or two about hemorrhoids after days of sitting on a tractor seat) is to chop up a cabbage, lay it on a towel, and sit on it. Don't forget to take your pants off first! Chopped up well, the cabbage soothes the pain and the cabbage juice lessens the swelling.

Hiccups

They're probably not gonna kill you, but hiccups sure can be annoying. I'm talking about hiccups or "he-coughs," as Grand-ma Putt used to call them. Here are a few of her remedies.

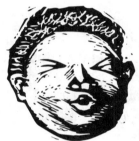

◆ HOLD IT

Here's a surefire cure that doesn't require anything but the ability to hold your breath. Take a deep breath and hold it for as long as you can. When you can't hold it any longer, let it out and take another deep breath and hold that one, too. By the time you let that one go, the hiccups should be gone with it. The buildup of the un-exhaled carbon dioxide relaxes your diaphragm and stops the hiccups.

◆ BE A SOUR PUSS

Here's another hiccup remedy: Cut a small slice of lemon and put it under your tongue. Suck it once and hold the juice in your mouth for 10 seconds. Then swallow the lemon juice, and your hiccups will be gone.

Indigestion

Too much pizza? One too many meatball hoagies? Lots of onions? Shame on you! But once in a while we all overindulge and end up with a stomachache. The remedy? Fresh

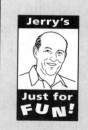

Jerry's
Just for FUN!

Feeling Eel?

Times have changed—back in 18th-century Europe, doctors cured colic (acute abdominal pain) by placing live eels on the patient's stomach. Yuck!

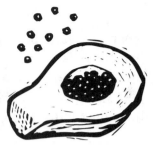

papaya or a little papaya juice. It contains an enzyme called papain, which aids digestion and works just as well as those over-the-counter preparations.

Itching

What's an itch? It's your skin's way of telling you that something's bugging it. Lots of things can cause you to itch: a brush with poison ivy, a mosquito bite, sunburn, or even prickly heat. No matter what the cause, here's how to soothe that troubled skin.

◆ MINTY MANEUVERS

To ease an itch, brew up a cup of fresh mint tea. Let the mint leaves steep for 10 minutes, then allow the tea to cool for another minute or so. Now don't drink it. Instead, take a soft cloth or cotton ball, dip it into the tea, and apply it as a compress to the affected area to relieve the itching.

If you don't have a mint plant in your garden or window box (and shame on you if you don't!), you can get some fresh mint leaves at your local produce stand or farmers' market, or look for dried mint or mint tea in your supermarket.

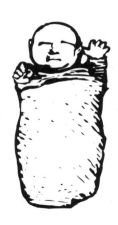

◆ SOOTHING RASH RELIEF

Another tactic you can use when dealing with persistent itchy rashes like diaper rash or hives is to apply some aloe vera juice to the affected area. If you look at the label of many commercial diaper rash and skin care preparations, you'll see that aloe vera is often a main ingredient.

But you don't need to go buy aloe vera juice or gel if, like many folks (myself included), you're already growing an aloe vera plant at home. Just break off a leaf or two and apply the juice directly to the inflamed area. The juice from this amazing aloe plant will provide soothing relief in no time at all.

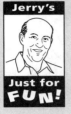

Jerry's Just for FUN!

Bottoms Up

All this talk of itching reminds me of the proud young papa who noticed a mysterious rash around his neck. At first he thought it was a sunburn, but knew he hadn't been out in the sun much. And besides, that part of his body was mostly covered up because he had gotten into the habit of carrying his young son around town on his shoulders. Fortunately, his wife knew how to treat a diaper rash when she saw one!

Laryngitis

If you're like me, one of the worst things that can happen to you is to come down with a case of laryngitis. It's not the pain, it's just that I like to talk so darn much!

Whenever a case of laryngitis has got you down, give yourself a treat—try a little candy. I like good, hard lemon candies that feel syrupy when they dissolve in my mouth and coat my throat. Another of my favorites is licorice, famous for its soothing properties. Make sure you choose a candy made with natural licorice oil and not one of those artificially flavored kinds, unless you've got an artificial throat.

Motion Sickness

I've got a granddaughter, Emily, who gets queasy at the mere mention of a road trip. So if you, too, suffer from motion sickness, do what we do for Emily—prepare yourself ahead of time by drinking a cup of peppermint tea just before you start your trip. The peppermint will keep your stomach calm. The only drawback to this cure is that you may need to make a few extra pit stops along the way if it's a long ride!

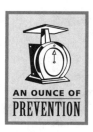

Call a Copper (or Two)

AN OUNCE OF PREVENTION

When I was a kid, I used to get awfully car sick. One hot day, we were driving around some bumpy country roads, and I got that feeling. We pulled over to the side of the road, and I proceeded to lose my lunch. Just as I was heaving my last, a car pulled over. Inside was an old country doctor. He asked if I was car sick. I nodded feebly. Then he gave me two pennies.

He said that anytime I was in a car and felt sick, I should put a penny in each hand and hold them tight and that would make me feel better. I have no idea whether it had something to do with the copper or if my concentrating on something other than my queasy stomach did the trick, but I followed his advice and was never car sick again!

Nausea

If your stomach is upset and you're afraid that your lunch is about to make an unwelcome reappearance, then get your hands on some fresh ginger. Chewing it will calm your stomach. If you can't get hold of fresh ginger (or you can't get your young patient to chew on a root), then try sipping warm, flat ginger ale. With all that sugar in the soda pop, it's not a particularly healthy substitute, but it'll still do in a pinch.

Poison Ivy

Sure enough, as spring turns to summer, someone gets too busy enjoying their romp through the woods to pay much attention to how many leaves were on the plants they've been romping through. Along with brightly colored flowers and thunderstorms, poison ivy is just one of Mother Nature's ways of saying, "Pay attention to me!" For those unfortunates who learn the expression "Leaves of three, let it be," a little too late, try one of these remedies.

◆ BAKING SODA SOLUTION

For a skin-soothing solution for poison-ivy itch, make a paste of baking soda and water. Apply this to the affected areas to relieve the itching and reduce blistering.

◆ ALOE VERA TO THE RESCUE

You've heard the expression, "Fight fire with fire." Well, when it comes to poison ivy, you might say, "Fight a plant with another plant." What do I mean? I'm talking about aloe vera. Lots of folks (including yours truly) have an aloe plant growing in a pot on the windowsill. If you do, too, then simply break off one of the leaves and apply the juice directly to the irritated areas. If you're really covered in blisters from poison ivy, high-tail it to your local health food store and buy a bottle (or two) of aloe vera gel.

Rheumatism

There are lots of folks who can tell that a change in the weather is due because their toes or maybe their elbows ache. But weather prediction aside, most of us would rather not have aches and pains in our joints. To reduce the swelling and ease the discomfort of occasional bouts of rheumatism, I like to soak in a warm bath with Grandma Putt's bath salt formula. For a full bath, mix 2 cups of Epsom salts with a cup of sea salt and a cup of baking soda. Add these to the bath as the tub fills. Then settle in for a soothing soak.

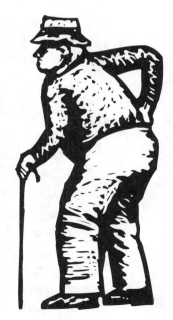

To soak your foot or elbow in a basin, or to make enough for a compress, add the same ingredients in the same proportions, but just use 1 or 2 tablespoons per gallon of water.

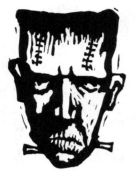

Scars

Believe it or not, you can actually reduce the appearance of certain scars with some homemade potions. Here's how.

◆ CODDLE YOUR SKIN

I know that some of you grew up hating to hear the words "cod liver oil." It usually meant you were going to get something awful smelling and tasting, just because it was good for you. Well, I've got news for you. It still smells and tastes bad, but it's still good for you—at least when it comes to scars. If you have a scar that you want to lighten, rub a drop of cod liver oil on it. The oil is high in vitamin E, and not only will it help lighten your scar, but it'll also improve the scar's elasticity as well.

◆ AN E-ZY SOLUTION

If you really can't stand the smell of cod liver oil, or your pharmacy doesn't carry it, you can use a vitamin E capsule instead to lighten the appearance of scars. Just poke a hole in the capsule with a pin and squeeze out a few drops of the oil. Use it the same way as cod liver oil (see above).

Sleeplessness

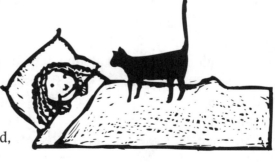

If you can't get to sleep, it could be for lots of reasons. In addition to having a lot on your mind, are you drinking coffee, tea, or some other kind of caffeinated beverage late in the day? Are you getting enough exercise? Maybe there's something particularly upsetting that's keeping you up.

The worst part about not getting enough sleep is that you

lay there worrying about it, instead of relaxing, and then you don't fall asleep until
you're absolutely exhausted—usually a few
minutes before the alarm goes off. If you are
having trouble falling asleep, try some of
these remarkable remedies.

> *Goe to bed with the lambe
> and rise with the larke.*
>
> JOHN LYLY

◆ EAT LIKE POPEYE

During the day, eat plenty of foods rich in iron and potassium
like spinach (iron) and bananas (potassium) or take a supplement. Both of these minerals are known to encourage a deep,
restful sleep.

◆ TAKE A SOOTHING SOAK

Try soaking in a nice relaxing, warm bath before you go to bed.
Add a few basil leaves to the bath water. Then after your bath
go right to bed so you don't have a chance to un-relax.

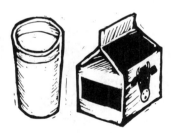

◆ WARM YOUR INNARDS

Drinking a cup of warm milk before
going to bed sends me off with
Winkin', Blinkin', and Nod every
time. But if that doesn't sound appetizing to you, try a cup of warm
chamomile tea. Chamomile, available in most health food
stores, is known to bring on sleepiness.

◆ SMELLS SO GOOD

If your nighttime routine involves lying wide-eyed in bed,
counting sheep, try this fragrant remedy. Visit the local health
food store and get yourself some chamomile essential oil and
dab four or five drops on a cotton ball. Put that cotton ball
under or near your pillow. The relaxing scent of the oil will
send you off to dreamland like that!

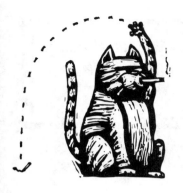

Smoking

Finally decided to quit cigarettes? Good for you and everyone else around you. It's not easy. As you may know, it's not just the desire for nicotine that makes quitting tough, but also what to do with yourself when you would otherwise be smoking. Here are some old-time ways to help the process along. Yes, even way back in Grandma Putt's day, folks were trying to kick the habit.

◆ DO THE PEPPERMINT TWIST

When you feel like smoking, start chewing. I don't mean chewing tobacco (which is no better for you than cigarettes), but gum. It's basically trading a bad habit for a not-so-bad one. Chew the gum only when you crave a cigarette. Any brand will do, but for an added benefit, choose one that is flavored with real peppermint. Peppermint has been known to lessen the desire for nicotine. And do your teeth a favor by only chewing sugarless gum.

◆ SIP, DON'T SMOKE

While you're kicking the smoking habit, start drinking—herbal tea, that is. Choose one containing catnip, chamomile, hops, lobelia, peppermint, skullcap, or valerian. Each of these herbs is known to lessen the urge for nicotine and help you relax.

Sore Throat

They say a strand of garlic tied around the throat will ward off vampires. Well, I don't know about that, but it will certainly help you get a seat on the bus! And garlic also helps get rid of a sore throat. Gargle with a mixture of warm salt water (a teaspoon of salt in a drinking glass) with a tiny pinch of cayenne pepper and a clove of garlic crushed in it.

Toothaches

Your tooth starts aching, and your dentist can't see you until tomorrow. Don't sit there in agony, try one of these natural painkillers.

◆ A SPICY SOLUTION

One way to ease the pain of a toothache is as close as your spice rack. But not just any spice will do—you need allspice. Put 1 or 2 teaspoons of allspice powder in a cup of boiling water. Steep it for 10 to 20 minutes and strain. Gargle with the tea while it's warm, swishing it around your mouth and spitting it out.

◆ CALM PAIN WITH CLOVES

Another effective temporary treatment for a toothache that you may already have in your cupboard is clove oil. A few drops applied with a cotton swab directly to the tooth can ease the pain until you get to see the dentist. If you don't already have clove oil, it's available in most pharmacies and health food stores. Or, you can place a whole clove between the aching tooth and your cheek to ease the pain.

Cloves, and to a lesser degree allspice, contain eugenol, the same ingredient that appears in over-the-counter toothache remedies. It's also in the local anesthetic your dentist may use.

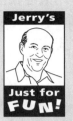

Jerry's Just for FUN!

What's That Stuck Between Your Teeth?

Here are two unbelievable, but true, toothy tales from antiquity. Remember, I'm relating these just for fun—don't give them a try!

It's well known that the ancient Egyptians were great cat worshipers. But did you know that they also had a high opinion of mice? As a matter of fact, the observant Egyptians noticed that mice have very good teeth, so they put a live mouse in the mouth of a toothache victim.

Meanwhile, the ancient Romans thought that if you tied a frog to your teeth, they (the teeth—not the frogs) would stay hard. Don't ask me how it was done!

Warts

One old cure for warts was to bury a black cat at midnight. Yikes! Another old cure that kitty won't mind as much is to rub the wart with a pumice stone to rough up the surface, and then apply a few drops of oil of wintergreen. Cover the wart with a bandage strip. The wintergreen contains methyl salicylate, which is similar to the main ingredient in most commercial wart and corn removers—salicylic acid. Repeat this treatment every other day until the wart dissolves.

Look Your Best: Personal Care

My Grandma Putt wasn't a fancy woman, and she had a word or two to say (under her breath, of course) about those "painted ladies." But she did know a few tricks for how to show off to best advantage what God gave us in the looks department. Here are some of my favorites.

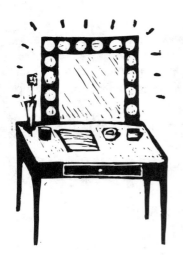

The Eyes Have It

Your eyes can say a lot about you—especially if they're tired looking or black and blue! Here are a few tips on having the best-looking peepers around.

◆ LOOK CUKE

I'm not the kind of guy who worries much, and when I do have something on my mind, I try not to let it keep me up at night. But if you're losing sleep over something and wake up with dark circles under your eyes, here's a little something you can try that'll get rid of those rings and will make you feel relaxed for a while.

Cucumbers have been used since ancient times as a skin cleanser; they're also an ingredient in many skin care products today. Cut two slices from a fresh cucumber. Find a nice, quiet place to lie back, and place one slice of cucumber over each eye. For a cool treat on a hot day, use a cuke that's been in the refrigerator. Not only is this great for dark circles, but if your eyes are irritated from smoke or dust in the air, this'll soothe them better than any eyedrops will.

◆ FINER THAN A SHINER

I'm a peaceable sort and never have been given a black eye in anger. But there was that time or two when the wind caught the door, and the door caught me by surprise, right in the eye. It gave me a shiner a prizefighter would have been proud of. What did I do? Why naturally, I turned to an ancient Native American remedy for soothing cuts and bruises—witch hazel.

Now, I'm fortunate enough to have had a witch hazel shrub on hand to brew a tea from the bark and leaves. I applied this tea, cooled down, as a compress over the black eye with a towel. It reduced the swelling and helped the cut heal. If you don't have your own witch hazel bush, the commercial preparation of witch hazel is the next best thing. Apply it as a compress, but make sure you don't get any in your eye. The alcohol in it will sting like crazy and really get you fighting mad.

> ### Send Those Crows Feet a Walkin'
>
> Eventually, everybody winds up with those little wrinkles, called crow's feet, at the corners of their eyes. I like to think of them as the result of a lifetime of smiling, so I tend not to worry too much about them. But if your face is accumulating "character" a little too quickly for your liking, then try this.
>
> Use a pin to prick a tiny hole in a vitamin E capsule. Squeeze a drop of the vitamin oil onto your fingertip and massage it into the creases. Be careful not to get any of the stuff in your eye. This ought to help keep the skin around your eyes softer and less likely to wrinkle—for a little while longer, anyway. So keep on smiling!

Face and Skin Care

Before you run off and spend every last dime on those high-priced creams, gels, and serums that crowd the department store shelves, try some of my Grandma Putt's old-time skin care techniques. They'll not only keep your skin looking its best, they'll save you a bundle, too!

◆ A HEALTHY MEAL FOR YOUR FACE

Ben Franklin said, "Early to bed and early to rise, makes a man healthy, wealthy, and wise." And I say, when it comes to keeping your face looking young and healthy, you should rise early and invite your face to a hearty breakfast!

Give yourself a facial with any one (or a mixture) of the following ingredients: chamomile tea, oatmeal, puréed fresh strawberries, sunflower oil, or wheat germ oil. Leave it on your skin for 15 minutes or so, and rinse it off with cold water. *Mmmmm* good.

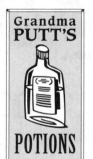

Sunburn Salad

When it comes to sunburn, the best remedy is prevention. Grandma Putt never let us play in the sun without some kind of covering—especially between the hours of 10:00 A.M. and 2:00 P.M. when the sun's rays are the strongest.

Sometimes I didn't listen, though, and ended up looking more like a rock lobster than a little boy. When that happened, Grandma didn't scold me, she just reached for two of her favorite remedies, both of which she kept in the icebox.

The first was white vinegar. She kept some in a spray bottle in the refrigerator and when she sprayed it on...well, first of all, it was nice and cool, but something in the vinegar really soothed the pain.

Other times, she'd apply a little cold, plain yogurt. That was my favorite because not only was it cold, but it also took away the pain—and I didn't end up smelling like salad dressing!

◆ THE FACE OF MILK AND HONEY

For a delightful milk-and-honey facial cleanser, mix 2 teaspoons of warmed (not hot) honey with 2 tablespoons of whole milk. This mixture doesn't keep very well, so make it as you need it. Rinse your face, massage the cleanser in for a couple of minutes, then rinse it off, and pat your face dry.

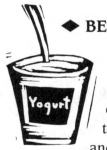

◆ BE A MASKED (WO)MAN

Natural yogurt (unflavored, of course) makes a terrific facial mask and cleanser for your skin—the gentle acids in the yogurt clean and tone your skin. If you're the abrasive type (I didn't say that), or rather, if you like a little scrubbing action, grind a little dry, uncooked oatmeal in your coffee grinder until it's a fine powder. Mix that into the yogurt (along with some honey, if you like) before you apply it to your face. Wash it all off with warm water.

◆ TAKE A SPICY SOAK

There's nothing like a good, hot bath after a long, hard day to soothe those tired muscles and help you relax. Another great thing about a hot bath is that it opens the pores and rids the body of toxins. Sure, you can use hot water alone, but to really add some spice to your life...add some spice to your bath!

Grate about 4 tablespoons of fresh ginger (that's about a quarter of a cup), and add it to the bath water while the tub is filling. Not only does this make the water (and you) smell great, but the ginger also promotes perspiration, which is your skin's way of getting rid of some of the poisons your body has absorbed. And it sure beats those perfumy, soapy bubbles that can dry out your skin!

◆ GIVE YOURSELF A HOTFOOT

If you suffer from cold feet (and I don't mean the kind that leave the groom at the altar), then here's a hot tip. Before you slip into your snuggly slippers, sprinkle a little cayenne pepper into your socks. This works great at bedtime, or when you need to go out in the cold, too. If you're worried about the pepper staining them, use an old pair of socks.

Hair Care

You probably have a favorite shampoo, conditioner, mousse, gel, or what-have-you, that you use all the time. And I'm not here to make you switch to something different. But here are a few old-fashioned hair-care tips that you may not have heard of before that still work wonders today.

◆ CLEAN RINSE

Believe it or not: Shampoo makes your hair dirty! Like every-one else, you probably use shampoo to clean your hair. But shampoo doesn't rinse away entirely, and it can build up in your hair, making it harder to clean. Not to worry—you've got

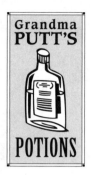

Mother Nature's Hair Care

There are a million products in the stores that will "fix" whatever's wrong with your hair. And about another million to buy even if there's nothing wrong. I buy my hair-care products in the supermarket produce section. Here's why:

☑ If your hair is oily, it needs something that will absorb the excess oil without drying out your scalp. Chop up three good-sized **raw carrots,** and then purée them in a blender. Apply this to your scalp and leave it on for 15 minutes. Rinse it off with cool water.

☑ Dry hair your problem? It makes sense to me that if your hair is dry, it's crying out for something oily. The cure? A ripe (or overripe is even better!) **avocado,** skinned and mashed. Apply it to your hair and leave it on for 15 minutes, then rinse it out with cool water. Holy guacamole! Your dry hair will be rich with moisture after you try that a few times.

☑ So what about the rest of you who have what the shampoo companies like to call "normal" hair? That is, hair that's not too oily or too dry. Even normal folks need TLC, too. Peel and then purée two **cucumbers** in a blender. Massage the mixture into your hair and leave it there for 15 minutes. Rinse it away with cool water. Feel how good it is on your scalp? Almost makes you glad you're normal.

something in your cupboard that'll solve that problem in a jiffy. The next time you wash your hair, use a little white vinegar instead of shampoo. If you do this every so often, you'll rinse away any shampoo residue still in your hair, and your favorite shampoo will work better.

◆ A NATURAL HIGH(LIGHTER)

One of the biggest trends in commercial shampoo formulas is botanicals. But you don't need to buy a fancy, expensive, trendy bottle of suds to give your hair a natural treat. If you drink chamomile tea, brew an extra cup and set it aside for the next time you wash your hair. After you shampoo, rinse your hair with the tea to add a luxurious shine to it.

CHAPTER 6

Man's Best Friends

So you have a pet, or you're thinking about getting one. Well, join the club! Most households in this country include at least one pet—and many of them have two, three, four, or even more!

Americans love pets, and for good reason. They provide unconditional love and companionship—and science is now proving that owning a pet has real health benefits. Holding a kitty or petting a dog can measurably lower your blood pressure and help you live longer. Heck, who needs medicine when you can just hug your cat?

Let's say you've made up your mind to get yourself a pet. You simply drive to the pet store or breeder, plunk down your cash, and head home with your new friend, right? Not so fast! There's a bit of legwork to do, questions to ask (and answer) before you even choose your pet. Or maybe you already have a pet—a dog who barks all day long and is driving you (and your neighbors) absolutely nuts. The solution is to keep shouting at him to quiet down, right? Nope.

As you can see, the joys of pet ownership also bring responsibility. I've written this chapter to help you deal with some of the more common issues that come with owning a pet, whether you're just now thinking of getting one, or if you've had your best friend for a long time.

One word of apology: throughout this chapter, I refer to dogs as "he" and cats as "she." I certainly don't mean to discriminate, so please bear with me (and offer my apologies to your female dog and male cat).

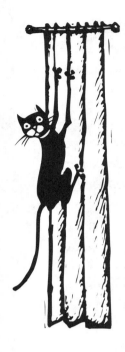

Are You Ready for a Pet?

The decision to bring a pet into your home is a mighty big one, and one that you and your family shouldn't make lightly. You've heard all the stories about the thousands and thousands of unwanted pets languishing in shelters all over the country. That news always breaks my heart, and I'd hate for my readers to in any way contribute to that problem.

So before you make the leap into pet ownership, think long and hard—especially if the reason you want one is because you have kids who are begging and pleading for a pet. Little ones will promise to feed, care for, walk, pet, and play with a new puppy or kitty, but kids will be kids, and sometimes those chores are either taken care of by parents or neglected altogether. And that can mean one more pet ends up in a shelter.

Ponder This

So how can you be sure you're really ready for a pet? Well, you've got to do a lot of thinking and a little research. To make things easier, I've come up with the questions you need to ask yourself when you're trying to decide if a pet is right for you.

Why Do I Want a Pet? Sounds like a silly question? Not at all! People get pets for all sorts of reasons. Some folks want a lap companion; others want a protector; still others want a hiking friend. If you know why you want a pet, you can narrow down the type of pet that's best for you.

Have I Ever Had a Pet Before? If the answer's no, perhaps you'd best start small, say with a hamster or a goldfish. If I were brand-new to the world of pet ownership, I probably wouldn't want to start with a hard-to-care-for pet such as an expensive macaw or an iguana. Makes sense, huh?

Do We Have Enough Room? The size of your home plays a big role in the kind of pet you might get. A 30-acre farm would make a terrific home for a big dog who likes to run around, or for an outdoor cat. Even birds need space, at least inside your home (that means the largest cage you can afford, and with some kinds of birds, flying room outside his cage as well).

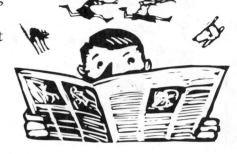

But what if you live in a tiny apartment? Not to worry; there are plenty of pets that would be perfectly happy living in a small space. All a hamster, gerbil, or other "pocket pet" needs is a cage. A cat would be perfectly happy in a small space, as would a small dog like a Chihuahua.

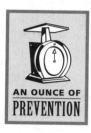

AN OUNCE OF
PREVENTION

Don't Get Your Dander Up!

Here's a little fable I like to tell folks who are thinking about getting a pet. It's about a family named the Smiths. Mrs. Smith really wanted a purebred standard poodle. She used the excuse that it would teach the kids responsibility—but the real reason was that a friend of hers had a dog that she was always bragging about and Mrs. Smith wanted one of her own.

So Mr. and Mrs. Smith shopped around, visiting all the most exclusive breeders in town, and finally, they plopped down more than $1,000 for a poodle. And that was without the rhinestone collar!

Well, they got that doggie home and everyone immediately fell in love with her. And Mrs. Smith had gone all out. She bought the dog an expensive leather leash, a handmade pottery dog dish, and a fancy grooming kit. Only there was one thing that Mrs. Smith hadn't planned for. About three days after Pinky (that's what they named her) arrived, one of the kids started sneezing and wheezing and coughing and hacking. Uh-oh. Turns out that little Billy Smith was allergic to pet dander, only no one knew that until they brought Pinky home.

Poor Pinky ended up being sold—for less than half of what the family originally paid for her. Everyone was heartbroken, especially the kids.

The moral? Don't let this happen to you! Before you bring a pet home, make sure that no one in your family is allergic to animals. One way to do that is to visit an animal shelter over a period of days and take a pet to the "get acquainted" room (all shelters have one). Let everyone play with the animal and watch carefully for any allergic reactions.

Can You Afford a Pet?

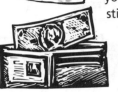

Even after you've considered how much time and energy you can spend with a pet and how much room you have to offer, you still need to consider the cost of being a pet owner. Up-front costs for a pet can vary widely—a hamster will cost a couple of bucks, while fish can be anywhere from a few bucks to a few hundred bucks and more. Dogs and cats, depending on the breed and whether or not they're purebred, can set you back from less than $100 to thousands of dollars.

If it's a bird that tickles your fancy, costs vary depending on the kind of bird that you're interested in. Finches and budgies are at the low end of the price scale, around $20 each. Cockatiels can cost four or five times as much as that and parrots four or five times as much as cockatiels. Certain exotic types, like the hyacinth macaw, can cost several thousand dollars.

But keep in mind that no matter how inexpensive the pet may be, you still have to account for expenses like cages, water bottles, food dishes, leashes, collars, toys, and, of course, food. You know, just like with kids, the costs of pets don't stop when you get them home. Oh, no—you'll be paying expenses for a very long time.

And it's important to calculate those weekly, monthly or annual costs when you decide to get a pet to make sure you really can afford one. Use this checklist as a general guide.

☑ **Food.** Oh, but you knew that, right? Your new best friend will eat every single day of his or her life (unless you get an animal like a snake, which doesn't eat that frequently at all). And don't forget miscellaneous treats, too.

☑ **Veterinary care.** Your pet is going to continue to need annual exams and shots over the course of his or her life. And even though no one likes to think in these terms, your pet will probably need at least one emergency visit to the vet, too.

☑ **Kennels or pet-sitting services.** What happens when you go on vacation or on a business trip and your pet can't accompany you? You'll have to board your pet or hire a pet sitter to come to your home to take care of him or her.

☑ **Grooming.** Some pets (hamsters, for instance) don't need to be groomed. But some dogs and cats that have fussy coats may need this service fairly frequently.

☑ **Liability.** What happens if Fido takes a bite out of the neighbor's cat—or worse—his child? Does your insurance cover this?

How Much Energy Do I Have? If the extent of your exercise plan is changing channels, well, I'd advise you not to get a dog that needs lots of activity. Take a beagle, for instance. Cute? You bet. 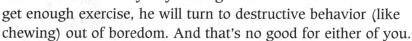 Sedate? Not on your life. Beagles are hunting dogs that need to run around for at least an hour a day. If your dog doesn't get enough exercise, he will turn to destructive behavior (like chewing) out of boredom. And that's no good for either of you.

Now, if you're kind of sedentary and you've got your heart set on a dog, you might want to get a toy poodle or some other small, less hyper dog. Another way to go is to get a non-active pet like a fish.

Some pets don't need you to be active, just interested. The most important thing to consider when choosing a bird, for instance, is if you want a pet that needs to be fussed over. Most birds are social, intelligent animals that require lots of attention and stimulation. They like to play, just like puppies, though you probably won't get your heart rate up. Of course, the opposite applies, too. If you're looking for a friend to go along with you on your daily 3-mile run, you don't want a canary, but a beagle might be perfect.

How Often Am I Away from Home? Are you one of those folks who leaves for work at 7:00 A.M. and doesn't get back home until 8:00 P.M.? You wouldn't want to inflict that schedule on a dog, would you? Of course not. Dogs are social animals and need companionship and attention—so are birds. On the other hand, a cat (or a fish) won't mind (and probably won't even notice) that you're not around.

Choices, Choices

Once you've decided that you're ready for a pet, you've got a lot of choices. No matter if you've got your heart set on a tank full of fish, a bird or two, or a furry friend, take a look at the tips below before you get going.

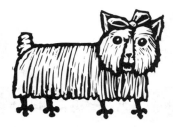

◆ THE SHORT AND THE LONG OF IT

If you can't bear the thought of pet hair all over your furniture and carpeting, you may want to consider a "pocket pet" (such as a hamster or gerbil), a bird, or a short-haired dog or cat. All dogs shed to a certain extent, as do most cats, but you're going to notice long strands of pet fur around the house a lot more than little short ones. Some cats and dogs are hairless, or nearly so, and have the added bonus of being suitable for (some) folks with allergies! Long-haired dogs and cats need a lot more grooming and regular brushing than short-haired pets, so be prepared.

◆ QUIET OR LOUD?

Fish are really, really quiet. Kitties can be quiet, but some meow to beat the band. Dogs, well, you know. And birds? Suffice it to say that while some (budgies and cockatiels) are relatively quiet, most birds' songs and calls are intended by nature to carry for great distances. Now, you might not mind a loudish pet, but what about your neighbors?

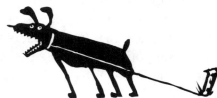

◆ GIMME SHELTER

I know they're cuter than cute, but do you really, truly need to bring home a puppy or kitten, or would an adult animal better fit into your home and lifestyle?

It's true that most folks prefer a young animal so that they can get to know and train their pet from the start. But I'm going to make my pitch for shelter animals. Shelters are full to bursting with beautiful, lovable, housetrained dogs and cats that are in desperate need of a good home. So please, if you're in the market for a pet, consider adopting one of them.

Of course, you need to take time to get to know a shelter dog or cat before you bring him or her home. Make sure to quiz the staff about the animal's temperament and why it was given up for adoption.

◆ IT'S IN THE BLOOD

Owning a purebred dog—complete with papers—is a point of pride with many folks, and rightly so. A purebred dog is beautiful. And since particular breeds have (generally speaking) predictable personality traits, their temperaments are easier to predict. But purebred dogs aren't for everyone. For one thing, they can cost thousands of dollars. And finding a reliable breeder can be a problem. And be aware that some dogs are so overbred that they're prone to health problems.

But what about a mutt? They're not called lovable for nothing! Mutts are easier (and less expensive) to come by, too, especially if you scout your local shelters. Just remember: A mutt will love you just as much as a purebred dog will—and isn't that what really counts?

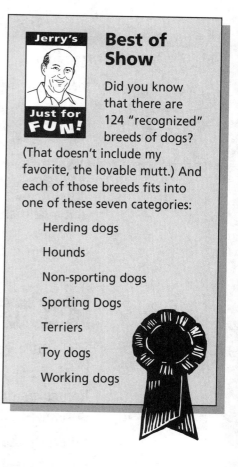

Jerry's Just for FUN!

Best of Show

Did you know that there are 124 "recognized" breeds of dogs? (That doesn't include my favorite, the lovable mutt.) And each of those breeds fits into one of these seven categories:

Herding dogs

Hounds

Non-sporting dogs

Sporting Dogs

Terriers

Toy dogs

Working dogs

◆ THE CAT'S MEOW

Most of the cats you see around you are mixed-breed cats, but there are purebred kitties to be had, too. And just as with purebred dogs, they can cost a whole lot, too. Particular breeds have fairly predictable personality traits (independent or affectionate or vocal, for instance). There are lots of terrific sources you can use if you have your heart set on a purebred—I'd start with your local vet and library.

◆ LET ME ASK YOU THIS

Let's face it, there are challenges to be met when you're a pet owner, and for some folks, they simply don't outweigh the (myriad) benefits. Are you really ready to walk your dog four

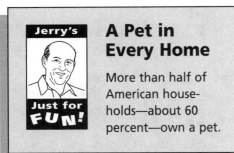

Jerry's Just for FUN!

A Pet in Every Home

More than half of American house-holds—about 60 percent—own a pet.

or five times a day, in driving rain, sleet, snow, cold, and heat? Do you mind the smell of a litter box? How about pet hair on the furniture? Or bird poop? If you live in the city, you're going to have to pick up the dog doo. Can you bear a pet saying "Polly want a cracker" all night? Paper training a puppy requires a substantial effort. Ever smelled a wet dog on a hot day? Ever tried to bathe a dog that just didn't want to get bathed? Ever try to trim a skittish cat's claws? Or give it a pill when it was sick?

Now, I'm a real animal lover, and I hate doing some of this stuff—but to me, it's all worth it. Is it for you?

Finding the Perfect Pet (for You)

Once you've decided what kind of pet you want to bring home, it's time to take a look at what's out there. Don't be taken by the very first fuzzy 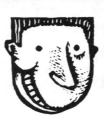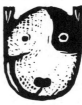 critter you see. Read on for some pointers on what to keep in mind when the "adoption" day arrives.

Where, Oh Where, Do I Get a Pet?

As you've probably guessed by now, my most favorite place to pick out a new feline or canine companion is the local humane shelter. But there are lots of other terrific places to find a new pet, too.

◆ RESCUE ME

Have you heard about rescue groups? These are organizations that take in unwanted dogs, cats, and birds of particular breeds.

For instance, greyhound rescue groups take in greyhounds that have retired from racing. The group then makes those dogs available to loving families.

If you're interested in a dog or a cat of a particular breed or a particular kind of bird, find out if the breed you're interested in is represented by a rescue group. The easiest ways to find out are to ask a veterinarian or to search the Internet. (For instance, if you'd like to own a Persian cat, search under "Persian cat rescue.")

◆ NEAT AS A PEN

A local veterinarian is a terrific resource for finding pets. He or she can steer you in the right direction and can help you from making mistakes. Whether you're sent to a breeder, a rescue operation, or a private home, once you arrive there, take a good, hard look around. Do the doggies or kitties seem healthy and happy? Are the bottoms of the bird cages neat? Are the surroundings clean? Is there plenty of food and water available for the animals? If the answers are no, you should take your business elsewhere.

> *To a dog, you're family.*
> *To a cat, you're staff.*
>
> JERRY BAKER

Puppy Love

I'm a softy—always have been, especially when I was a little kid. I remember when I was 10 years old, and Grandma Putt told me that I could get a puppy.

Now, I was the kind of kid who always wanted to get the straggliest little Christmas tree because I felt sorry for it, sure that no one else would buy it.

Grandma Putt knew that about me, and so before we left to pick out my new puppy, she gave me these words of advice. "I know you're going to see the runt, the littlest guy, the one that seems shy and frightened, and you're going to want to rescue him. But remember that a shy and frightened puppy will probably grow up to be a shy and frightened dog, and a frightened dog can be aggressive. So be careful, Jerry. Play with all the puppies and pick one that's friendly and alert—it'll be better for the both of you."

You know, she was right. And that advice goes for kittens, too; a healthy kitten won't be overly shy—but she shouldn't attack you, either!

Take Him for a Test Drive

You wouldn't buy a used car without having your mechanic look at it first, would you? Well, the same goes for a pet from a pet store or a private seller. No, I'm not suggesting that you take your kitten or puppy to the local garage. Rather, take him to visit your vet before you buy him—any reputable pet store will allow you to do that. And if a private seller won't agree to a pre-purchase checkup, go someplace else. Your vet can make sure the animal is absolutely healthy and warn you about any health problems that may develop later on. The small cost of the exam will certainly outweigh the cost (and pain) of purchasing a sick animal.

◆ DON'T ROB THE CRADLE

Make sure that the adorable, alert, friendly, and frisky little puppy or kitten you picked out is ready to leave the litter. Puppies should be at least 10 weeks old and kittens at least 12 weeks old before they are taken from their mothers.

◆ IT'S IN THE GENES

Wondering just how big that puppy you have your eye on will be in a few years? Take a look at his parents. It's a safe bet that the puppy, when full grown, will be no bigger than his largest parent.

Bring in the Birds!

Whether they're sweet singers or downright chatty, birds are truly interesting and beautiful pets for those willing to devote the time and attention. If you think a bird is for you, here's a little help to get you started.

◆ HEY, GOOD LOOKIN'

When you're ready to purchase a bird from a breeder or dealer, you should know what a healthy bird looks like. Birds are beautiful animals and seem to take pride in their appearance. So, just as you may not want to fuss with your hair on a day you wake up with a cold, a messy bird is probably sick. Healthy birds, on the other hand, spend a lot of time grooming themselves (you know, like teenagers). Their feathers should look unruffled and intact (except when they're molting, when they can look a little scruffy). There should also be no secretions near the nostrils or ears.

◆ A BUNDLE OF ENERGY

A healthy bird is active and alert. While they do take naps, most birds are usually bundles of energy. So any bird you're observing should be observing you. In addition, it should be continuously watching and responding to its environment, as well as grooming itself, moving around the cage, and playing with its toys.

Bird Basics

Here's a short introduction to some different kinds of birds suitable for first-time bird owners:

Finches. Their unique song can be quite beautiful. They get along with other finches, but love being around their owner.

Canaries. These pretty birds have lots of personality. They like lots of room to move around, and they're good with other canaries in the cage.

Budgerigars. That's a tongue-twister, eh? Budgies, as these small parrots are called, are tame and sociable. They're known to be friendly and very talkative.

Cockatiels. These mid-sized birds are intelligent, amusing, and lovable.

Lovebirds. They're not big talkers, but they can be very affectionate.

Call Me Methuselah

Cats may have nine lives, but birds only have one life that can last for a very long time. A cockatiel can live up to 20 years. An Amazon or African grey parrot can live 50 or 60 years, and there are cases of some birds living to be 100 or more! Are you ready for that kind of commitment?

As you can imagine, it's not unusual for birds to be passed down from one generation to another. So if you have a breed of bird that has a particularly long lifespan, be sure to make arrangements for your pet's care after you're gone.

◆ SOUNDS GOOD TO ME

A healthy bird breathes easily, with no wheezing or clicking sounds. If you hear anything strange, the bird is most likely sick.

There's Something Fishy Going On!

Freshwater tropical fish and goldfish are great first pets. And like all pets, they require a certain amount of attention. But once you set up your aquarium, aside from regular maintenance like keeping the water filter clean and feedings, fish are practically pure enjoyment. Here's what to look for when you're shopping for a pet fish.

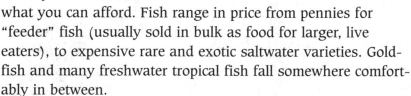

◆ HOW MUCH IS THAT FISHY IN THE WINDOW?

If you're thinking of buying a fish, first visit the pet store and see what's available. Then check your bank account to see what you can afford. Fish range in price from pennies for "feeder" fish (usually sold in bulk as food for larger, live eaters), to expensive rare and exotic saltwater varieties. Goldfish and many freshwater tropical fish fall somewhere comfortably in between.

◆ GOOD NEIGHBORS

Be sure to select fish that will get along with each other in the confines of their tank. For instance, Mollies and Plattys are bosom buddies, but a medium-sized Jack Dempsey will go through that school of Neons like a bear coming out of hibernation. And two males will fight over territory and females. (Men!) Make sure that the salesperson knows that the fish you're purchasing are going in the same tank. He or she will let you know if they're compatible.

◆ MAKE ROOM

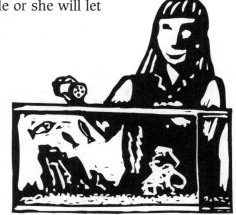

Overcrowding the tank is a common error that first-time fish owners make. Here's how to prevent that mistake: Allow 1 gallon of water per 1 inch of fish. Keep this rule in mind as you make your selections at the pet store. Some types of fish actually require less room than others, but this is a good place to start.

◆ LOCATION, LOCATION, LOCATION

Remember this old saying when trying to decide where to place the fish tank: A pint's a pound the world around—a pint of water weighs 1 pound. So a 10-gallon tank weighs more than 80 pounds when filled with water, gravel, plants, and fish. It may look like it fits on that bookshelf, but you'd be better off placing it on something more sturdy, like a tabletop or a tank stand.

I used to keep a 20-gallon tank on top of an old dresser I purchased at a garage sale. The drawers underneath were the perfect place to keep my fish supplies—food, extra filter materials, and cleaning supplies.

◆ DON'T GET INTO HOT WATER

Another factor to consider when placing the fish tank in your home is if anything immediately outside the tank will affect the environment inside of it. This, in turn, will affect the fish. Windows can affect the temperature of the tank. So can direct sunlight, which will also promote the growth of algae. And steer clear of areas near radiators and hot water risers, as they can affect the temperature of the tank as well.

◆ THERE'S NO PLACE LIKE HOME

Set up your aquarium entirely, including water, plants, filter, gravel, and ornaments, before bringing your new charges home. Do this about 48 hours before your guests arrive so that the entire tank environment will be stabilized by the time you add the fish.

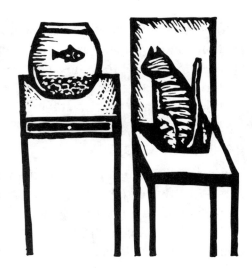

◆ MAKE A FRUGAL FILTER

If your filter uses an activated charcoal-and-polyester cartridge, you may be able to save some money by making your own filter with activated charcoal bought in bulk from the pet store and polyester pillow stuffing purchased at a craft store. Here's how:

1. Fill a clean, old nylon stocking with about 3 tablespoons of activated charcoal. Knot it and run it under cool, running water until the dust is removed.

2. Place this sack of charcoal in the cartridge compartment of the filter, along with two or three good-sized pinches of the poly stuffing.

3. Change the poly stuffing whenever it gets soiled (usually after a couple of weeks). At that time, run the charcoal stocking under cool running water to rinse it. Replace the charcoal once a month and replace the stocking once it starts to wear out.

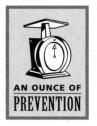

AN OUNCE OF PREVENTION

Hold Your Water

When you finally bring you new fish home, don't just open the bag and dump them into the tank. Let the closed bag float in the water for about an hour before releasing the fish into the aquarium. That'll get them used to any difference in the water temperatures.

Making Your Pet Feel at Home

You know it's going to be wonderful having a new pal around, but there are bound to be a few challenges, too. You can pave the way for an easy homecoming by being prepared for your pet's arrival *before* the big day. Here are some of my favorite ways to adjust to having a new pet around the house.

Before the Homecoming

OK, you've decided that you've got the room in your home and your heart for that new pet. So you run right out and buy one, right? Wrong! It's not that simple. You must first make sure that everything's ready before you bring home your companion. Here's what you need to know.

◆ FIND THE VET, *THEN* GET THE PET

Once you've made the commitment to adopt a new companion, you need to decide on one of the most important people in your pet's life (next to you, of course)—the veterinarian. Think of it as a kind of family planning. Your vet can help you decide just what kind of pet is right for you, and a local vet may suggest the best place to adopt a pet. Your vet will also tell you what shots your pet will need in order to stay healthy and strong.

You're going to be seeing a lot of that guy or gal, especially throughout your pet's first year, so choose a vet you feel comfortable with. The most reliable way to find a vet is by word of mouth. Ask your pet-owning neighbors and friends who they use, and that'll put you on the right track.

◆ POINTS TO PONDER

Of course, you want a veterinarian who will answer all of your questions and has a good kennel-side manner, too. Here are a few more points to consider when you're in search of a vet:

☞ Will your vet make house calls, or do you need to bring the pet in?

☞ Is his or her waiting room large enough to accommodate both dogs and cats—so they can't fight like cats and dogs?

☞ Does the vet provide long-term care and 24-hour emergency care? If not, where is the nearest animal clinic or hospital, and is the vet affiliated?

☞ Sure, the vet's an expert with dogs and cats, but what if you've got a bird, or a reptile, or a pot-bellied pig? Will he or she know how to treat it?

◆ PET-PROOF THE PREMISES

Just as you wouldn't allow a toddler in your home without making your home toddler-proof, you need to make your home safe for your new pet, as well. Put away anything chewable or breakable—like your favorite leather shoes or that expensive porcelain floor vase or even those heirloom champagne flutes that you keep on top of your refrigerator (remember, kitties are good jumpers and birds can fly).

◆ WOULDN'T CHEW KNOW IT

Both cats and dogs and some birds like to chew, so you need to put anything you don't want chewed up and sopping with pet spit out of reach. Your velvet slippers now belong in the closet (and keep that door closed!), and not under your bed.

◆ HOW SHOCKING!

Electrical wires can pose a real danger to pets, so they need to be put out of reach. You can tape them down or spray them with a wonderful concoction called Bitter Apple—which you can get at any pet store. Bitter Apple is a harmless liquid that you can spray on anything that you don't want your animal to chew. It tastes nasty, and so your pet will avoid it like the plague. The best part is that you can spray it on almost anything, from wood to fabric to leather, without harming it (or your pet).

And speaking of nasty-tasting stuff, you'll want to clean up any insect repellent or pest poison that may be on the floors or in crevices. Also, promptly clean up spills of detergent, floor cleaner, and so on before your curious pet has a chance to get a taste.

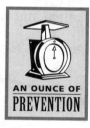

AN OUNCE OF PREVENTION

Strictly Forbidden

There are lurking dangers in your home and yard that can make your dog or cat very ill if he or she eats them. Here are just a few that you should be aware of. If you suspect that your animal has been poisoned, call your vet immediately.

- ☑ After-shave
- ☑ Alcoholic beverages
- ☑ Antifreeze; even a very tiny amount can be fatal
- ☑ Artificial-snow spray
- ☑ Bubbling holiday lights
- ☑ Cement used for plastic models
- ☑ Chocolate; dark chocolate is more toxic than milk chocolate, but don't give either to your pet
- ☑ Christmas tree-preservative chemicals
- ☑ Crayons/paints
- ☑ Epoxy

- ☑ Holly berries and leaves
- ☑ Icicles, tinsel (the kind you drape on Christmas tree branches)
- ☑ Liquid from snow globes
- ☑ Mistletoe, especially the berries
- ☑ Needles or leaves from your Christmas tree (balsam, pine or cedar)
- ☑ Perfumes
- ☑ Poinsettia leaves and stems
- ☑ Styrofoam
- ☑ Super glue

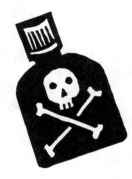

Safety First!

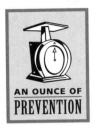

AN OUNCE OF
PREVENTION

So many of us consider our pet to be a part of the family, and they are. But there are some areas of family life your furry (or feathered) friend shouldn't participate in. Here are some do's and don'ts:

☞ Don't wash your cat's or dog's food dish with yours—it's best to wash pet dishes separately and rinse them in boiling water to kill any lingering germs.

☞ Don't kiss your pet. I know it's tempting, but it's dangerous, too. Dogs and cats eat some pretty awful stuff as they roam around, and both use their mouths to clean themselves you-know-where. Kissing your pet or letting him lick you on the mouth can lead to some big-time diseases.

☞ Always wash your hands—and make sure your kids do the same—after you touch or play with your pets.

◆ DON'T PLAY HIDE AND SEEK

Close all your closet doors and shut off any other nook that your new pet could (and, take my word for it, *would*) get into: heating vents, washers, dryers, unpatched holes in walls, crawl spaces, attics; these are all nifty pet hiding places. And take a look at the undersides of your upholstered furniture—believe it or not, some cats and other small pets find holes in the fabric that covers the bottom and will crawl up into the furniture!

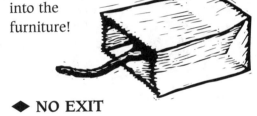

◆ NO EXIT

If you live in an apartment building or even if you have a second story on your house, make sure that your windows stay closed—and if you do open them, make absolutely sure that the screens are secure. Better yet, make it a habit to only open windows from the top, and don't push them down too far.

Bringing Puppies and Kittens Home

Moving into a new home can be a traumatic experience for a young pet. Sure, you're gonna lavish lots of love and attention on your new "baby", but until that puppy or kitten comes to think of you as family, it is going to be unsure of its new surroundings and miss his or her real mommy. Here are a couple of ways to help ease that transition.

◆ MAKE WAY FOR FIDO

Before you bring your new doggie home, you should already have the following supplies:

Brush. You want to look your best, why shouldn't he?

Chew toys. Better a bone than your loafers, right?

Collar. Make sure it's an adjustable one so that it can grow as your dog does.

Crate. If your new dog is a puppy, a crate gives him someplace den-like to hide and sleep.

Food and water dishes and dog food. You don't want the poor pup to go hungry while you run out for food, so have some on hand.

Leash. Many experts recommend the adjustable-length leashes.

Nail clippers. To reduce that "click, click, click" of your new pup walking across a hardwood, vinyl, or tile floor.

◆ GET READY FOR KITTY

Before you bring your new kitty home, you should already have the following supplies:

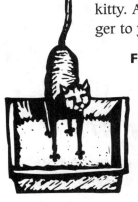

Cat carrier. You'll need this to transport your kitty. A cat running loose in the car poses a danger to you and others on the road.

Food and water dishes and cat food. Have the dishes filled when you bring kitty home.

Litter box and litter. Be sure to put the litter box in a quiet place and introduce your kitty to it as soon as you get home. And don't forget a **scoop**—you'll need it to clean out the litter box.

Scratching post. If your kitty hasn't been declawed, this is a must, or your upholstery will be ruined in no time.

◆ THERE'S THE RUB

If you got your new puppy or kitten from a breeder, take along a clean piece of fabric or a clean, old sock. When you pick out a puppy or kitten, rub the fabric on the fur of your new pet's mother, picking up her scent. Leave the sock in your new one's bed, and he will sleep dreaming of mom. (Don't be envious, you'll use this same trick to remind your pet of *you* when you leave him or her behind the first few times.)

◆ JUST LIKE CLOCKWORK

When your new little guy or gal beds down for the night, you want your pet to feel like mom is still nearby. Try the old trick of wrapping a ticking clock in a towel (just make sure the alarm won't go off!) to mimic mom's heartbeat. You can also try a hot water bottle (not too hot, please!) wrapped in a soft towel, to comfort your new arrival.

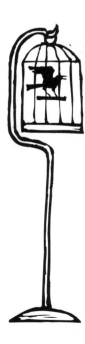

Bringing Birds Home

You know you'll need a cage and some food before you bring your new bird home. Here's what else you need to know to make your bird feel right at home.

◆ BE CAGEY

Don't let the different sizes and styles of birdcages confuse you. Just look for these features and you won't go wrong:

A slide out tray at the bottom. This'll make it easier to clean the cage. You can line the tray with newspaper or commercial liner paper—just make sure your bird doesn't eat it. A grid that separates the liner tray from the bottom of the cage is a good feature to look for.

Size matters. The cage needs to be at least as large as an adult bird can spread its wings. How big is that going to be? Do some homework on your particular species, and ask the breeder. And just like fish gotta swim, birds gotta fly—or at least have lots of room to roam around, climb, and hop from perch to perch. Get the largest cage that you can afford and have room for.

Don't forget perches. Offer your bird at least two different kinds of perches. Different sizes, shapes, and textures will allow your bird to exercise the muscles in its claws and help keep its beak and nails trim. You can buy perches, or (as I would certainly recommend) you can make them yourself (see "Build Your Bird a Perch," at right).

◆ EAT, DRINK, AND BE CHIRPY

When you get your containers for food and water, make sure they are made from a material that can be washed and sterilized regularly. And then, please remember to wash and sterilize them often in boiling water.

Build Your Bird a Perch

Wood, plastic, or rope all work fine as perch material. Just make sure the surface is something the bird can grip, will support its weight, and will attach to the cage securely. If you use wood from your yard, make sure it's sturdy enough to support your bird, is free of bugs, and hasn't been treated with pesticides. Leave the bark on; your bird will love to peel it off.

Place the perches far enough apart so your pet can stand on one upright, without hitting his or her little head on the next one (ouch!).

◆ NIGHTY, NIGHT

By covering your bird's cage at night, your feathered friend will get undisturbed sleep. But you don't have to run out and buy anything fancy—an old blanket or curtain will do. As long as it keeps the cage warm during the cooler weather, and can act as a shade if the cage is in a particularly sunny spot, it'll do the trick. But there's another reason why you should cover the cage—*your* undisturbed sleep.

A cover will prevent sunrise squawking, allowing you and the neighbors to get in a few more hours of shut-eye. Uncover the cage when you get up.

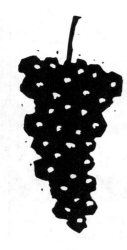

◆ POLLY WANT A PELLET...AND A GRAPE

Some birds, like finches and canaries, eat mostly seeds, but most birds will be healthier on a diet of commercially prepared food pellets. Ideally, birds should be fed twice a day, and you need to remove the uneaten food after an hour or so. This keeps the food from spoiling and your pet from overeating.

Regularly supplement your bird's diet with natural goodies like fruits and vegetables, as well as a little cooked rice and pasta. Birds love to eat foods that are entertaining as well as nutritious. For a bird, peeling a grape or a banana is a double treat—and it's a treat to watch him do it, too!

Bringing Tropical Fish Home

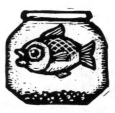

Ready to buy some tropical fish? Here's all you need to know to set up a tropical aquarium and have your fish settling in swimmingly.

◆ TANKS A LOT!

First and foremost, you'll need a tank. The kind you buy largely depends on how much room you have. A typical 10-gallon tank is about 20 inches long, 12 inches high, and 12 inches deep. Of course, you can get a wall-sized, custom-made tank if you've got the budget—and if your floor will support the weight!(See "Location, Location, Location" on page 187.)

◆ HOT STUFF

Tropical fish need to have water that's a constant 78°F to 80°F. The way to maintain these temperatures is with a small electric heater specially designed for aquariums.

◆ COVER ME

A well-designed cover will keep dust out of the tank and evaporation to a minimum. Most covers come with built-in light fixtures. Fluorescent light is best, but incandescent bulbs work well and cost less to buy.

◆ BOTTOMS UP!

You'll need to cover the bottom of the tank with something, and that something is usually gravel. Aquarium gravel is inexpensive and is available in a wide assortment of colors and styles at the pet store.

◆ KEEP IT CLEAN

In nature, fish wastes, decaying food, and plant matter are washed away by moving tides and currents. But in the closed system of an aquarium, these waste products have nowhere to go, so they need to be removed by a filtering system. Some filters fit inside the tank, while others operate from the outside. All require some form of regular maintenance, like changing a filter cartridge. Be sure to talk with the salesperson at the pet shop and get the right-sized filter for your tank.

Into the Cooler

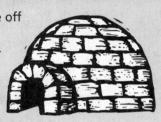

So you're off to the pet store to purchase a brand-new tropical fish. Problem is, it's about 30°F outside with a wind-chill factor of about 15°F. Now, you don't need to be a fishologist to know tropical fish (think palm trees and sandy beaches) and 15°F weather (think igloos and penguins) don't mix.

So how do you get your fishy friend from the store to your car to go home? Simple. Dig around the storage areas in your house, and grab the cooler that you take to the beach. Take it to the pet store with you and let it come to room temperature inside the store. Then, when you get your bag of fish, put it inside the cooler. I know, it's called a cooler, but it's really an insulator, and it will protect your fish from the cold outside.

◆ AQUARIUM DÉCOR

One of my favorite aquarium elements (other than my fish) are the plants. There are almost as many to choose from as there are fish! They provide color to the environment and places for shy fish to hide.

The same goes for rocks and stones. You can buy them

ready to place in the tank at the pet store. If you choose to include ones you've found yourself, be sure to sterilize them in boiling water, or you may end up poisoning your fish.

◆ PUMP ME UP!

Don't forget the pump. Aquarium pumps are small electric devices that add oxygen to the water. Some in-tank filters are also powered by a pump. And pumps drive those air-powered, moving fish tank ornaments that I love so much.

Housetraining How-To

Now that the welcome party is over, it's time to settle in with your new pet. While fish and birds need attention, they don't need housetraining. But we all know that puppies and kittens sure need to know the rules of the house! Here's a rundown of the do's and don'ts for housetraining your pets.

Dogs

In a perfect world, when your puppy had to go potty, he'd scamper off to the toilet, do his business, flush, wash his little paws, and remember to put the seat back down. Alas, it's not a perfect world, and housetraining a dog can take a lot of time. Here are some tips that can make the process a lot easier.

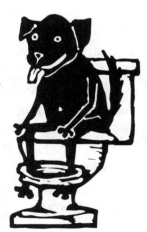

◆ DON'T RUB HIS NOSE IN IT

If there's one thing that drives me crazy, it's seeing someone rubbing a puppy's nose in a pile of poop or urine. What the heck good is that? It certainly doesn't work. To teach a dog you have to think like a dog. And for the best results, consistent and positive reinforcement are two important keys.

If you want to paper-train your pup, keep this in mind. To keep him from going on the carpet, you absolutely, positively must catch him in the act. That means when you see him starting to pee or poop on the rug, you give him *one* stern "NO!", pick him up, and move him to the newspaper. Never say "no" more than once—you don't want your puppy to think he has a choice.

There is no point in yelling at a puppy an hour after he's already made the mistake. Let's say you come home from work, and see that he's peed on the rug. You start to yell. All he knows is that he gets yelled at when you come home, even if you "show" him the mistake. On the other hand, if, when you catch him starting to pee on the rug, you say "no" in a stern voice, but praise him when he

goes on the paper, he learns, "Oh, mom loves me when I pee here." Now you're cooking with gas.

Dog-Gone Trivia

Jerry's Just for FUN!

If you're a dog lover, you probably love to hear about all kinds of obscure doggie facts. Well, here's a collection that will have you saying "hot diggity dog!"

☞ The fastest kind of dog, the Greyhound, can reach speeds of over 40 miles per hour. And not only are they fast, but Greyhounds also have the best eyesight of any breed.

☞ At the end of the Beatles' song "A Day in the Life," Paul McCartney recorded an ultrasonic whistle, audible only to dogs, for his Shetland sheep dog, Martha.

☞ The "poodle cut" was originally developed to increase the dog's swimming ability as a retriever. The haircut allowed for faster swimming while the pom-poms kept the dog's joints warm.

☞ Newfoundland dogs have webbed feet, making them strong swimmers.

☞ Sled dogs running in Alaska's annual 1,149-mile Iditarod race burn an average of 10,000 calories daily.

◆ AFTER THE FACT

So what do you do when you get home from work and find your puppy has gone on the rug? Absolutely nothing—your opportunity to correct him has passed. All you can do now is clean it up. I'll repeat: The only way to get your pup trained is to pick him up and put him on the newspaper the minute he starts to go to the bathroom. Expect this to take a while if no one is home during the day to keep an eye out.

◆ GOTTA GO!

Now there are some clues that your puppy is about to let loose. Puppies go potty very soon after they eat or drink, so that's the time to put him on the paper. If your dog is in your lap and starts to squirm, put him on the paper. When he does go on the paper, praise him like crazy—maybe even give him a treat. Consistently give your pup one firm "no" when he misses the paper, and put him on the paper when he does go. Give him consistent praise when he goes on the paper, and in time you'll have a paper-trained pup.

◆ TIME FOR SCHOOL

Once your puppy is about six months old, you may want to enroll him (and yourself) in obedience training. It's a fun way to learn the basics of training and to get your dog used to being around other dogs. And since dogs think in terms of social hierarchies, training will reinforce your dog's view of you as the one in charge.

But where do you find a school? Check the Yellow Pages; talk to your vet; get recommendations from friends, the humane society, or trusted breeders; or even check your local YMCA, which sometimes offers classes.

◆ SHHHH, QUIET PLEASE

Dogs may not be sophisticated conversationalists (like yours truly), but they definitely have something to say. And sometimes you (and the neighbors) might just wish your dog would keep it to himself. But before you scold that noisy dog, try to figure out what he's trying to say. If he barks while you're away, ask a neighbor what he sounds like. By changing his circumstances, you'll have a good chance of keeping him quiet.

Animal behaviorists say dogs have about 10 different vocalizations. Here are two that may help you figure out what's on his mind:

Long, repetitive barks may mean that your pup's bored. Get out there and play with him! He needs some excitement. If you haven't taken him already, enroll him in obedience or agility training (sort of advanced obedience training). Take him to a local park and let him meet other dogs—anything to keep him interested in life!

Excited barking means he's excited about something—maybe it's the mailman, maybe it's a burglar, or maybe it's just time for a walk.

◆ FIGHT NOISE WITH NOISE

If your dog is skittish and easily spooked by noises outside, think how scared he might be while you're away. That could be why he barks so much. To camouflage the din of the outside world, plug in one of those "white noise" machines.

What the heck are they? They're about the size of a clock radio, and they play electronic sounds resembling a babbling brook, rainfall, or the ocean, as well as a kind of a soft static, which is called white noise. Folks use them at night to help them sleep; the soothing sounds help them relax. It'll work for your pup, too. They're

---

Be a Puppy Pro

One of the easiest—and most fun—ways to make sure your puppy grows up to be friendly and easy to handle is to make sure you give him lots and lots of physical attention when he's young.

Play with and rub your pup all over. Handle him a lot, gently rubbing his face, mouth, and ears. Always be exceedingly gentle. By doing this very frequently, you will help him get used to being bathed, having his teeth brushed, and seeing the vet without much fuss.

Don't play rough games with your puppy. I know tug-of-war sounds like fun, but it will just teach your pet to be aggressive. You surely don't want that, do you?

sold in electronics stores as well as some larger drugstores and department stores.

◆ THAT'S ENTERTAINMENT!

Another trick you can try to occupy a bored or scared dog is to leave the television or radio on while you're away. The idea is not to drown out your pup, but to give him something to listen to instead of the scary outside noises. Keep the volume down so the neighbors don't have something else to complain about.

◆ I'M STILL HERE—IN SPIRIT

The great thing about dogs is they miss you while you're away. But sometimes they miss you so much that they may bark or do something destructive like digging or chewing. To take your dog's mind off the fact that you're not around, try this: Just before you leave, rub your hands all over your dog's favorite toy or bone. He'll like it even more now that it reminds him of you.

◆ HELLO...HELLO...

If your dog barks at you constantly, one way to get him to stop may be to acknowledge him. He's trying to tell you something. Once he's sure *you* know, he might stop.

◆ CRATES ARE GREAT

I know that from a human's perspective, the thought of being in a crate is awful. But let's face it—as much as we'd like them to be, and no matter how much we treat them as if they were, dogs aren't humans. They're, well, dogs! And in nature, dogs live in small dens, and those dens are places of comfort. What's my point? Well, when you bring home a new puppy, it's a wonderful idea to have a crate waiting for him. It's a place where he can sleep and hang out and, most important, feel safe.

Crates are great for a number of reasons:

☞ The crate is a safety zone for your puppy. While he's in there, your puppy won't be able to chew your slippers or electrical cords (or anything else).

☞ Your puppy will feel safe in a crate. That means he'll be less frightened when you're not around.

☞ Dogs don't like to go to the bathroom in the same spot where they sleep. That means if you're trying to housetrain your puppy, he's likely to "hold" it a little longer when he's in his crate. (Though you must keep in mind that puppies don't have terrific control over their bodily functions and have to go to the toilet very frequently.) You can put a 12-week-old puppy in a crate for two hours and expect him to hold it. Check with your vet to find out how long your puppy can stay in the crate.

AN OUNCE OF PREVENTION

Just Say No

Ah, mealtime—yours, that is. But what's this? A cute face looking up at you, begging for a small morsel, a crumb, a tasty castoff.

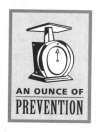

Wait! Here's your perfect opportunity to keep your pet from ever begging: Never, EVER give your animal table scraps, and he'll never expect to get them. I know it's tempting (just look at that face!), but once you give him a taste, he'll associate your dinnertime with treat time for the rest of his life. Plus, table scraps are not healthy for your pet, so please, be firm and just say no.

◆ HOW MUCH CRATE DOES A DOG NEED?

Sure, you want your dog's crate to be cozy, but not confining. When you pick one out, make sure it's large enough for your dog to stand up, turn around, and lay down in.

◆ TAKE A BITE OUT OF BITING

Here's my favorite way to stop a puppy from biting. (If you have an adult dog that bites, well that's a whole other kettle of fish; call a reputable obedience trainer right away.) Now, as far as your puppy is concerned, you are the world, and he counts on your love, affection, and attention. You can use this to your advantage to train your puppy—without resorting to any type of unkind punishment.

As soon as the little nipper bites your hand, give him one stern "NO!", put him in his crate, and ignore him for five minutes or so. Never say "no" more than once—you don't want him to learn that he can keep biting until you say "no" the fifth time. By being put in the cage alone, he's learning that biting is not a good way to get your attention. You must be consistent, though, and do this *every single time* your puppy bites.

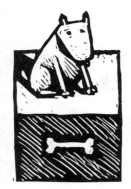

◆ DE-CHEWIFY THE ROOM

Puppies chew. Especially when they're teething. Period. But you can help reduce destructive chewing by putting away things that he shouldn't chew on. Of course, the best way to help this is to give him toys that he *is* allowed to chew—a great one is a new, sterilized bone filled with cheese. When you find your pup chewing your shoe, give him the old "NO!" and put a bone in front of him instead.

Older dogs sometimes chew because they're bored (you know, the way you bite your nails or nibble on potato chips when you're bored). What's that mean for you? Get him moving! Play with him, take him to the park, get him some obedience training—if he's active and stimulated, he'll likely give up the chewing.

Cats

Lucky for cat owners, there isn't a whole lot involved in training a cat to use the litter box. Simply make it available, fill it with an inch or two of clean litter, show it to her, and that's usually it. Unfortunately, people do make some fairly common mistakes that cause Fluffy to "miss" the box. Here's what to avoid.

◆ WHERE'S THE BATHROOM?

First of all, don't go moving the litter box around. It's important to keep it in one place, otherwise your cat may become confused. And make sure the spot is a low-traffic area—felines like their privacy, after all.

Now this may sound a bit odd, but make it obvious. When Grandma Putt first brought her kitten home, she made the mistake of putting a large potted plant in the same room as the litter box. Guess which one the kitten used? The moral of this story: Remove any other type of container from the litter box area so there is no doubt in kitty's mind.

◆ OOOH, STINKY

Keep the litter box clean. Your cat will not use a litter box that's not kept impeccably clean. Keep it scooped out and, at least once a week, rinse it with hot water. I tell folks that they can keep the box smelling a little better by putting a layer of baking soda in the bottom of the box before adding the litter.

You can make your life easier by investing in litter box liners. These are heavy plastic drawstring bags that fit into the box. Then you fill the lined box with litter. You still need to scoop daily, but at the end of the week, you simply gather up the drawstring and put the bag in the trash. It keeps the box itself clean, and you won't have to scrub it out.

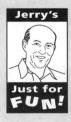

Catalog of Cat Facts

Cat lovers rejoice. Here's a sampling of feline facts that will make you purr:

☑ Cats respond better to names that end in an "ee" sound.

☑ Only 80% of all cats respond to the effects of catnip. If the cat doesn't have a specific gene, it won't even notice the herb.

☑ A cat can jump five times as high as it is tall.

☑ A cat spends nearly 30% of its life grooming itself.

☑ The Maine coon cat is America's only native breed of domestic feline.

☑ A domestic cat can run at the speed of about 31 miles per hour over short distances.

☑ Cats step with both left legs then both right legs when they walk or run.

☑ A Colonial-era superstition held that a person who kicked a cat would develop rheumatism in that leg.

Bad Kitty!

If you think you're going to train your cat to sit or come, you're barking up the wrong tree, my friend. In fact, in the end, your cat will probably train you. Of course, you may have to put an end to some destructive behaviors, and that's what we're talking about here.

◆ SCRATCH HER ITCH

Uh, oh. Is kitty scratching up that chair leg pretty bad? Well, this is a toughie, but not impossible to deal with. First off, you need to get your kitty a sturdy scratching post that's high enough for her to stretch to her full height. Then introduce her to it by gently taking her paws and showing her how to stretch and scratch. This just may save your furniture.

◆ WATCH IT, MISTER

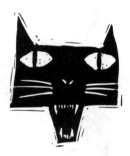

If your cat's acting aggressive, give her a spritz with a plant mister or a water pistol. It's a safe and effective way to curb all sorts of problems. But be sure that the spray bottle contained no chemicals before using it on your pet.

◆ HEY! THAT'S MY RUBBER PLANT!

Why is it that kitties like to eat plants? Is it to annoy us? Now, you all know that I'm very proud and particular about my houseplants, so you can be sure I know how to keep kitties from eating them.

Dab the plants with Bitter Apple (which you can get at pet stores). It's a foul-tasting liquid that will hurt neither your plants nor your cat, but that will keep her from feasting on your favorite greenery.

Pet Care on the Cheap

From veterinary care to pet toys to food and cleaning supplies, pet ownership can be an expensive proposition. But read on for some super ways to reduce those expenses.

Is There a Doctor in the House?

Veterinary care can really add up over time, but here are a few alternatives you may not have known about.

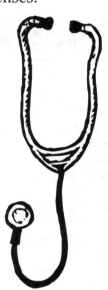

◆ GO TO VET U

If you live near a university that has a veterinary school, you may be able to get care for all kinds of pets at a greatly reduced cost. And that can mean health care, vaccinations, flea dips, even grooming, so be sure to check it out.

◆ LEAD A SHELTERED EXISTENCE

Animal shelters sometimes offer pet care like spaying, neutering, and vaccinations for a greatly reduced cost. Call your local shelter to see if it offers those services. And don't overlook pet stores. They often hold clinics and offer reduced-fee vaccinations or tests.

◆ SNIP, SNIP!

When is it time to have your pet spayed or neutered? Dogs and cats can be as young as 10 to 12 weeks old.

◆ A CRUNCHY BREATH SWEETENER

Is Fido's breath a little, um, ripe? Do your kitty's kisses make you a bit dizzy? Well, it may not be time to go to the vet just yet. Instead of tossing your pet outside, toss some raw carrot in his or her food dish—shredded for your cat and small sliced rounds for your dog. As your pet crunches, the carrot helps scrape some of the plaque from his teeth—and that can help sweeten breath.

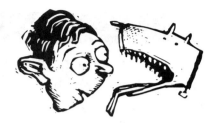

Vaccination Schedule for Dogs

DISEASE	AGE (IN WEEKS) AT 1ST, 2ND, 3RD VACCINATIONS	FOLLOW-UP VACCINATIONS NEEDED EVERY
Bordetellosis	6-8; 10-12; 14-16	12 months
Coronavirus	6-8; 10-12; 14-16	12 months
Distemper	6-8; 10-12; 14-16	12 months
Infectious canine hepatitis	6-8; 10-12; 14-16	12 months
Leptospirosis	10-12; 14-16; —	12 months
Parainfluenza	6-8; 10-12; 14-16	12 months
Parvovirus infection	6-8; 10-12; 14-16	12 months
Rabies	12; 64; —	12 or 26 months (depends on type of vaccine)

Vaccination Schedule for Cats

DISEASE	AGE (IN WEEKS) AT 1ST, 2ND VACCINATIONS	FOLLOW-UP VACCINATIONS NEEDED EVERY
Caliciviral disease	8-10; 12-16	12 months
Feline leukemia	10-12 or 13-14	24 months (depends on type of vaccine)
Panleukopenia	8-10; 12-16	12 months
Pneumonitis (chlamydiosis)	8-10; 12-16	12 months
Rabies	12; 64	12 or 36 months (depends on type of vaccine)
Viral rhinotracheitis	8-10; 12-16	12 months

Grooming for Less

Your pet can use a helping hand when it comes to keeping clean and neat, especially if it goes outdoors. But don't think you have to spend a fortune at the dog or cat groomer's. Try some of these at-home techniques first.

◆ POOCH, MEET MR. SKUNK

You're out on that evening stroll with your dog and he pokes his nose around that bush and...oh no! What's that smell? You know very well what that smell is: Your pal has just been sprayed by a skunk. That encounter is no fun for anyone, skunk included, but now you and your dog have a real mess to deal with.

First, make sure your dog wasn't injured by the skunk. If he's been bitten and is bleeding, get him to an emergency vet immediately. Skunks can carry rabies. If your dog has been vaccinated, he's safe from the rabies virus—but you're not.

Next, you'll want to get rid of that odor. Now, I know you've all heard of the tomato juice solution, but frankly, that leaves your pup pink and your hands red, and it doesn't always work. See Grandma Putt's Potion above for a solution that should do the trick.

◆ FLEE, FLEAS!

Oh, those nasty fleas. What do you do? Well, you don't have to rely solely on harsh chemicals to avoid them. Here's a flea repellent that Grandma Putt liked to recommend to her dog-owning friends. Mix a drop or two of oil of eucalyptus in your pet's shampoo. Be careful not to get it into his eyes. Also, be aware of

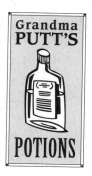

Doggie Deodorizer

Grandma Putt always used this de-skunking solution whenever my pooch got himself in a stinky situation.

2 cups of hydrogen peroxide
¼ to ½ cup of baking soda
1 tablespoon of mild dish-
    washing liquid

Mix the ingredients together, and apply to your dog's coat (but don't get it on his head or near his eyes or ears). Rub it in, then wash it out. After this deodorizing rubdown, your best friend should smell fresh and clean.

any irritated skin; the eucalyptus might make it worse. The odor, which smells good to us, keeps those pesky fleas away.

If you don't have any oil of eucalyptus on hand, grab the bottle of garlic powder that you keep in your spice rack, and mix a little into your pet's food. The aroma of the garlic will come out of Fluffy's or Spot's skin, and repel the fleas.

◆ A LOW-TECH FLEA CATCHER

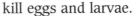

Here's a solution to flea problems that doesn't require a change in your pet's diet or bathing habits. It's a flea comb, available at most pet stores. If your pet has a problem with fleas, you'll initially need to comb your pet's coat several times a day. After about a month, once a week ought to do it to keep fleas at bay.

◆ HIT 'EM WHERE THEY LIVE

When you're fighting fleas, don't forget to clean all around the area where your pet spends most of his time, mainly pet beds, favorite rugs, and upholstery. Steam clean the areas if possible, and wash what you can in really hot soapy water to kill eggs and larvae.

Speedy Shampoo

Cornstarch, rubbed into your pet's fur and brushed out, will make his or her coat fluffy and clean when there's just no time to shampoo!

◆ SHED YOUR INHIBITIONS

It's completely normal for your dog or cat to shed—but there is one easy step you can take to reduce the amount of hair you find on your sofa and your rug and your bedspread and your...

Brush him! Too good to be true? Not at all. Regular brushing, with a good-quality brush, is the easiest way to get the hair out of your dog or cat before it falls out. Especially if you have a long-haired pet, try to give him a good going over once a day. The energy you expend brushing him will more than be made up for in the time you save not having to vacuum up the mess.

And by the way, don't buy one of those fancy gizmos they sell to get pet hair off the furniture. Rub a damp sponge over the furniture (and your clothing, too). It works just as well— and it's free!

◆ SCRUB THOSE PEARLY WHITES

It's true that many tonics you use for grooming and taking care of your dog should be specifically designed for dogs (doggie toothpaste, for instance). But if you brush your dog's teeth, you certainly don't need to purchase a special doggie toothbrush. A soft-bristled brush (child size for smaller breeds) works just fine and will probably cost less. Oh yes, one thing: Just make sure you don't mix up Fido's toothbrush with the rest of the family's!

Penny-Pinching Pet Supplies

You don't have to spend a bundle on collars, catnip, doggie treats, and toys. Here are some thrifty ways to supply your pets with the fun stuff.

◆ CHEAP CAT TOYS

Cats love to play, and fortunately, they're easily amused. The best part is that you don't need to spend a small fortune to entertain your small friend. Here are some of my favorite cat toys for cats (and owners!) on a budget:

Ping-pong balls and plastic practice golf balls, sold in any sporting goods store, are cheap and will keep kitty amused for hours. In fact, anything a cat can bat around with its paws, like a plastic bottle cap or a balled-up sock, will suit her just fine.

A do-it-yourself scratching post made out of a 12-inch piece of two-by-four wrapped in a scrap of carpeting or sisal rope. You can *really* get kitty's attention by scenting the scratching post with a little catnip—just rub it into the material. Catnip is a kind of mint that makes most cats act just silly. Like any drug, it should be given in small doses.

Catnip in a sock. Don't waste money on those expensive store-bought catnip toys that come in all shapes and sizes. Believe me, your cat doesn't care if the toy looks like a cute pink pig! It's what's inside that counts, so do your cat a favor and place some catnip in the toe of an old, clean sock. Knot the sock to keep the catnip in, and let kitty go wild with her new toy.

◆ CUT-RATE COLLAR

Do you have a leather belt that no longer fits you? Well, it might just fit another member of the family. If the leather and buckle are still sound, make a present for your pooch. First, try the belt on around his neck. Don't make it too tight (he may not be able to breathe), yet don't make it too loose, either (Fido might slip out of it or get caught on something). Trim the end of the belt with a pair of scissors, leaving enough to fit through the loop behind the buckle. Use a pen to mark the spot where the arm on the buckle will pass through the belt, and make the hole with an awl or nail.

Now, before you put the new collar around old poochie's neck, slide the belt through a key ring. This is where you'll hang his ID and vaccination tags.

◆ GROW YOUR OWN CATNIP

You can buy catnip in any pet store, but it's an easy herb to grow in your garden or in a sunny window box. You can buy the seeds from any good nursery or seed catalog.

Plant the seeds in sandy soil about 10 inches deep. The catnip will grow quickly. When it's over a foot tall with nickel-sized leaves, cut down the stalks and hang them to dry, out of kitty's reach.

Homemade Dog Biscuits

There's nothing like a home-baked treat, even if you're a dog. Here's my recipe for homemade dog biscuits that's so easy, Bowser could almost bake them himself!

²/₃ cup of water or chicken/beef stock or bullion
6 tablespoons of vegetable oil
½ cup of cornmeal
2 cups of whole wheat flour

1. Preheat the oven to 350°F. In a medium bowl, combine the water or bullion and the vegetable oil. Add the cornmeal and flour. Mix well until a dough forms, adding more flour if necessary.

2. Turn the dough out onto a lightly floured surface, and roll it out to a ¼-inch thickness.

3. Using a cookie cutter, cut the dough into shapes, re-rolling scraps as you go. If you're feeling creative, form the biscuits into shapes your pooch will love to munch on, like bones or little mailmen. Remember to keep them on the small side if your dog is little.

4. Transfer the cut-out biscuits to a nonstick cookie sheet, and bake 35 to 40 minutes, until golden brown. Let the biscuits cool on a rack, out of Fido's reach. They'll keep for a couple of weeks if you store them in a tightly sealed container or plastic bag.

Yield: At least a dozen biscuits, depending on size.

◆ PUP-SICLES

It's hot. It's humid. And everybody, including your canine companion, is as uncomfortable as all get out. What hits the spot on a day like this? How about a homemade, frozen confection—one for you and another for your pal? No, don't give your dog a popsicle—give him a *pup*sicle!

The next time you stop by your local butcher's, ask him for any lamb or beef soup bones he has on hand (they'll be cheap or maybe even free). Throw the bones in a pot of water, and let everything simmer slowly for about an hour. Cut any remaining meat off of the bones and throw it back into the pot. Let it cool completely, then pour the "soup" into several old ice cube trays and freeze them.

When the pupsicles are frozen solid, transfer them to heavy freezer bags. Then, on those hot, sultry summer days when your pup is ready for a treat, toss him one of these while you enjoy your ice cream.

◆ CHEAP TREATS

Nothin' says lovin' like somethin' from the oven, right? Well, believe you me, your canine companion feels exactly the same way. So the next time you're whipping up a batch of cookies for your family, don't turn the oven off until you've whipped up a batch of goodies for your four-legged friend.

Here's a recipe I turned up in my travels. Your dog ought to love them! Just to be on the safe side, though, you may want to show this recipe to your vet to make sure your dog doesn't have any allergies or sensitivities to any of the ingredients.

1. Preheat your oven to 350°F.

2. In a large bowl, combine 1 pound of canned dog food with 1½ cups of unsweetened wheat germ, 1¼ cups of cornmeal (*not* cornbread mix, which contains ingredients other than just cornmeal), 3 large eggs, and 1 teaspoon of powdered garlic.

3. Mix this all together very well and spread the mixture in a greased baking pan. Pop it into the oven and bake for 20 minutes.

4. Let cool completely, cut into squares, and serve to Fido.

◆ AW, SHOOT!

You're out for a walk on a hot day and Fido's getting pretty thirsty (you can tell because he's panting like mad), but there's not a water fountain in sight. First off, shame on you! In hot weather, your dog needs lots of water to keep from becoming dehydrated, just as you do. Second, you don't have to tote around a big, heavy water bottle. A better idea is to bring along a water pistol or two.

When your dog gets thirsty, you can shoot some water in his mouth. A pistol is small enough to tuck in your pocket or fanny pack and, let's face it, it's fun to use! Plan ahead—about an hour before you go for your walk, load your "weapon" and put it into the freezer or refriger-ator to keep it cool.

◆ WALL-TO-CRATE CARPETING

Sometimes you've just gotta put your dog or cat in a traveling crate and let's face it, those things aren't exactly cozy. Now, you could put some of your good towels in there to make it more comfy, but I've got an even bet-ter idea. Stop by the carpet store,

Glow-in-the-Dark Pets

How can you be sure that your dog or cat is safe outdoors after the sun goes down? Go down to your basement or out to the garage, grab the small reflectors off that old bike, and attach one to your pet's collar. Then if your cat or dog should wander out onto the street at night, passing motorists will be able to spot—and avoid—your pet.

and find yourself a scrap or two of carpet that will fit in the bottom of the crate. Since the piece will be so very small, the merchant just might give you a piece for free. (I'd wash the scrap just because the smell of new carpeting isn't very pleasant.) Now put that in the traveling crate, and your pet will thank you every time he uses the cage.

◆ BARKIN' IN THE RAIN

Maybe your furry friend hates to go out into the rain. Or perhaps it's just that you don't care for the aroma of wet dog throughout the house. Either way, there is a simple solution: a raincoat. Now, you could spend your hard-earned cash and buy one from the pet store, but here's a better, and cheaper, alternative.

Make a trip to your local thrift shop or Salvation

Army and head for the children's section. A child's small plastic rain slicker should be just about the right size for a medium-sized dog. Of course, you may have to do a few small alterations, but it's a heck of a lot better than spending a fortune on designer doggie raingear!

First-Aid for Dogs and Cats

At one time or another, most dogs and cats will put a paw or nose somewhere it doesn't belong. And when that happens, your pet will probably end up with a cut or scrape. A mere flesh wound, perhaps, but if left untreated, the cut could get infected. Along with cuts and scrapes, pets can suffer, just like us, from heat exhaustion and intestinal gas. Read on for my first-aid and health care tips for your pets.

◆ KEEP CALM

Just like you, when an animal gets a wound, if it's not too bad, he'll give it a lick, say the animal equivalent of "oh darn," and continue on his way. But if your animal gets hurt and is frightened, you need to calm him down before you can treat the wound. This not only helps you treat your pet, but it also makes treating him safer for you.

If your dog is injured and you think you're in danger of being bitten, improvise a muzzle out of a roll of gauze or an athletic bandage. Loosely wrap the dog's snout. Be sure not to cover his nostrils. For a very small dog or a cat, wrap the animal securely in a towel or blanket to keep him calm.

◆ STOP THE BLEEDING

To stop the bleeding, apply direct pressure to the wound with a square of gauze, clean fabric, or handkerchief. The bleeding should stop in a minute or two. If it doesn't, tie a bandage loosely (we're not talking tourniquet here) to hold the cloth in place. If the gauze soaks with blood, don't change it; the gauze

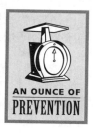

AN OUNCE OF
PREVENTION

Cat's Up a Tree!

Don't call the fire department. As one veteran fire fighter wryly observed, "How many cat skeletons do find in trees?" Usually the only time you need to assist a cat out of a tree is if it's injured or night is approaching.

Most cats, even young ones, can figure out how to get down without any help—when they're good and ready. Standing around the base of the tree, calling to her, and causing a commotion will probably only serve to keep her up there longer.

So what should you do? Place a bowl of cat food (or even some tuna) at the base of the tree. A hungry cat will be more inclined to come back down if she knows her favorite food is nearby.

If you decide that your cat isn't coming down without help, and you want to try to rescue her yourself, be prepared. Use a sturdy extension ladder—it'll be easier to get down while you're holding your scaredy cat. And dress for the part. Wear heavy work gloves and a long-sleeved shirt. Cats aren't always grateful, even when you're rescuing them, so be prepared for your frightened kitty to take a swipe at you. When it's time to grab her, pick her up by the scruff of the neck, just like a mama cat would; she probably won't resist.

If you do need to call for help, opt for the local humane society (its number's in the Yellow Pages), rather than the fire department. The humane society is more likely to have experience in this area.

---

will actually help the wound to close. Pulling it away may reopen the clot that's forming. If you must, add more gauze or cloth on top, until you can get to the vet.

◆ A LICK IN TIME

Most dogs and cats will lick their wounds. Let them. It's nature's way of allowing them to clean out their wounds. After your pet is done, you can step in and wash the wound. Flush the wound with a stream of clean, warm water. Make sure there's nothing lodged in there like a thorn, splinter, or a piece of glass.

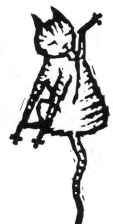

◆ SOCK IT TO HIM

If your dog has a cut paw pad, it's hard to come up with a bandage that poochie won't tear off the minute you get it on him so try this: After you clean the wound and cover it with gauze (see "Play Dress Up", below) use a clean, old cotton sock to keep the gauze covered. Just slip your pooch's paw right in.

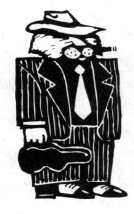

◆ PLAY DRESS UP

If the wound isn't bleeding too badly, and you've cleaned it well, you can dress it with an over-the-counter antibiotic ointment, the same that you'd use on yourself. Apply it with a cotton swab. Keep the wound covered with gauze to keep it clean. Once a day, remove the gauze to clean the wound with warm water, and then reapply the antibiotic cream. Rewrap the cut, making sure the bandage is not too tight.

◆ A CHANGE IN THE WIND

Some dogs just love to roll around in stinky stuff—usually just after they've had a bath! But if your dog has a peculiar body odor, and he hasn't been rolling around in anything, it could be an indication of trouble. For instance, it could be a sign of an infected wound. Look your pet over for any trouble spots.

◆ MY DOG HAS...GAS

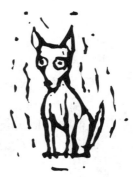

Pheeew, Rover! People aren't the only one's who suffer from flatulence, but believe you me, it's no better when it's your pet who's the offending family member. So how do you alleviate this problem? First of all, a good romp should help move the gas out of your pet's intestines. Just make sure you're not standing downwind!

◆ CHARCOAL CHEW

Another cure for gas is activated charcoal, which you can buy at any pharmacy (it's used as a remedy for poisoning). Give your pet some of the charcoal ($\frac{1}{8}$ to $\frac{1}{4}$ teaspoon for small dogs and cats and ½ teaspoon for larger dogs). Then make sure your pet drinks lots of fresh water. Don't continue this treatment for more than two days.

◆ AVOID THE HOT STUFF

Just like people, pets can suffer from heat exhaustion and heat stroke when the temperature shoots up. Here are some ways to protect your pal during hot weather:

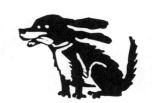

☞ Don't ever leave your pet in the car on a hot day. It can be fatal to your pet much more quickly than you'd imagine—even if you leave a window open.

☞ Exercise in the early morning and evening, when it's cooler. Always carry water when you go for a walk—and not just for yourself. Carry enough for your dog, too. And every single time you drink, give your dog some water, too.

☞ If your dog enjoys the water, fill a kiddie pool and place it in the yard. Then let Rover go for a swim.

☞ If, in hot weather, your dog begins to stagger, pant loudly, or to breathe rapidly, he probably is suffering from heatstroke. Immediately take him indoors to a cool room or to a shady spot. Pour cool water on him and offer him water, then get to a vet ASAP.

◆ GOTTA GO!

Older dogs (as well as some younger ones) often develop bladder-control problems. If your dog seems to be urinating a lot more frequently lately and in the places you'd rather he didn't, it could be a sign of something serious like a bladder infection,

> ## Hear Ye, Hear Ye
>
> As some dogs grow older, they can lose their hearing, just like some older people. You can help your old buddy out by adding simple gestures to your voice commands. For instance, let him know it's time to eat by pointing toward your mouth. Do it consistently, and he'll begin to associate that motion with mealtime.

diabetes, or kidney problems. Get your vet's opinion if symptoms last more than a few days. In the meantime, here are a few things you can try:

☞ Strive to keep a regular feeding schedule. While you may feel comfortable eating at different times on different days, your pet's potty habits are geared to his eating habits. The more regular and predictable those times are, the more predictable his other needs will be.

☞ Increase the frequency of time outside. Add an extra walk or time in the yard if at all possible, and reward him for "a job well done."

In Case of Emergency

✚ If you have dogs or cats that have the run of the house, don't use rat or ant poisons to control household pests. Your pet could get into it, and the ingredients are as highly toxic to them as they are to the pests they were intended for.

If you suspect that your pet has accidentally ingested poison, call your vet or the nearest animal emergency clinic immediately. If there is none available (for instance, if you're on vacation in an unfamiliar city) call the local poison control center's emergency number. Look for the number in the White Pages of the local phone directory, usually on the first page. Be prepared to identify the poison you think your pet has ingested.

When you take your pet to the clinic or vet, bring along the container of pesticide. The information on the box or bottle will help the vet determine a course of treatment.

☞ If your dog is alone most of the day, you may want to consider a crate. When he's home alone all day, he may be lonely or frightened, and that's when accidents can happen. If he spends most of his day in a good-sized crate that's big enough for him to stand up, turn around, and lie down in, he'll feel more secure, and a dog is less likely to make a mess where he spends most of his time. Just be sure to give him a good long walk before you leave and the minute you get home.

☞ Consider using disposable diapers especially designed for your dog. Most pet stores carry them. Of course, you can try to modify baby diapers, but remember to make room for the tail. Make sure you change the diapers often; you don't want your pet to come down with a case of canine diaper rash.

First Aid for Birds and Fish

Your bird or fish may not fall down and scrape their little knees, but from time to time, they may need a little first-aid, just like you. Here are some basic tips.

◆ JUST DROPPING IN

A healthy bird's droppings are a key to just how he's doing. Bird droppings consist of a dark portion (non-digestible matter), a white or off-white part (the nitrogenous waste called urates), and a fluid part that varies in amount depending on how much water the bird has ingested. Colorful foods will affect the color of the droppings, so don't be alarmed.

Very watery droppings (not due to diet change) or food particles in the stool are signs of potential trouble, so call the vet.

◆ BIRD 911

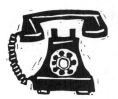

Even big birds like parrots are pretty delicate. If your bird suffers any kind of trauma (appears to have a broken bone, is attacked by the neighbor's cat or dog, suffers a puncture wound, ingests a poison) there's not much you can do about it yourself in the way of first aid. The best bet is to get the bird to a vet or animal clinic, pronto.

Place the bird in a box just large enough to hold it, with a few holes cut out for ventilation, and some paper towels on the bottom to collect droppings for the vet to examine. Make sure the bird is kept warm or cool enough.

If you must take your bird to the vet in a cage, try to limit the bird's instinct to fly by keeping the cage covered (birds are less inclined to fly in the dark).

◆ SCRATCH CONTROL

If your bird suffers a simple bleeding scratch on its beak or foot, perhaps from getting nipped by a cage mate, apply a little flour or cornstarch to the wound to aid in coagulation. If it doesn't stop bleeding in a minute or two, get thee to a vet.

◆ CALL IN THE MAIDS

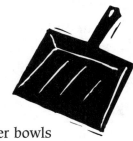

Birds are experts at grooming themselves; after all, they spend a lot of time doing it. But they're not great housekeepers. That's where you come in. Keep the cage clean by washing food and water bowls daily, before refilling. Sterilize them once a week with boiling water. Clean and occasionally sterilize any toys that are covered with food or droppings.

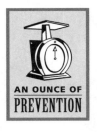

Polly Want a Checkup?

Sure, you'd take a dog or cat for an annual checkup, but what about a bird? Of course! And the more your bird is used to handling, the less stressful the trip to the vet will be.

AN OUNCE OF PREVENTION

◆ ICH!? WHAT'S THAT?

If your tropical fish are under stress, they can develop white, fuzzy-looking spots known as "ich." Fish get stressed for lots of reasons: fluctuating temperature; a crowded tank; an aggressive tank mate; or water that's too acidic, alkaline, hard, or soft. And it's contagious, so you may see more than one fish in your tank with ich.

Your best bet for dealing with an outbreak of ich is to buy a commercially prepared medication from your pet store. But be careful to read all of the directions before you use it. Like most medications, the dose required is based on the size of your tank and the number of fish in it. And as with many fish treatments, you may need to remove the activated charcoal from your filter, so the medication doesn't get removed before it gets a chance to do some good. Here's to good fishin'.

CHAPTER 7

Outside the House

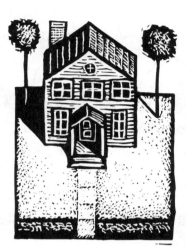

Back in Medieval times, some folks—the rich people, anyway—lived in castles. Sounds like the life, right? Well, back in those days, all anybody had to protect themselves and their homes from the elements was a moat (with maybe a few scary alligators swimming around in it). We're lucky—now we've got stuff like clapboard and aluminum siding. But that stuff needs a lot more care than a moat does!

And we've got other stuff to care for these days, too, like patios, decks, lawn furniture, and firewood. Heck, makes me tired just thinking about it! Well, if it makes you tired, too, you've come to the right place, because in this chapter, I'm going to give you some tried-and-true advice to make caring for your castle a whole lot easier.

I'll show you a bunch of clever ways to clean everything from siding to side-walks. (I even found an ingenious way to put cat litter to use!) Hate cleaning out your gutters? Well, I've got a quick and easy method for you to try—using something from your kitchen cupboard!

Then we'll take a spin around the backyard, where I'll let you in on some secrets for keeping your lawn furniture shipshape and I'll answer that age-old question, exactly how do you get in and out of a hammock?

When you have guests over for a patio party, you want to spiff up the place, right? I'll give you some dandy ideas for that! There's more, too. But you'll have to keep reading…

Beyond the Front Door

There's a whole world outside your front door—and I'm not talking about traveling. I'm talking about what's *right* outside your front door, namely the sidewalk, driveway, decks, patios—even the gutters, downspouts, and house siding itself. It all needs care and attention from time to time. Keep on top of things, and you'll be rewarded with a house that looks just as good on the outside as it does once you step through the door.

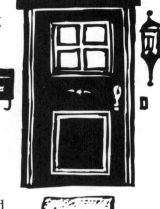

Keep It Clean

Just as you clean the inside of your house, once in a while, you've gotta clean up some of the things outside your house: the driveway, walkways, walls, siding, and so forth. Here are some of my favorite hints and tips for doing just that.

◆ SPIC AND SPAN SIDEWALKS

The next time you think your concrete sidewalks and/or patio are due for a general cleaning, don't go to the home center or garden supply store for a fancy cleaning concoction. No, siree. Instead, march right into your laundry room, and grab your powdered laundry detergent. Mix the detergent in hot water (as hot as you can get it) at the ratio of 1 tablespoon of detergent per gallon of water. Wet the concrete and use a stiff push broom to scrub it with the soapy water, then hose it down with a good rinse. Voilà! Clean concrete for just pennies a wash!

◆ BRICK A BRACK

Is there an area of brick around your house that needs to be cleaned? (Perhaps your barbecue pit is starting to look a bit grungy.) Well, here's how to clean it up so that it looks like new. Into a bucket of really hot water—as hot as you can get it—add about 1/2 cup of trisodium phosphate, a.k.a. TSP, which you can get at any hardware store. Now get yourself a pair of rubber gloves and a stiff-bristled brush, and scrub the heck out of the brick. (Hey, I never said this cleaning business would be fun!) When you've finished, rinse the brick off well with water.

◆ BE THE BOSS OF MOSS

And what have we here? Moss growing on a brick or stone wall? Some folks like the way that looks, but sometimes it's

---

Ah, Those Awnings

One of my favorite childhood memories is sitting on my neighbor's back deck during a summer shower. The deck had a canvas awning that my neighbors would roll out when the drops started to fall. I still can hear the *tap, tap, tap* sound that the rain made on the canvas. If you're lucky enough to have an awning on your deck or over your patio, you should know that it needs to be cleaned regularly so that it will last a good long time. Here's what I recommend:

Don't leaf it alone. If your awning is near a tree, brush off any leaves that stay on it. Leaves trap moisture, and moisture is the enemy of canvas—it allows mildew to develop, and mildew rots the canvas. Use your garden hose to wash off the leaves and any surface dirt about once a week. Do it early, on a day that's clear, so that the awning has a chance to dry thoroughly before you roll it back up.

Hit the spot. Don't use harsh detergents to clean your awning because they can break down the fabric much more quickly than just water. Instead, treat individual spots with a mild soap such as Ivory and a clean, old, soft toothbrush.

Skip the power wash. The rest of the house might be able to withstand it, but if you spray-wash your house using one of those power-wash attachments and your garden hose, turn down the pressure when you get to the awnings. That powerful spray can weaken the weave of the fabric—and nobody, but nobody, likes a leaky awning!

just ugly. I find that the easiest way to get rid of pesky moss is to spray it with a little weed killer. One solution I use is 2 tablespoons of rubbing alcohol in about a pint of water. Another is 2 tablespoons of gin and 2 tablespoons of vinegar in a pint of water.

Take it from me, this stuff is toxic to moss, but it's also toxic to other plants, so keep it well clear of your garden.

◆ OIL'S WELL THAT ENDS WELL

Tired of that oil stain on the driveway (or garage floor)? Well, the best solution to this pesky problem is not to let it happen in the first place. If you keep your car in a garage, pour a bit of sand or sawdust, enough to make a small pile, in the area under the car. Leave it there, and the sand or sawdust will absorb the grease and protect the floor. And once it's saturated, you can sweep it up and dump it out. Another solution is to put an old baking pan underneath your car to collect the oil.

Of course, hindsight is 20/20, and if there's already a big old grease spot on your driveway or garage floor, here' s how to handle it. First off, get yourself a bag of old-fashioned clay cat litter; don't use the new-fangled clumping litter. (Even if you don't have a kitty, you should have a bag of this stuff in your garage because it comes in handy for so many things.) Anyway, dump a small pile of the litter onto the greasy stain, let it sit for several hours, then sweep it up and throw it away. The litter will absorb most of the oil or grease.

Next, into a big bucket, pour about a gallon of really hot water and add about 1 cup of trisodium phosphate (TSP). Pour a little of the mixture onto the stain and with a stiff-bristled brush (of course, you're wearing rubber gloves), scrub the heck out of it. Then pour on a little more of the TSP solution, let it sit for about a half hour, and then rinse the area well. That should get rid of the stain—and encourage you to get that leak fixed!

By the way, this method works well on any greasy stain on concrete or cement.

◆ GREASE GETTER

Another way to take greasy stains out of concrete is to first pour a pile of clay cat litter on the stain (see "Oil's Well That Ends Well," at left). Let it sit for several hours, then sweep it up. Then spread some powdered dishwashing detergent (the kind you put in the dishwasher) on the spot, and let it sit for about 15 minutes. Next, pour a little boiling water over the detergent, scrub it with a stiff-bristled brush, and rinse well.

This solution isn't just for car grease—it'll work if you spill something oily on the concrete while you're barbecuing, too!

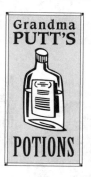

All-Purpose Clean-Up Solution

Looking for a general, all-purpose solution for cleaning the outside of your house? Here's a handy recipe that'll clean almost anything—be it stucco, siding, or a concrete patio. You should have everything you need in your garage or basement, or even under your kitchen sink!

⅓ cup of powdered laundry detergent
⅔ cup of powdered household detergent
1 gallon of water

Mix it all together, put on a pair of rubber gloves, and you're good to go. That's all there is to it! I like to apply this solution with a bristle brush to scrub out the stains. If you're cleaning something that's mildewed, use less water and add about a pint of household bleach.

◆ MOLDY OLDIES

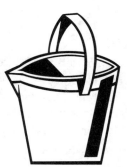

Ick! There's mold and mildew growing all over the siding on your home! The thing to do is to paint right over it, right? Not on your life. A fresh coat of paint might hide the mold for a while, but it will almost certainly reappear. To get rid of mold and mildew permanently, you need to kill it.

Now, you could go to the nearest home center and buy an expensive mildewicide, but if you wash clothes, you most certainly have something far less expensive in your laundry room: household bleach.

Into a gallon of very hot water, add about 3 pints of household bleach, and wash down the siding with it. You may have to scrub a bit, but that should take care of the foul fungi. Now you can prep the surface and repaint, but I suspect that after this treatment, you won't have to!

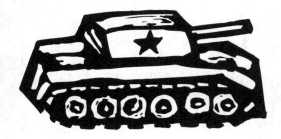

◆ THE HEAVY ARTILLERY

You're walking along the outside of your house and you notice what looks like ugly fly specks all over it. What the heck? Well, those black specks may have absolutely nothing to do with flies or any other insects. It may be what the experts call artillery fungus. How can you tell? Artillery fungus spots are between 1 and 2 millimeters in diameter and are slightly raised. If you break one open, inside it's off-white and gummy. Sound like what you've got?

The culprit, believe it or not, may be your garden mulch. Artillery fungus grows on rotting wood chips, so the best solution to this spotty problem is to replace your mulch every year with fresh wood—or switch to gravel.

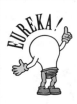

Soft Touch

Worried about your ladder putting a dent or a scratch in your siding? Try this hint: Grab a pair of old, heavy socks or heavy, puffy mittens, and slip them over the tops of the ladder rails. The mittens will cushion the ladder so that it won't mark up your house!

◆ I'M BE-SIDING MYSELF

You put siding on your home because it's low-maintenance, right? Well, low-maintenance doesn't mean no-maintenance, and so you're going to have to clean it once in a while. (Sorry—I don't make the rules!) Here's my favorite solution for cleaning aluminum and vinyl siding. Into each gallon of warm water, mix a couple of tablespoons of powdered dishwashing detergent. If you haven't cleaned the siding in a while (shame on you), you may have to use a soft brush; otherwise, a sponge should do the trick. But no matter which you use, make sure to wear rubber gloves. Take the time to do this once a season, and your house will look just like new!

P.S. This solution works on painted surfaces, too.

Great Gutters

Gutter. Even the word conjures images of yuckiness—old leaves, the dirt from the roof, and maybe even something worse. (You remember that favorite little squirrel friend of yours that disappeared last summer? Well...) I've got some bad news and some good news. The bad news is that if you don't keep your gutters clear, they'll fill up with leaves. Then, when it rains, water will run straight down the side of the house and soak into the foundation (that's really, really bad). Or, the leaves will dam the water and the gutters may get so heavy that they'll break and come down, pulling the fascia with them (that's really, really bad, too).

The good news is that caring for your gutters (and down-spouts, too) doesn't require major surgery; it's easy enough for almost anyone to do.

◆ HERE'S THE SCOOP

To keep gutters in good working order, you need to clean them twice a year—in late spring and again in autumn. Now I know that cleaning your gutters may not be the worst thing in the world, but I'm sure you can certainly think of other ways you'd rather be spending your afternoons than up to your elbows in gunky, wet leaves. So to make the job a little less yucky, try using a scoop of some sort to clean out the leaves. Some folks cut a U-shaped paddle out of a piece of plastic, like the bottom of an old plastic container, and use that to scoop the leaves.

A while back, my wife came home with a rice cooker that came with not one rice paddle, but two. So I nabbed one and now I use it to scrape the leaves. The moral? Use your imagination and hunt through the house for a usable scoop.

◆ DOWN AND OUT

Downspouts blocked? Don't worry—it happens to the best of us at one time or another. You may be able to clear them out from below with a good blast from your garden hose. Just push the hose up the downspout and turn the water on full force. The pressure should work the blockage loose. Of course, if it does, you may get a little wet, so wear your rain hat! If the garden hose doesn't do the trick, try using a plumber's snake.

◆ GO TUBING

After you've cleared the gutters and downspouts of leaves and debris, give them a good rinse with your garden hose. Now if you don't like the thought of climbing up the ladder with your hose, try this idea. Dig around in the attic for an old, rigid vacuum cleaner tube. Remove the spray head from the hose, and feed the hose through the tube so that 12 to 15 inches extends out of the tube. The idea is to create a rigid cuff for the hose that allows you to extend your reach to the gutter. The hose will flop over the end of the tube and aim itself into the gutter. If you don't have an old vacuum cleaner tube, a piece of PVC pipe will work just as well. Now you don't have to go all the way up on the ladder!

◆ LOOK FOR LEAKS

So now you know how to clean your gutters a couple of times a year, but you'll want to inspect them once in a while, too. The next time you hear the pitter-patter of tiny raindrops, put on

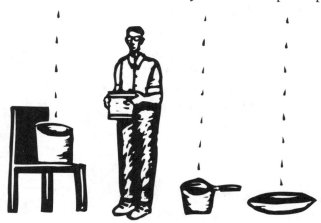

your raincoat, go outside, and look up at your gutters. (If you look *between* the raindrops, you won't get any water in your eyes. Just kidding!) See any water overflowing from the gutters? See any noticeable leaks? If you do, make note of where they are. Then, wait for a dry day, get out the old ladder, climb up, and take a look.

◆ DO-IT-YOURSELF GUTTER REPAIR

Most gutter repairs are fairly easy to do yourself, even if you're all thumbs like I am a lot of the time! The worst part of the whole operation is getting up on the ladder—please, please be careful up there—and make sure to read "Ladder Safety" on page 247. I must say, if your roof is really high or if you're at all nervous about heights, ask someone else to do these simple repairs for you.

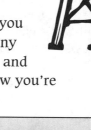

Once you find out where the leak is, but before you try to repair it, you need to prepare the area. Clear any debris from around the leak, and then sand it down and rub it with a little paint thinner to really clean it. Now you're ready to repair.

◆ STOP LEAKY JOINTS

The most common type of gutter leak is where two pieces meet, at a joint. This is really easy to fix. All you need is a tube of silicone sealant, which you can buy at any hardware store. Just coat the area where the two pieces of gutter meet with the silicone, making sure to apply it to both the inside and the outside of the gutter. Keep in mind that some silicone sealants need to dry for up to two days, so make the repair during a stretch of dry weather.

◆ HOLE-Y GUTTERS!

If it's a small hole (½ inch or smaller) that's making your gutter leak, head to the hardware store and ask for some roofing cement. Apply it right in and around the hole and spread it with a popsicle stick or a putty knife. Make sure to spread the cement beyond the hole by at least an inch.

Now if the hole in your gutter is bigger than ½ inch, things

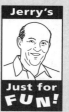

Jerry's Just for FUN!

A Little Gutter Humor

Just when you think you've heard them all, here's a joke about those rain troughs under your roof:

Q. What do you call a bird that sits on the roof?
A. A gutta percha!

Get it? No! Okay, maybe you didn't know that gutta percha is a natural latex that comes from the sap of a Malaysian rubber tree—they used to make galoshes from it. Now do you get it? Good!

get just a little more complicated. You're still going to cover the whole area with roofing cement, but you'll also need to use a thin piece of rustproof metal to cover the hole. Here's my can't-fail method:

1. Gather up the following very high-tech equipment: an empty soda pop can, some tin snips (or even an old pair of heavy-duty scissors), a little sandpaper, and some roofing cement. Remove the top and bottom of the pop can and flatten it so that you have a sheet of aluminum.

They Do It with Mirrors

If you have problems with birds nesting in your gutters, try this old-time trick. After you've cleared away an old nest, replace it with a small mirror. The next bird that wants to build a home in that spot will be discouraged when he sees that it's already occupied. That mirror works just like a "no vacancy" sign!

---

2. Wait for a dry day, then climb up on a ladder to scope out the leak and clear out any debris from the gutter.

3. Fit the aluminum to the hole from the inside of the gutter (so that it will be invisible from the ground). You may need to trim the can, using the snips or scissors, to get a good fit. Remove the aluminum.

4. Now sand the area around the hole and brush away any dirt. Cover the hole from inside the gutter with roofing cement and embed the aluminum patch in the cement. Apply another coat of cement over the patch, and there you have it, a gutter as good as new!

◆ BEFORE YOU PAINT...

...Mix up a sour. No, not a whiskey sour, silly! Before you paint brand-new galvanized gutters, run to the grocery store and purchase the biggest, cheapest bottle of lemon juice and the biggest, cheapest bottle of vinegar that you can find. Soak a sponge with the lemon juice and give the gutters a good going over. Then do the same thing with the vinegar. This treatment will prep the surface and your paint will adhere to the metal a whole heck of a lot better.

◆ GET WIRED

Gee, wouldn't it be nice if you never had to clean out your gutters in the first place? Well, I can't guarantee that this idea will allow you to ignore your gutters altogether, but it will reduce the frequency that you have to be up there. And all you'll need is a little chicken wire—maybe you already have some in the garage.

With your trusty tin snips or heavy-duty pair of old scissors (don't use the "good" scissors!), cut the chicken wire into 6-inch-wide strips. Now bend the strips in half lengthwise, like you're making really long tents. Fit the chicken wire tents into your gutters and the downspout opening, too. Now, when it rains, the leaves will get caught up on the tents, and not in your gutter. And because the tents have holes in them, the water can still drain out. You're still going to have to get rid of the leaves, but your gutters won't clog up as much.

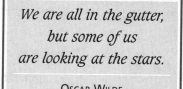

◆ RAIN, RAIN *DON'T* GO AWAY

If you live in an area that's subject to drought and occasional water-use restrictions, here's a way to get the most out of your gutters and downspouts. Make sure they empty into good old-fashioned rain barrels. Any watertight container will do; if you use smaller containers, such as buckets or gallon milk jugs, be sure to empty them into a larger barrel from time to time. Then, next time the sky refuses to give up any water, you'll already have plenty on hand!

All Decked Out

As you've probably figured out by now, I'm the sort of guy who doesn't mind relaxing. And one of my favorite places to relax is on my deck. You, too? Well, here are some tips to keep yours looking as good as new.

◆ SWABBING THE OL' DECK

A clean deck is a happy deck, and you want yours to be delirious! The best part is that you don't have to buy any fancy concoctions to keep yours shipshape. Here's a good cleaning solution you can make yourself. (This is best done in late afternoon or evening, out of the sun's direct rays.) First, sweep the deck well and cover any plants around or under the deck. Then fill a bucket with a couple of gallons of hot water, about a quart of household bleach, and about a ½ cup of powdered laundry detergent. Scrub the deck with a brush (such as a push broom), and then rinse it well with water. If you're cleaning the

Now You See Me, Now You Don't!

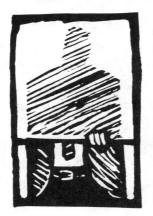

Want a little more privacy on your deck or patio, but hate the thought of closing it in? Set up a simple, beautiful, natural screen—for less than $20! Here's how it's done.

Zig-zag nylon fishing line between large bamboo tomato plant stakes that you've put in the ground around the perimeter of the deck or patio. Make sure the stakes are buried about a foot, so they'll be secure. Place several 8- to 10-inch pots, each containing several morning glory seedlings, along the perimeter of each nylon "wall," every foot or so. In a few weeks the vines will be as high as a nosy neighbor's eye.

Do you like to snack on your deck—literally? Plant nasturtiums instead of morning glories. They'll climb just as fast, and the young leaves are edible! (They're terrific in salads.)

deck because you're planning to seal or stain it, make sure to let it dry for several days before you do.

◆ NO SLIP, NO SKID

Getting ready to repaint your deck? Here's an old-fashioned way to give it a non-slip surface: Just add a little sand to the paint and when it dries, there will be no more slippin' and a slidin'!

◆ BEAD OR SOAK?

Here's a surefire way to tell if it's time to reseal your deck. The next time it rains, take a look at the deck's surface. If the water is beading up, you're fine for at least another season. If, on the other hand, the water soaks in, get ready for a re-sealing party.

If you're going through a dry spell or you just can't bear to wait until it rains again, hose off the deck or even pour a glass of water on it and see if the water beads off or soaks in.

Housepainting Primer

Nothing can quite match a new paint job for giving the exterior of your house an instant facelift. But let's face it, it's an enormous job and one, quite frankly, I'd rather leave to the pros. Still, if you decide to do it yourself, there are some basic hints and tips to make the job a little easier. And even if you do hire a pro, it's better to have a little knowledge under your belt so you'll know the job is getting done right.

Not Too Hot, Not Too Cold

Planning to paint your house? Save it for a warm, dry day. The temperature of the paint, the surface of your house, and the air should all be between 50°F and 90°F and the humidity should be below 85%.

◆ I'VE GOT YOU COVERED

Just how much paint you need to paint your house depends a lot on the surface you're painting. For instance, if your house is stucco (a very rough, uneven surface), you're going to need more paint than the formula on the side of the can might indi-

The House of Many Colors

Wish you lived in a taller house? A bigger house? A wider house? Well you can, and it won't take lots of construction or buying a new house! Here's how to trick the eye with color.

The White House is really a one-bedroom. Painting your house with light colors gives the illusion that it's larger than it really is.

The Jolly Green Giant lives here. To make your home look taller than it is, paint vertical trim in a contrasting color to the rest of the house. For instance, if you paint the house yellow, choose a darker color for the vertical trim. (Of course, this won't make a ranch look like a skyscraper!)

Put on a few pounds. If you want to make your narrow home look wider, paint horizontal trim in a contrasting color to the rest of your house.

Show it off. If you're especially proud of the trim on your house—maybe it's ornately carved—and you want to emphasize it, paint it in a highly contrasting color from the rest of the house. Experts say that light-colored trim shows up best against a dark-colored house.

Be a smoothie. Does your house include several textures, such as siding and brick? If you want that contrast to be less noticeable, paint the entire house one color for a smoother look.

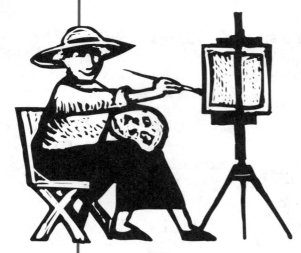

Blend into the background. Perhaps you live in a wooded area and you want the house to blend in. What color works best? You guessed it, green. The same goes anytime you want your home to blend into the surroundings. Choose a color that isn't obtrusive, and one that goes well with what's around the house.

cate. This is especially important to know because to match colors, you should buy all of your paint at once. And if you're buying specially mixed colors and you don't buy enough, well, you're going to have a heck of a time trying to match colors. So remember, any time you're painting uneven or rough surfaces, add about 20 percent more to your paint total.

◆ BUG OFF!

You're getting ready to paint the outside of your house, but you want some way to keep dive-bombing mosquitoes and other insects from embedding themselves in the paint. Are you out of luck? Not at all. Just add a couple of drops of citronella oil to every gallon of paint. It won't affect the paint, but it will keep bugs out of your paint job.

◆ DO A TEST RUN

Here's a clever tip a friend told me about a couple of years back. It's such a terrific idea, I want to share it with you. Let's say you've painted the outside of your house, but you're having trouble deciding on a trim color. Those tiny chip samples from the paint store just seem to get lost when they're up against house siding. So instead, get yourself some large pieces of cardboard—like the sides of a refrigerator box—and paint them with your potential trim color. Now prop up the board in a window frame, step back, and see how you like the color. It's a great way to test different colors without having the headache of repainting over and over again.

Outdoor Living

If you're like me, you love spending time outdoors. And when I'm not puttering around in my gardens or doing lawn work, I'm relaxing on my patio, enjoying Mother

Nature, taking a snooze in my hammock, or stoking a fire for a barbecue. Of course, it's not all play and no work—even outdoor stuff, like patio furniture, lighting, and the good ol' wood pile, needs some attention and maintenance from time to time. Read on for my favorite tips.

Caring for Patio Furniture

I love lazing around on my patio furniture. I cherish my chaise and love my lounger, and I'd bet you do, too! Here are some simple ways to give your patio and lawn furniture longer life.

◆ RUST-OFF

Are you finding rust on your wrought-iron patio furniture (or even your iron railings)? Not to worry. Just rub the rusty spots with some kerosene, then lightly scour them with some very fine steel wool. If the rust is stubborn, let a kerosene-soaked rag sit against it for awhile. Now, to keep that rust from making a comeback, give the furniture a good going over with some car wax. Yep, car wax. It's designed to protect the finish of cars and works just as well on all kinds of patio furniture, too.

◆ EASY CLEANING

Almost any patio furniture—from metal to plastic to wood—can be cleaned with a little dishwashing liquid in warm water. Scrub it with a soft brush if necessary, and then rinse it well.

◆ CUSHION THE BLOW

Follow these few easy steps and your patio furniture cushions will last a long time:

1. If you wear sunscreen (and I hope the heck you do), put a towel on the cushion before you sit down. That will protect the cushion from staining.

2. Always bring your cushions in during wet weather.

3. Give your cushions a good cleaning once a season. I like to use a mild dish detergent and a sponge, then I rinse them well with a hose. Most important, make sure the cushions are completely dry before you store them for the winter because damp cushions are the perfect home for wayward mildew.

> **Jerry's Just for FUN!**
>
> **Aprés Ski**
>
> There's a company in Massachusetts that sells Adirondack chairs—made from recycled skis! Now that's what I call a tush schuss!

◆ UMBRELLAS ARE US

Do you have a patio umbrella? You know, the big kind that goes in the middle of a table and lets you enjoy your lunch on the patio without getting sun in your eyes? Well, it needs tender loving care just as much as the rest of your patio furniture does.

First off, make sure to take the umbrella down (or at least close it) during storms—but make sure to open it again after the storm so that any dirt or debris that gets caught in the creases can fall out and not wear away the fabric or vinyl.

My secret weapon for caring for a vinyl umbrella comes from the automotive supply store. First, I clean it with the cheapest car vinyl top cleaner I can buy, and then I protect it against the elements with a finish for vinyl car tops, again, the least expensive one I can find. It works like a charm!

Hammock How-Tos

Is there anything better than kicking back on a lazy summer afternoon, gently swaying in a backyard hammock? Many folks own hammocks, but they don't know how to string 'em up. Here's the low-down on all you need to know so you can get started on that much-deserved nap.

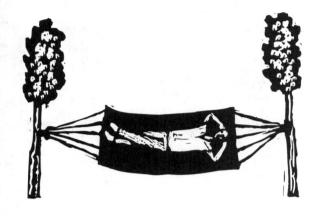

◆ MADE IN THE SHADE

First, you need to find the right location for you hammock. If you have some trees in your backyard, find two that are about 12 to 15 feet apart. That's the ideal distance for most hammocks. If you have only one good-sized tree, a wall of your house or a sturdy fence post will do just fine for the other anchor.

◆ KNOT SO BAD

OK, you've found the perfect site for your hammock. Now what? Well, you've got to tie the rope around the tree or pole, about 5 feet above the ground. The best knot to use is the bowline. This old favorite of sailors and campers is a simple knot to learn and handy to know. Go to the library and check a book on knots to see how to make this knot step-by-step, or find a Boy Scout who can show you how!

◆ GET SCREWY

If you don't trust your knot-tying ability or you can't tie the end rope around a support because you're using the side of a building, don't worry. You can use large screw-eyes, driven into the tree or a stud in the wall. Just make sure the tree is large enough to handle it.

◆ TAKE A STAND

What if you're yearning for a hammock, but your yard doesn't have any trees? Don't fret—you can purchase a hammock stand from your local home center or department store, or you can put up your own supports. You can use aluminum fence posts or wooden ones; just make sure they are buried at least 2 feet into the ground and extend at least 6 feet above the ground.

◆ A LITTLE SAG IS A GOOD THING

Don't tie up your hammock too taut between its supports. In fact, it's important to leave some slack in the hammock. This way, there'll be a little give when you get into it, and then you won't bounce right out!

Let There Be Light

Don't you just love having people over for an evening party in the summertime? Maybe it's a barbecue, or perhaps it's something a bit more elegant (ooh la la). Heck, maybe it's just you and your better half enjoying a beer on the back porch! No matter how you entertain, here are some fun lighting ideas that will add a little atmosphere to the occasion.

◆ VOTIVE IN A BAG

Having folks over for an evening soirée? Looking for an interesting way to light up the house for the holidays? Light the way in style (and for pennies) with this great decorative idea: luminaries made from votive candles and

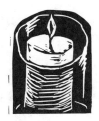

The Ins and Outs of Hammocks

Guess what happened to me the first time I tried to get into and out of a hammock? Let's just say it wasn't very elegant. To save you the embarrassment that I suffered at the hands of my hammock, I offer these bits of advice (you may want to practice a few times by yourself before you invite the gang over):

To get into a hammock: Sit down on the edge, like you would sit on a chair, but first reach behind you and spread out the edge of the hammock underneath you before putting your full weight down. Sit down and lay back, then swing your legs up and in. If you don't want to get dumped before you get in, never climb in feet first.

To get out of a hammock: Well, now that you're in there, you'd love a glass of lemonade, but there's nobody around to get it for you. You've got to get out again. It's a little tricky for a first-timer. Swing your legs over the side and sit up. Then, stand up and hold the edges of the hammock, and push yourself up and off.

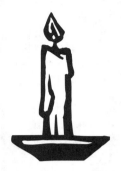

small paper bags. Plan out in advance where you want your lights to go. A great system is to line driveways or walkways with the candle holders. For an extra-special effect, line both sides of your path with them.

Luminaries should be spaced about 2 feet apart. Be sure they will not be placed anywhere they could accidentally get knocked over and start a fire. Once you know where you want to put them, and how many you'll need, purchase small paper lunch bags and small votive candles. To be really fancy, you could spend a little more money and buy colorful bags at the art supply store. I like to use white bags because they glow more brightly than their brown cousins, but any kind will do. If you're feeling especially creative, you can cut a small design out of the side of the bag with a craft knife, or trace a design on the outside and punch some holes in the bag along the outline with a pin.

> There are two ways of spreading light: to be the candle or the mirror that reflects it.
>
> EDITH WHARTON

For the next step, you'll need some sand or even some potting soil. Place about 2 inches (about 2 cups) of sand or soil in the bottom of each bag, or enough to weigh it down. Push the candle down into the sand in the center of each bag to make sure it's securely in place.

When the sun begins to set, light the candles with a long taper or a barbecue lighter and enjoy the show. Don't forget to blow out the candles before turning in for the night. If you burn the candles for about four hours each evening, they should last about four days.

◆ CAN IT!

Here's a longer-lasting way to decoratively light up an outdoor area like a patio or porch. All you need is an aluminum can, a nail, a hammer, paper, a pencil, and some masking tape. The idea is to punch holes in the can to let the candlelight shine through. But hammering on an empty can will end up flattening it out, that is, unless you know this trick.

Wash and dry the can, and remove the label. Make sure there are no sharp edges where the lid was attached. Fill the can with water and place it in the freezer until it's frozen solid. The ice that fills the can will help it retain its shape while you pound away at it. (Neat trick, eh?)

While you're waiting for the water to freeze, design a pattern on paper with the pencil. Start with simple geometric shapes or perhaps a flower design, anything you can render in a simple line drawing.

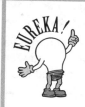

All Strung Out

Umbrella lights that attach to the ribs of patio umbrellas provide attractive patio lighting. Problem is, they sure are pricey! So save yourself a bundle by purchasing mini Christmas tree lights during the after-Christmas sales. String them under the umbrella for a copycat look at a fraction of the price.

Once the water is frozen, stick your design to the side of the can with the masking tape. Using the nail and hammer, drive small, evenly spaced holes along the lines of the pattern and through the wall of the can. You can vary the hole sizes occasionally to make the design more interesting. Once you're finished punching out the design, let the ice melt and you're ready to put a candle inside!

Wooden It Be Nice

Back in the really old days, wood was the only fuel around. These days, most of us don't rely solely on it for heat, but many of us do have outdoor and/or indoor fireplaces or wood stoves. Here are some of my favorite hints and tips to help you get the most from the old wood pile out back.

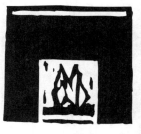

◆ JUST WHAT IS A CORD, ANYWAY?

Well, a cord is a measure of volume, not a measure of weight. It's 128 cubic feet to be exact. More simply put, a cord of wood is a rectangular stack of wood that is 2 feet wide, 4 feet high, and 16 feet long. A face cord is really half a cord, 2 feet wide, 4 feet high, and 8 feet long.

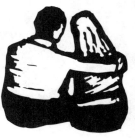

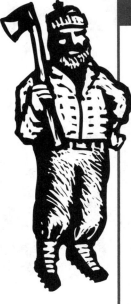

Wood Wisdom

Wondering what kinds of wood make for the best firewood? Wonder no more! The United States Forest Products Laboratory developed this chart, which explains the merits of all kinds of wood.

NAME	RELATIVE AMOUNT OF HEAT	EASY TO BURN?
HARDWOODS		
Ash, red oak, white oak	high	yes
Beech, birch, hickory	high	yes
Hard maple, pecan, dogwood	high	yes
Soft maple, cherry, walnut	medium	yes
Elm, sycamore, gum	medium	medium
Mesquite	high	medium
Aspen, basswood, cottonwood	low	yes
Chestnut, yellow poplar	low	yes
SOFTWOODS		
Southern yellow pine, Douglas fir	high	yes
Cypress, redwood	medium	yes
White cedar, western red cedar	medium	yes
Eastern red cedar, juniper, piñon cedar	medium	yes
Eastern white pine, western white pine	low	medium
Sugar pine, ponderosa pine, true firs	low	medium
Tamarack, larch	medium	yes
Spruce	low	yes

EASY TO SPLIT?	SMOKY?	DOES IT POP OR THROW SPARKS?	COMMENTS
yes	no	no	excellent
yes	no	no	excellent
yes	no	no	good
yes	no	no	fair
no	medium	no	good
no	medium	no	fair, good for kindling
yes	medium	no	excellent
yes	medium	yes	poor
yes	yes	no	good, but smoky
yes	medium	no	fair
yes	medium	yes	good, excellent for kindling
yes	medium	yes	good, excellent for kindling
yes	medium	no	fair, good for kindling
yes	no	fair	good for kindling
yes	medium	yes	fair
yes	medium	yes	poor

◆ HOW MUCH IS ENOUGH?

Wondering how much wood you need to buy? If you heat your home with wood, a cord should get you though a heating season. If you build fires just for atmosphere (like most of us do) or for summer barbecuing, a third of a cord should do the trick.

◆ STACK IT RIGHT

Moisture and bugs: the two reasons you should never stack your firewood right up against your house. Instead, stack firewood at least 15 feet away from the nearest building. This will ensure that bugs like ants and termites can't get into your home, plus it will allow the firewood to dry out well.

Some folks make the mistake of stacking the wood right on the ground. That's a no-no, too, because air can't circulate well around the logs, and those bottom logs will never dry out. Keep the wood a good 6 inches off the ground. The easiest way to do that is to stack it on pallets or in a firewood rack.

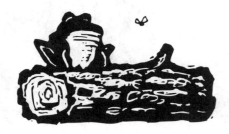

◆ KNOCK ON WOOD

Here's my surefire way to tell if your firewood is really, truly dry. Knock two pieces together. If the wood is seasoned (dry), you'll hear a sharp crack. If you hear a heavy thump, the wood is too green to burn efficiently.

Puttering Around

I've got so many great tips for making things easy for you as you putter around your property. Read on for a potpourri of outdoor-related hints and tips.

◆ EXTEND YOURSELF

You know that for safety's sake you should always keep one hand on the ladder. But if you're on an aluminum extension ladder, how the heck are you supposed to hold on to, say, a bucket, while you're washing the windows? Here's how: Cut a small notch near the end of an old broom handle. Then slip the broom handle through the rung nearest your chest height. (The rungs on an aluminum ladder are usually hollow.) The notch will hold the handle of the bucket.

Now before you climb up with broom handle in hand, first practice on a lower rung to see how far you need to slide the broom handle through to support the weight of the bucket.

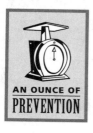

AN OUNCE OF
PREVENTION

Ladder Safety

Sometimes, there's just no getting around the fact that you have to get up on a ladder. I'm not crazy about it myself, and I'd hate for one of my readers to take a tumble. Here are some tips I've gathered to make your next trip up on the roof a little bit safer.

☑ Before you climb up on a ladder, take a minute to inspect it. Lay it flat on the ground. Check for loose rungs and, if it's wooden, large cracks. If your ladder has "feet," check to make sure they're securely attached.

☑ When you set up the ladder against the house, make sure the bottom is no less than one-quarter of the ladder's overall length away from the wall. So, for instance, if the ladder is 12 feet tall, the base of the ladder should be at least 3 feet from the house.

☑ Always make sure your ladder is standing on firm, level, compact ground.

☑ The ladder should extend at least 2 feet past the highest point you're trying to reach.

☑ When you're on the ladder, keep your hips between the rails.

☑ Always keep one hand on the ladder, and never reach out to the side more than arm's length.

☑ This may sound obvious, but by all means, stay off of the ladder in bad weather!

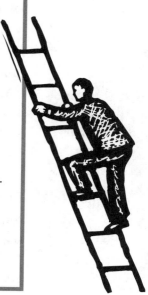

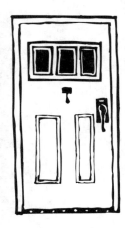

◆ KEEP THE GREAT OUTDOORS...OUTDOORS

Grandma Putt always said that a house with a solid front door always made her feel extra safe. If yours has a flimsy front door, it's about time you changed it.

Replace a hollow-core exterior door with a solid wood core door, or a steel-shelled door with a foam core. That fragile, hollow-core door is made from 1/8-inch plywood with some cardboard stiffeners thrown in to give it some body, and a little reinforcement near the doorknob. Now, I won't say that Grandma Putt could have put her foot through one of those...she was too much of a lady, but it sure won't stop a thug.

Here's something else: In some areas, solid-core doors are required by the local building code, especially between an attached garage and the main house.

◆ GREATER INSULATOR

Need another reason to replace your hollow-core door? Here's one: Solid-core doors insulate better than hollow-core ones, cutting down outside noises as well as frosty temperatures.

◆ GATE WAYS

If you have a wooden gate that closes with a latch, you may have noticed that the latch hardware gets loose occasionally from constant closing. Every time the gate closes, the screws that hold the latch on the gate get pulled loose a bit. Now, you might be tempted to replace the old screws with longer or wider ones, and that might work for a little while, anyway, but here are some better solutions.

Stuff it. Remove the screws, then get some wooden matchsticks or small dowels from the hardware store. Coat them with some waterproof glue and stuff them into the screw hole. Now, go ahead and replace the latch and attach it with larger screws. The dowel or matchsticks give the screw something more to hold onto, and that should keep your latch attached tightly.

Screw it. For an even more secure fit, remove the old screws and, using the old holes as guides, drill all the way through the gate post. Then replace the latch and attach it with screws that go all the way through the post, using a lock washer and nut to secure it.

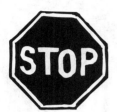

Stop it. Another way to keep your gate's hardware from loosening every time it slams shut is to install a gate stop. That's a block of wood attached to the stile on the latch side. The block of wood takes some of the force of the closing gate so that the latch isn't doing all of the work. Install it with the gate closed so it's flush with the face of the gate. And don't make it too big, or you might hit your leg on it as you leave.

◆ SQUARE DEAL

If your wooden gate is out of square, use a wire and a turnbuckle to pull it into shape. Attach the wire to screw-eyes at the top left and bottom right corners (or vice versa).

◆ HOW DRY I AM

You know those weeds that pop up through the cracks in a garden path or patio? They can be annoying, but you don't want to poison the entire lawn just to get to one or two isolated plants! Pour some rubbing alcohol into a hand-held

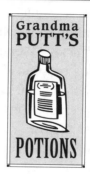

Grandma
PUTT'S

POTIONS

Mossy Mixtures

If you like the aged, weathered look of moss growing on walls or containers, give these mixtures a try. Use the Moss Mix on stone walls and the Moss Slurry on planters or other containers.

MOSS MIX

½ quart of buttermilk
1 tsp. of corn syrup
1 cup of moss

Mix all ingredients in a blender, then paint the mixture on the area where you want the moss to grow.

MOSS SLURRY

½ can of beer
½ tsp. of sugar
1 cup of moss

Mix all ingredients in a blender on low speed. Evenly paint the mixture on the outside of containers. Set in your plants and then sit back and wait for the moss to grow.

spray bottle. Drench any unwanted weed directly. The alcohol will dehydrate the plant almost immediately, killing the weed right where it stands. Just be sure not to spray any other plants, or they'll suffer the same consequences.

◆ PUT A LID ON IT

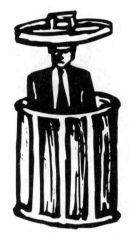

I hate to let anything go to waste. And that includes the last little bit of caulk in the tube. Whether you're just taking a break from caulking around windows or finished for the day, if you leave the top exposed, the remaining caulk will dry out and become unusable. Some tubes of caulk come with a cap, but if yours doesn't—or if you lost the one that did—then here's a good replacement. Screw a large wire connector over the tip. Those little do-dads cost next to nothing at the local hardware store, so you may want to buy one when you're picking up the caulk. Or, root around the garage or workshop; you just might have one around from your last electrical project.

Tools of the Trade

We sure wouldn't be successful do-it-yourselfers without our tools. They help us do so much, inside and outside of our homes. My number one tool tip of all time is this: Buy the best you can afford. Skimping isn't worth the few dollars you'll save because over the years, you'll find yourself replacing cheap tools over and over again. So do it right the first time and go for quality goods.

And now, on to my hints and tips for making the most of your tools.

Keep 'Em Sharp

You know that garden tools are cutting tools, and just like any other cutting tools, they'll work more easily (and be safer to use) when they're sharp. Dull tools make you work harder, and take it from me, it's no fun to work any harder than you have to! Read on for my advice on how to keep your tools sharp as a whistle. (For tips on sharpening lawnmower blades, see page 259.)

One word of caution: Always wear a pair of work gloves any time you sharpen your tools.

> *A sharp tongue is the only edge tool that grows keener with constant use.*
>
> WASHINGTON IRVING

◆ WHICH EDGE IS WHICH?

When sharpening any type of garden tool, whether it's a hoe, tiller, Edge Hounds, or whatever, you only want to sharpen one edge of the blade—the cutting edge. How do you know which edge is the cutting edge? Look at the blade; the edge you'll want to sharpen is the one that *isn't* straight.

◆ SHOVELS, SPADES, AND TROWELS, OH MY!

To sharpen these tools, use a single-cut bench file. Don't worry, the guy at the hardware store will help you find one. Hold the tool against something solid, like your work bench. Work along the underside of the edge of the shovel, matching its 45-degree angle. And use the file to knock off the burrs that form on the tool when you strike a rock.

◆ CHOOSE YOUR WEAPONS WISELY

Sharpen tools by using a file that matches the contour of the surface—a rounded file is best for a shovel, and a straight file is best for a flat-faced garden spade.

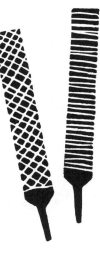

◆ IT'S SHEAR MADNESS

Here's how to sharpen garden shears, including hedge clippers, edge trimmers, bud clippers, and the like. First off, if it looks as though you can take them apart without an engineering degree, go ahead (and congratulations!). Then, sharpen the beveled edges with a whetstone. Use a single-cut file if there are any bad dings. A few strokes will generally be enough. Sharpen these tools every third time you use them and once before you store them away for the winter.

◆ STRAIGHT AND SMOOTH—AND SHARP!

At a loss for how to hold that favorite tool in place without cutting yourself to ribbons? My solution is to clamp the tool in a vise. Then hold the file in both hands, and push it across the edge of the tool. Only push in one direction, never back and forth in a sawing motion. Keep filing until the tool has a nice, sharp edge.

Clean and Neat

Clean tools don't rust. Why is this important? Because rusty tools don't keep their sharp edges and rusty tools have a pretty short lifespan. So keep your tools nice and clean, and in good repair. Here's how.

◆ A SANDY SOLUTION

This is about as close to effortless cleaning as you can get. Fill a bucket or an old washtub with sand, and saturate it with clean motor oil. Put that bucket near where you keep your garden tools. After a day's work in the garden, dip the blade of the shovel, spade, or shears into the oily sand, stir it around, then remove it and wipe it down with a rag. The sand scrapes off any remaining soil and the light coating of oil that's left will lubricate and rust-proof the tool. Now that was easy, wasn't it?

◆ MILK DOES YOUR TOOLS GOOD

An old metal milk delivery box—the kind that the milkman used to leave home-delivered milk bottles in—makes a great weather-proof storage bin for hand-held garden tools. If you don't have one handy, you can usually find one at a garage sale.

◆ PAINT YOUR HANDLE

One way to avoid leaving and losing your tools in the garden or the grass is to paint a bright red or yellow stripe on the handle. You could use some leftover house paint, but even better choices are model paint and nail polish, which will make the tool stand out against the greenery. While you're at it, mark every 6 inches or so along the handle so the next time you need to take a measurement in the yard, you've got a convenient ruler in hand!

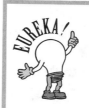

Rub Out Rust

If your favorite trowel got left out in the rain and develops a little rust, don't worry, it's not ready for the scrap heap. Remove surface rust by rubbing the tool with some fine emery paper. Stop sanding once the rust is gone, then coat the entire metal surface of the tool with some light household oil such as sewing machine oil, or (in a pinch) vegetable oil.

◆ JUST HANDLE IT!

A broken wooden handle is an easy problem to, er, handle —if you know how. For larger tools like shovels, spades, and hoes, a trip to any home center will provide a replacement. But you may have a more difficult time finding replacements for smaller tools such as hand trowels. For those, I use ¾-inch dowels (from the lumberyard) or an old mop handle that I cut down to size.

Whichever I use, I shave down one end so that it fits into the head of the tool. Then I secure it by drilling a hole clear through the part of the head that holds the handle, and the handle itself once it's in place. Then I put a bolt all the way through the hole and secure it with a nut on the other side. There...good as new!

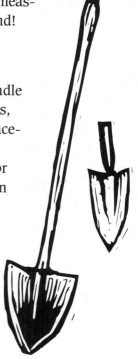

◆ SAND 'EM DOWN

Moisture affects more than just the metal parts of your garden tools. It also causes the grain in wooden handles to expand, making it easier for the wood to split and cause splinters (ouch!). Give the wooden handles of your tools (and don't forget the handles on your wheelbarrows) special treatment. Sand down the entire length of the handles with medium- or light-grade sandpaper to smooth the roughness, then coat the handles with a wood preservative such as linseed oil or a light coat of polyurethane.

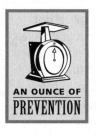

AN OUNCE OF PREVENTION

Lock, Sock and Waterproof

Do you find that the padlock on the garden shed gets too rusty to use? Protect it with a sleeve cut from an old bicycle inner tube. Cut a section that's an inch or so longer than the lock, and roll it over the padlock like a sock to keep it safe from the elements.

◆ WIRE NOT?

One tool I find invaluable for maintaining the rest of my garden tools is a wire brush, the kind sold in paint and hardware stores that's used for stripping paint. There's nothing better for scraping off dried old clumps of soil. And cheap? You bet!

◆ THAT'S RUST, BUSTER

Dampness is a funny thing—it can creep up on you when you least expect it. Here's a little story about a friend of mine, and what he did about dampness.

One winter several years ago, he stored his tools leaning against the side wall inside his garden shed. He felt secure in the knowledge that the tools were protected from the elements. But when he was ready to start planting the following spring, he discovered that all of the metal parts on his tools that were touching the concrete floor had rusted. Yep, the concrete floor of the shed was damp enough to rust the metal.

The following autumn he had a better idea—or at least he

thought he did. He hung the tools up on the wall, off of the floor. But the same thing happened! It seems that the moisture seeped through the uninsulated cinder block walls.

Well, he finally got around to asking me my not-so-humble opinion. It just so happened that I had some leftover carpeting in my garage. We fastened a 2-foot strip along the wall with some construction adhesive, right where the metal parts of the tools touched the wall. This provided just enough insulation to keep the tools from rusting over the winter. Problem solved!

Mower Madness

I remember the big day—it finally came in my gardening career. I needed more power—a power mower, that is. Now, I'd always been partial to push mowers for a whole host of reasons. But between my own lawn and the ones I was helping friends with, well, it was getting to be an awful lot of mowing. And let's face it; I wasn't getting any younger. So anyway, I finally decided to buy a power mower. Are you thinking of doing the same, or thinking of trading in your old power mower for a new one? Here are some helpful hints and tips to keep in mind.

◆ KNOW YOUR MOWER

When you're in the market for a walk-behind mower (that's the kind most folks use) you have three choices to consider:

Push mowers. This is my personal favorite—you know, the manual, person-powered (if you're lucky, teenager-powered) mower, also known as a rotary mower or reel mower. If you have a small lawn—about 1,500 square feet or less—I really feel it's the way to go. Keep in mind that push mowers aren't perfect, though. They sometimes have a hard time with really tall grass and some weeds. So it's not the tool to use to clear the back 40.

Electric mowers. Most electric mowers on the market these days are still the old-fashioned plug-in variety, which means you have a very long cord trailing behind you as you mow (having several exterior outlets to plug into can cut down on the length of cord you'll need). There are reliable battery-operated mowers on the market, too, but you may have to search for them. Look for the model that gives you the most mowing time before the battery needs to be recharged. If the battery price isn't too prohibitive, you may want to consider buying a second battery so you can keep mowing after the first one peters out.

Gas-powered mowers. These are what most folks are familiar with. They come in a range of horsepower choices with mulching or bagging options. If you don't want to regularly fill it with gas and change the oil, and then clean it all out at the end of the season, you may want to consider an electric mower.

◆ DO THE CAN-CAN

When I was selecting a power mower, I shopped carefully and came up with the best one I could afford. And, of course, when I got it home, I couldn't wait to gas it up and let it rip. That's when I discovered the one thing I forgot to buy: an approved gas can. You can't bring home fuel from the gas station in anything but an approved container. Now there was a gardening problem I'd never come across before! So when you buy your new mower, make sure to buy a gas can, too.

My choice? A plastic 1- or 2-gallon can. I prefer plastic because it's sturdy and won't rust. I recommend a 1- or 2-gallon container because anything bigger holds more gas than you're likely to use in a month, and gas that's older than 30 days can affect mower performance.

Jerry's Top 6 Reasons to Buy a Push Mower

Also known as a reel or rotary mower, a push mower is my very favorite grass-cutting tool. Here's why:

1. Noise. Push mowers make almost no noise, except for that very pleasant fluttering sound.

2. Cost. Push mowers are inexpensive. In fact, you can get a top-notch model for less than $200. And if you take good care of it, it could last you a lifetime. Now that's a bargain!

3. Weight. Push mowers are lightweight. Most are in the 15- to 30-pound range; and let me tell you, that's a lot lighter than the 60-pound monster Grandma Putt had me pushing around!

4. Exercise. A push mower will give you a little better upper body workout than a power mower and a lot better workout than one of those lazy-bones, sit-on-it riding mowers.

5. Fuss. With a push mower, there's no gasoline or motor oil to worry about. There's no tricky maintenance and no expensive parts to replace.

6. Effectiveness. Push mowers cause less damage (bruising and crushing) to your lawn than do power mowers.

◆ STROKE, STROKE, STROKE

Most gas-powered mowers are four-stroke. All that means is that the gasoline and motor oil are in separate receptacles, just like in your car. Some gas mowers (and some other gas-powered lawn tools) require a premixed solution of gasoline and oil. Those are two-stroke mowers. How can you tell what kind of mower you've got sitting out in your shed ? If there's a cap that says "oil" or "oil here," you've got yourself a four-stroke mower.

◆ SPOT CHECK

Before you get behind the mower, take a stroll through the area you plan to mow and keep your eyes peeled for large sticks, loose stones, or kid's or pet's toys. Pick up anything that could damage the mower or, even worse, become a projectile that injures you or someone nearby. (If you have kids or grandkids around, have them scout through the yard, and give them a nickel for anything they find and move out of the way.)

◆ BEWARE OF UFOS

No, not the kind carrying little green men! I'm talking about Upwardly Flying Objects. Since you won't be able to remove every little stone in your spot check (see above), there will most likely be a few objects remaining in your yard. Those can go flying, too, so always wear eye protection when pushing a mower. (Call me a nervous Nellie, but I've been nicked a few times by lawn mower UFOs.) A pair of shatter-proof sunglasses is better than nothing, but a pair of protective glasses are worth the investment. (Many professional gardeners wear a clear plastic face shield, especially when using a power mower.)

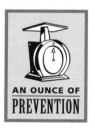

One Hill of a Job

AN OUNCE OF
PREVENTION

Does your backyard feature a steep slope? You know, one that makes for scary lawn mowing? Here's a tip: Mow that area by walking *across* the hill instead of up and down it. It's far safer, and easier, too.

◆ WATCH THOSE TOOTSIES!

Always wear "real" shoes when mowing the lawn. I like to wear my old golf shoes, the ones with the real metal spikes on the bottom. That way, I'm aerating the turf as I mow. I don't trust sneakers and just the idea of someone mowing the lawn in sandals, flip-flops, or bare feet makes me wince.

◆ NOT FOR THE KIDDIES

I'd be the first one to say that it's great to have the kids help out with yard work, but I would never, ever let anyone under the age of 12 use my power mower. And even then I'd use common sense. If your 12-year-old is easily distracted, I'd wait until he or she was older. Let 'em pull weeds instead.

◆ ONLY *YOU* CAN PREVENT A FIRE!

Never, ever start or refuel your lawn mower in your basement, garage, or garden shed. First, the gasoline fumes that collect in an enclosed area can knock you out. Second, those fumes can ignite if there's a spark of any kind, and that'll be all she wrote!

◆ TURN OFF, POWER UP

Make sure the mower's motor is turned off and cool to the touch before refueling. That goes for a lawn mower that's been sitting in the sun, too. It's better to be safe than sorry, so park your mower in the shade.

◆ A SHARP BLADE IS A WONDERFUL THING

Somewhere in the galaxy, there's a civilization—a whole lot more advanced than ours—that's invented a power mower blade that doesn't need to be sharpened. Dull blades never gum up the grass on that planet, and no one has to take a lawn mower apart. It's too bad that here on earth we're stuck with the not-so-fun job.

Now, I'm pretty comfortable working around engines, but it would take a lot more space than we have here to explain how to disassemble a lawn mower. So here are the bare-bones basics you need to keep in mind if you decide to tackle the job:

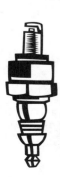

First things first. This is most important: You need to make *absolutely* sure that the lawn mower doesn't start up when you're trying to sharpen the blades. To do that, disconnect the spark plug and tie the wire back with a piece of garden twine or tape, or completely remove the spark plug. If you can't figure out how to do this, don't even think about playing with the mower blades. Take the whole shebang to a

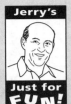

Jerry's Just for FUN!

The Kindest Cut

The man who invented the rotary lawn mower was inspired by a shearing machine that was used to trim the nap from cotton cloth. Edward Budding was a foreman in an English textile factory when he first saw the machine and wondered if the same principle could be applied to cutting grass. By 1830, he patented his machine, and while it wasn't an immediate success, it's still a favorite of gardeners everywhere.

professional or have someone who knows demonstrate how to do the job.

On or off? Next you need to decide whether or not to remove the blades to sharpen them. Removing the blades is usually a simple operation. But as with many things, the hard part is putting them back on properly. The easiest way to sharpen them is to set the blade height at its lowest or shortest setting (meaning fully extended away from the body of the mower) and tilt the mower back.

Empty the gas tank. If it's possible, remove it completely. Why? Because filing the blades can cause a spark. And when gasoline or gasoline fumes meet sparks, trouble is sure to follow.

Sharpen the blades. Use a whetstone or a fine-tooth file and work along the leading or forward edges of each blade. If you mow once a week (which you had better be doing!), sharpen the blades at least once every two months, more frequently if you have a large area to mow or if you tend to hit a lot of rocks and large sticks. (Hey! Be more careful!) A lawn mower blade doesn't need to be razor-sharp to do its job, so don't make yourself crazy trying to hone it to a scalpel-like edge.

◆ BALANCE YOUR BLADES

Here's where your counting skills come into play. When sharpening your lawn mower blades, give each blade edge the same number of strokes with the sharpening tool. If you go over one edge 10 times, go over the opposite edge 10 times, too. Why? To keep the blade in balance. A blade that's unbalanced can wreck your lawn mower; at the very least, it will leave you with a funny-looking lawn full of uneven cuts.

◆ A REAL BALANCING ACT

Now if you've already lost count, here's how you can check to see whether your mower blade is balanced, but you can do this test only if you've removed the blade to sharpen it. Get yourself a nail that's at least 1½ inches long, and drive it about a half inch into the wall in your garage or tool shed. Take the blade and slip it onto the nail (there should be a hole in the center of the blade). If the blade rotates at all, it's unbalanced. The heavier blade will want to roll down and that's the blade you should sharpen more. It's a good idea to try this with every blade before you sharpen anything.

◆ GETTING PUSHY

I love the sound a push mower (also known as a rotary mower or a reel mower) makes on a warm summer day. Now you do know what a push mower is, don't you? It's the old-fashioned kind that only moves when you do and it's the kind I recommend for small lawns. First, a quick lesson on how push mowers cut grass. They don't just chop it down the way a rotary mower does. Rather, they clip the grass with blades that rotate against a cutter bar, also known as a bed knife.

Push mowers don't need to be sharpened very often, only about once a season. If your yard is very small, the cutter bar is properly adjusted, and you're careful not to hit rocks and sticks, you may be able to get away with sharpening it only once every other season. That's good, because the action of the blades makes sharpening a push mower a bit of a challenge. But here's a trick I learned to hold those blades in place. Just wedge a piece of wood—like a scrap of lumber—into the blades to hold them still. Then put on those gloves, grab your whetstone or file and get to work!

If you have an old, rickety push mower and you're feeling flush, head to the local garden center and purchase one of the newer models—many are now designed to be self-sharpening!

CHAPTER 8

Around the Yard

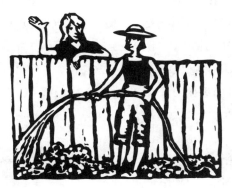

When you take a stroll around your yard, are you pleased with what you see? If not, then you've come to the right chapter! You probably already know that it's not enough to stick plants in the ground, water and feed them, and hope for the best. But what you may not realize is that creating a yard and garden that work as good as they look is not only an art, but also a craft. Like any craft, it's one you must learn from the ground up. And I do mean *ground*—otherwise known as soil.

Soil is to a gardener what a blank canvas is to a painter. It's the basis upon which all yards and gardens are built, and the better it is, the better your plants will be able to fend off trouble. So the more you know about your ground, the better off you'll be! That's why this chapter begins with my hints and tips for turning ho-hum dirt into super soil, so you're starting with the best the earth has to offer.

Once you've taken care of your soil, you can move on to my hard-won advice for planting things large and small, from long-lived trees to tiny seeds. (The trick is to head off problems before they start.) Then I'll let you in on my secrets for feeding and watering your plants so they keep growing the way that they should. And, no, you won't have to spend all your time tending your yard— most plants don't ask for much. Just follow my tips for treating them with kindness, and they'll repay you by growing like gang-busters. Before you know it, you'll have a yard that's the envy of the neighborhood.

Super Soil and Other Secrets

There is only one place to begin making a trouble-free yard, and that's the earth beneath your feet. You have to work from the ground up, because the foundation of any good lawn or garden is good, reliable soil. Or, as my Grandma Putt put it, even if you get a plant for free, give it a $10 hole! Here's how to make sure your green scene is growin' on a solid-gold foundation.

Setting the Groundwork

I like working in soil, because it's very responsive, pre-dictable stuff. I know that when I spend some time digging, cultivating, working in organic matter, and mixing in just the right timely tonics, the soil will become soft and porous, and my plants will be delighted. Yes, it's hard work, but the rewards are both immediate and long lasting. So what if it takes you an hour to prepare a planting hole for a crabapple tree and get it nicely situated in its new home? If you've done the job right, the tree will prosper for many years to come, and every time you look at it, you'll glow a little inside, knowing that you've done a small thing to make this great green world just a little bit more beautiful. So keep reading for my tips on developing great ground.

Put It to the Test

The easiest way to get a fix on soil type is to squeeze a ball of damp dirt in your hand. If it's so loose and unsticky that it won't form a ball, you've got sand. Clay soil will form a ball right away, and you can even flatten it into a pancake before it falls apart. Loam will form a ball, but the ball will shatter easily if you tap it with your finger.

◆ MAKE MINE ORGANIC

Anything you add to your soil to make it better is a soil amendment. But when gardeners use the phrase, they usually mean various sources of organic matter, such as compost, composted manure, humus, peat moss, or leaf mold. Lime and sulfur, used to adjust the soil's pH, are amendments, too.

◆ SANDY OR CLAY?

Both sand and clay soils are improved the same way: by adding air and organic matter. But understanding your soil texture tells you ahead of time how you can expect your soil to behave once you put it to work growing plants. Here's a look at the characteristics of each soil type:

Sandy soil drains fast and dries out quickly, so it tends to need more water and fertilizer. Gardeners with sandy soil are therefore destined to become big-time mulchers with a special interest in water conservation.

Clay soil is so tight that water moves through it much more slowly, which makes it more resistant to drought, yet more prone to staying wet when rains come too heavily and too often. If you've got clay, you'll soon long for the great drainage you get with raised beds.

◆ GET WET

If chipping away at subsoil with a sharp shovel and digging fork just doesn't work, call a halt to your struggle and run some water into the half-dug planting holes. After the water percolates in for a few hours, the digging gets much easier!

◆ THE MAGIC BULLET

Believe it or not, there is a way to get subsoil lighter and looser: Just keep pumping it full of organic matter. Like magic, it'll break down and fluff up those soil particles.

◆ GIVE IT A RAISE

Adjusting your soil's pH is easy. Here's all there is to it: To raise the pH of acid soil, add lime in the form of powdered limestone, which is sold at all garden centers. Because the amount of lime you need varies with your soil type and climate, either get expert local advice or start small, with a 50-pound bag per 1,000 square feet of soil area.

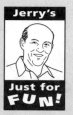

Sweet or Sour?

Care for a little taste of soil? I'm kidding, though back in Grandma Putt's day, many wise farmers decided whether or not they needed to lime their fields and gardens by taking a handful of soil, sniffing it, and touching their tongues to it to see if it tasted a little sweet or a little sour. This is a learned skill that's been all but forgotten, because today we have better ways to tell whether our soil is sweet (alkaline) or sour (acid).

So why should you care what your soil's pH is? I'll tell you why: The pH level determines, in part, how well nutrients in the soil can be absorbed into your plants' roots. If your soil is either too sweet or too sour to suit their needs, you'll wind up with malnourished plants. If your plants aren't well fed, they'll be easy prey for any pest or disease that comes their way. And that'll mean big-time trouble for you!

◆ GO LOW

To lower the pH of alkaline soil, use powdered soil sulfur. Start small (20 pounds per 1,000 square feet) or check with local master gardeners or your Cooperative Extension Service for guidance.

◆ KEEP TESTING

After adding either lime or sulfur, mix it in well, water the site, and test your soil again in a few months. Soils tend to revert to their natural pH over time. If you find that native soil in your area is either strongly acid or very alkaline, check your pH at least once a year, and keep a close watch on plants that have peculiar tastes in soil pH.

From Garbage to Black Gold

Believe you me, whatever ails your soil, adding plenty of compost is the best way I can think of to improve it! What's more, this "gold mine in a pile" is sort of like nature's garbage disposal: It takes leaves, sticks, banana peels, coffee grounds, tea bags, grass clippings, and just about any other type of plant material you toss into it, and transforms it all into soft, black humus, which plants crave like I crave chocolate. Here's the lowdown on making your own black gold.

◆ GREEN + BROWN = *COMPOST?*

It's important to get the right balance of high-nitrogen ingredients (what gardeners call "greens") and high-carbon ones (a.k.a. "browns") in your compost pile. That's because if your pile is too high in carbon, it'll take a coon's age to decompose. If it's too high in nitrogen, it'll smell to high heaven. Don't worry yourself into a frazzle over the equation, though. Just make sure you add roughly 3 parts of brown stuff (such as dried leaves, sawdust, wood chips, and sticks) for every 1 part of green (as in freshly pulled weeds, vegetable trimmings, fresh manure, and grass clippings).

Your Soil's Potential

The letters pH stand for "potential of hydrogen," and the pH scale runs from 1.0 to 14.0, with 7.0 being neutral. A measurement above that signifies alkaline soil; below is acid. You can test your own soil with an inexpensive kit from the garden center. Or, if you want a detailed analysis of the nutrients in your soil, as well as an accurate pH reading, send a soil sample to a private testing lab or your local Cooperative Extension Service. It'll take longer to get the results, but you'll wind up with some valuable information that could head off a lot of problems down the road.

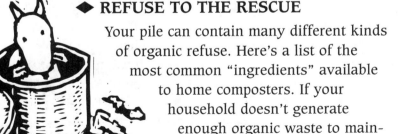

◆ REFUSE TO THE RESCUE

Your pile can contain many different kinds of organic refuse. Here's a list of the most common "ingredients" available to home composters. If your household doesn't generate enough organic waste to maintain your compost pile, ask a neighbor for help. You can also try to obtain some of these materials from local farmers and lawn and tree service companies:

☞ Cannery or winery wastes

☞ Chopped corncobs

☞ Chopped tobacco stalks

☞ Ground tree bark

☞ Manures

☞ Old produce

☞ Sawdust

☞ Spoiled hay

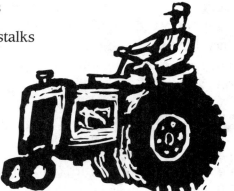

◆ COMPOST COCKTAIL

If you don't have the time, space, or energy to make your own compost, here's a quick compost cocktail that can still work wonders on your plants and in your garden. Save your table scraps each day—peels, shredded vegetables, eggshells, tea bags, and so on (but no fat or meat). If you have a small household, a crock or large ceramic bowl will work nicely for scrap saving, or you can simply toss everything into a plastic bag. Every day or two, place the scraps in a food processor or blender and cover them with water. Add a tablespoon of Epsom salts to the mix, and liquefy. Pour this cocktail onto the soil in your garden, lightly hoe it in, and you'll be as good as ("black") gold!

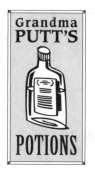

Grandma
PUTT'S

POTIONS

Compost Feeder Tonic

Grandma Putt knew that just like plants, a compost pile needs a boost now and then. So do what Grandma always did—once a month, spray yours with this tonic.

½ **can of beer**
½ **can of regular cola (not diet)**
½ **cup of dishwashing liquid**

Mix these ingredients in a bucket, pour into your 20 gallon hose-end sprayer, and apply generously to your compost pile.

◆ STOP THE STENCH

Too much nitrogen can turn a compost heap into a real nosesore, but so can lack of air: When the pile becomes too wet or too compacted, foul-smelling bacteria will give the heap a sewagelike aroma. To set things right, fluff the material with a pitchfork or digging fork, and work in some brown material, like dry leaves.

◆ QUICK FIX FOR SLOW COMPOST

It's normal for leaves, sticks, wood chips, and sawdust to take several months to decompose, but you can speed things along toward the end by mixing a little high-nitrogen organic fertilizer into your heap. Microorganisms that have been waiting for a good supply of nitrogen will get busy, and you should have finished compost in only a few weeks. And don't forget to feed your pile—Grandma's Compost Feeder Tonic (at left) works wonders.

◆ GIVE 'EM TIME

Sawdust, weathered mulch material, and wood chips are dandy soil amendments, too, but while they're decomposing, they tie up a lot of soil nutrients. So before you use them in your yard, let them mellow out in the compost heap for a while.

◆ HOLD THAT GOLD!

There are all kinds of ways to contain your black gold in the making, and they all serve the same purpose: To hold the stuff in while providing constant exposure to fresh air. You will also

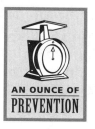

Do the Math

AN OUNCE OF PREVENTION

You never want your soil to end up being more than 50 percent amendment. So, if you are digging a 10-inch-deep bed, you would add no more than a 4- to 5-inch-deep layer of any soil amendment. Half that amount may do nicely if your soil is in pretty good shape. Use the same rule of thumb when preparing planting holes. Grandma Putt liked to dig out the soil, place it in a wheelbarrow, and mix it with a soil amendment, allowing about 2 parts soil to 1 part amendment. Then she'd use this mixture to line the bottom of the hole and backfill around the roots after the plant was in place.

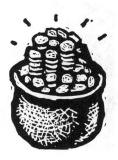

need a way to stir or turn the compost from time to time, so that everything gets a chance to be near the center and bottom of the mass, where decomposition tends to go fastest. Make sure you can easily add water, too. Here are some good compost container options:

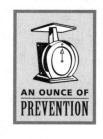

Compost Is a Must

Grandma Putt made sure that her plants had a steady supply of good compost. As little as a $1/2$-inch layer, worked into the soil in spring and fall, will ensure that your plants never run short of crucial nutrients such as zinc, selenium, and boron. Your soil will also drain better, and that's really important!

☞ A simple enclosure made from boards with hardware cloth or chicken wire nailed onto it. It's a snap to build, but it's usually not all that attractive.

☞ A special metal drum that you spin on a cylinder to mix the stuff. These things are convenient as all get-out, but they tend to rust over time.

☞ Plastic compost bins. In my book, this is the way to go if you care at all about appearances—they look like plastic trash cans, and they're easy to tuck out of sight or to screen with a vine-covered trellis. Plus, they last for years and keep your compost out of grabbing range of all kinds of pesky pests.

◆ KEEP COMPOST CLOSE AT HAND

You'll save a lot of time and effort by placing your compost bin close to your garden. Adding garden refuse to the pile and then using the resulting compost in your garden will be a heck of a lot easier and less time consuming if you don't have to trudge halfway across your yard

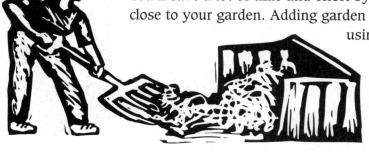

just to get to the bin. Remember, you want this to be fast, fun, and easy! Also, be sure to place your bin within easy reach of your garden hose, because you'll need to water your compost pile regularly. This'll help it keep growing.

◆ WHEN IN DOUBT, THROW IT OUT!

Many folks add all kinds of discarded vegetation and yard waste to their compost piles, in the hope of increasing their future supply of humus. They figure quantity is better than quality. Don't fall into this trap, because although at first glance this seems like a good idea, looks can be deceiving.

What these folks may be unknowingly adding to their compost piles are numerous insects and a whole host of diseases that carry through from year to year in the form of eggs, grubs, inactive spores, or what have you. Oftentimes, these carriers are on, in, or under some kind of plant growth, so adding infected plant material to the compost pile spells big trouble when you use the compost in your garden next year. How can you tell what's good to compost and what needs to be destroyed? You can't always be sure, unless you're a darned good scientist. But you'll be on the right track if you make it a point to burn any plants and plant parts that you know have been attacked by diseases or insects that bore or tunnel. Do not compost them. Remember: When in doubt, throw it out!

◆ IS IT DONE YET?

Compost is done, or finished, when it becomes dark and crumbly. When a batch nears this point, start a new one, and dole the good stuff out to your plants in generous servings. Compost is not a fertilizer, but it is very rich in enzymes and beneficial bacteria—and it's a first-class banquet of trace nutrients. That's why I call it black gold!

Planting Tips and Tricks

My Grandma Putt taught me that the best time to solve a problem in your yard is before it gets a toehold. And I'll let you in on a little secret: Every last one of your plants wants to grow and prosper in your yard. It's not hard to make that happen, but you do need to make sure your plants get started on the right root. In this section, I'll walk you through the whole process of planting, whether you're starting from seed or from container-grown plants.

Head Off Trouble

It may be but a short drive from the garden center to your yard, but if you want to head off problems before they start, there is much to know about selecting, planting, and caring for the plants you call your own. Let's start small, with seeds, and work our way up to long-lived trees and shrubs.

◆ SOW OR TRANSPLANT?

When you're setting out to grow annual flowers, most vegetables, and many herbs, you have two choices: You can start from seed or you can buy transplants at the garden center, all ready to be popped into the ground. There's no doubt about it, using transplants makes the job go more quickly, but to my way of thinking, there are three great reasons to start with seeds:

1. Broader choice. Seed catalogs offer a much greater variety than any garden center could hope to carry. For example, starting from seed may be the only way you can have a dozen hot pink zinnias, or grow beloved heirloom tomatoes like the ones you remember from your grandma's garden.

2. Rooting success. Some flowers, like morning glories, and a fair number of vegetables—including corn, beans, and all root crops—prefer to spend their lives right where they start out. In fact, some veggies resent root disturbance so much that you'll rarely, if ever, find them offered for sale as transplants.

3. Fun. Tinkering with seeds is great, because it's inexpensive, easy, and fun. In fact, some plants are so easily grown from seed that there is no reason to start them any other way.

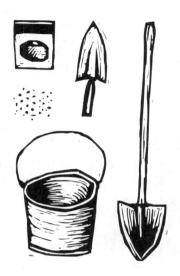

◆ MAKE 'EM SIZZLE

When you're getting a new site ready for planting, digging up weeds can be a real pain in the grass. So don't dig—cook 'em out. Just water the plot well, then stretch a sheet of clear plastic over it. (An old plastic drop cloth will work fine.) In about four weeks, with old Sol's cooperation, those weeds will be history!

◆ PICKING PACKETS

The larger the seeds, the easier they are to sow and grow. If you're new to gardening, the best plan is simply to learn the size of the seeds: Seeds that feel big and knobby are usually easy to handle, while tiny seeds require more time, patience, and know-how.

Hybrid How-To

Hybrid varieties are the result of carefully planned breeding projects, in which the pollen of one variety is used to fertilize the flowers of another. This crossing results in a single special generation of seeds, often coded as F1 on seed packets and in catalog descriptions. Hybrids are usually very vigorous plants, and often feature special colors, flavors, or resistance to disease. The downside is that, although F1 hybrids do produce seeds, those seeds won't have the same great characteristics as the parent plants. To get those, you'll have to buy more packaged F1 hybrid seeds from a garden center or catalog.

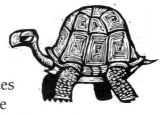

◆ SLOW GOING AHEAD

It is technically possible to start many flowering perennials, shrubs, and even trees from seed, but in most cases, it takes a lot of time and a lot of patience. Believe me, it's *not* a fast, easy route to a great-looking yard!

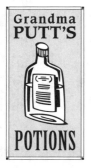

Seed and Soil Energizer

Grandma mixed up this potion to get her seeds off to a rip-roaring start.

1 tsp. of dishwashing liquid
1 tsp. of ammonia
1 tsp. of whiskey

Mix all of these ingredients in 1 quart of weak tea water*, pour into your mist-sprayer bottle, shake gently, then once a day, mist the surface of your seedbeds.

* To make weak tea water, soak a used tea bag in a solution of 1 gal. of warm water and 1 tsp. of dishwashing liquid until the mix is light brown. Store leftover liquid in a tightly capped jug or bottle for later use.

◆ SIZING UP SEEDS

The smaller the seeds, the easier it is for them to get lost in the rough-and-tumble world of the garden. Take it from me: You can avoid a lot of frustration by starting the little guys in the great indoors. Don't worry—it's easy to do, and a lot of fun, besides.

On the other hand, big seeds have no trouble muscling their way to the surface. In fact, many large seeds, such as beans, peas, corn, and squash, just hate having their roots tampered with. To get the best results, you need to plant them directly in the spots where you want them to grow up.

◆ DIRECT SOWING SAVVY

If you want to feel like a real down-and-dirty gardener, let yourself experience the excitement of sowing seeds directly into prepared ground. Nasturtiums, beans, and peas are great for beginners, and those beans and peas don't have to be the kind you eat. Scarlet runner beans and sweet peas will color up your yard and give you a chance to prove yourself as a champion sower of seeds. Here are a few tips to help you get growing:

Plant any seed at twice the depth of its size. Big beans go an inch deep, while smaller marigold seeds need shallower planting. Most seed packets list planting depth and spacing, along with the best time of year for sowing.

Plant promptly. You can plant seeds by poking them into the soil or by making shallow furrows with a hoe, stick, or your fingers. After that, I like to cover seeds with compost or potting soil, which doesn't form a crust at the surface the way regular soil often does. That way, you'll ensure that the little sprouts will have an easy time pushing themselves up to the sun.

Water well. To promote strong germination, keep the seeded spot constantly moist by hand watering or using a sprinkler. With luck, so many seeds will sprout that you will need to pull some of them out to give the others the room they need to grow. Usually, the best time to thin is about three weeks after planting.

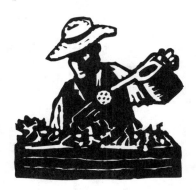

Start Seeds Indoors

You can get a head start by planting seeds indoors a few weeks to a month before the last spring frost. This is easy to do, especially if you have a grow light that you can suspend about 2 inches over the tops of your babies. Read on for more tips on how to ensure that your indoor-sown seeds start out strong and healthy.

◆ SKIP THE SOIL

To get your seeds growing on the right root, use a high-quality, professional seed-starting mix, not regular potting soil. Seed-starting mix is a very fine, light-textured, soilless planting medium that young roots can move through easily. The good brands have also been sterilized, so there's no way your baby plants can pick up pests or diseases.

◆ THE MATERNITY WARD

You can find all kinds of seed-starting containers, and even complete kits, at your local garden center or in gardening catalogs. They all work just fine. But they're not necessary. Anything that holds soil and has holes to let the extra water run out will work just as well. Here are some containers I like to use (after I've poked holes in the bottoms):

- ✔ Margarine, cottage cheese, and yogurt containers
- ✔ Milk cartons
- ✔ Paper, plastic, and foam drinking cups
- ✔ Pie and cake tins
- ✔ Plastic and plastic foam take-out boxes from delis and restaurants
- ✔ Plastic shoe boxes

◆ REFRIGERATE THE LEFTOVERS

If you find yourself with leftover seeds after the spring planting season, don't throw them out! You can store them for use next year. Seal them in their original packets, put the packets in small, airtight jars (like baby-food jars) with lids, and then tuck them away in your refrigerator. Be sure the temperature stays between 36°F and 45°F. (Check with a thermometer and adjust the fridge setting as needed.)

Hello, Jell-O!

To get your seeds off to a disease-free start, lightly sprinkle Jell-O® powder on 'em with a salt shaker. Any flavor works, but lemon is best, because it repels some bugs. As your plants grow, feed them more Jell-O—the gelatin helps the plants absorb water, and the sugar feeds the beneficial organisms in the soil.

◆ IT'S IN THE BAG

To help your seeds germinate better, save your plastic produce bags from the grocery store and turn them into mini-greenhouses. Just wrap them loosely around your seed flats; they'll hold in just the right amount of moisture. When seedlings appear, remove the bags and place the flats under lights.

◆ WINDOWSILL SALAD

For salad fixings in no time, plant radish, lettuce, and tomato seeds in containers and set them out on your windowsill. Plant radish seeds ¼ inch deep and 1 inch apart in a 9 × 12-inch cake pan. Scatter lettuce seeds on the surface of the soil in another cake pan, and cover with ⅛ inch of soil. Set the pans in a sunny windowsill, and keep the soil damp. The plants will be ready for your salad bowl in 8 to 10 weeks.

Grow 'Tiny Tim' tomatoes in clay pots on the windowsill, and they'll be ready in 12 to 14 weeks.

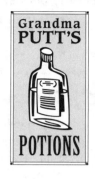

Seed Starter Tonic

Whether you start your seeds indoors or out, take Grandma Putt's advice and give 'em a good send-off with this timely tonic.

1 cup of white vinegar
1 tbsp. of dishwashing liquid
2 cups of warm water

Mix all of these ingredients together in a bowl, and let your seeds soak in it overnight before planting them in well-prepared soil.

◆ MOVE 'EM OUT

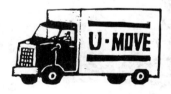

At transplant time, gradually get your seedlings ready for the outdoors by setting them outside in a protected place for a few hours a day for a day or two, working up to all day and night over a period of a week or so. Gardeners call this process "hardening off."

Easy Bedding Plants

Plants that come in six-packs are an incredible deal! For a dollar (more or less), you get seedlings that have been babied along in a greenhouse, given exactly the amount of light and diet they need, and are now ready to strut their stuff in your garden. I always buy begonias, geraniums, impatiens, and petunias as bedding plants, because growing them from tiny seeds takes forever! Here's how to make the most of these bedding beauties.

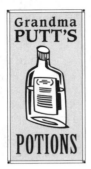

Damping-Off Prevention Tonic

Young seedlings are at risk for damping-off, a disease that causes their lower stems to rot. There's no cure, but you can prevent damping-off by using a sterile seed-starting medium and this quick tonic.

4 tsp. of chamomile tea
1 tsp. of dishwashing liquid

Mix these ingredients in 1 quart of boiling water. Let steep for at least an hour (the stronger the better), strain, then cool. Mist your seedlings as soon as their heads appear.

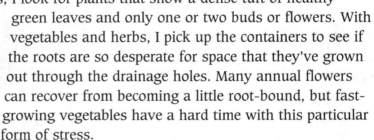

◆ SMART SHOPPING

Younger is always better when it comes to bedding plants. With flowers, I look for plants that show a dense tuft of healthy green leaves and only one or two buds or flowers. With vegetables and herbs, I pick up the containers to see if the roots are so desperate for space that they've grown out through the drainage holes. Many annual flowers can recover from becoming a little root-bound, but fast-growing vegetables have a hard time with this particular form of stress.

◆ BUYER BEWARE

Nurseries and garden centers offer many perennials for sale. Buying the plants (seedlings) instead of growing them from seed is a great way to get off to a fast start, but there are some things that you should look out for when purchasing perennials:

☞ Avoid plants that have been in warm areas for too long. You'll know them by their pale yellow stems and leaves.

☞ Choose plants that are short, compact, dark green, and that look healthy and strong.

☞ Buy only named varieties. They are bred to have specific characteristics, so you can easily research their disease resistance, heat and cold tolerance, and plant habits if you so desire.

◆ READY FOR TAKEOFF

Most bedding plants have already waited long enough to be planted, and they are eager for roomier quarters. Still, I like to give them a few days to prepare for their transplant operation, so I water them with my Seedling Starter Tonic (above) and busy myself getting their new home ready. This means cultivating a suitable bed and mixing an organic or timed-release fertilizer into the soil, or doing the same with planting holes, if that's what my planting plan requires.

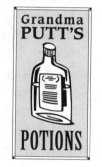

Grandma PUTT'S POTIONS

Seedling Starter Tonic

Don't let your bedding plants go hungry! While they're still in their six-packs, treat them to Grandma Putt's favorite nutritious mixture.

2 tsp. of fish emulsion
2 tsp. of dishwashing liquid
1 tsp. of whiskey

Mix all of these ingredients in one quart of water. Feed this brew to your adopted seedlings every other time you water them, and give them a good soak with it just before you set them out.

◆ SEEDLING TLC

Whatever you do, don't handle your seedlings by their stems or pull on them from the top. Twisting or bruising the main stem can cause serious injury to the tender young plants.

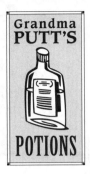

Seedling Strengthener

Until seedlings have a little time to stretch their roots a bit, they can't make use of the ready and waiting fertilizer you've mixed into the soil. To tide them over, Grandma Putt would mist-spray her bedding plants every few days with this elixir for two to three weeks after planting.

2 cups of manure
½ cup of instant tea granules
5 gal. of warm water

Put the manure and tea into an old nylon stocking, and let it steep in the warm water for several days. Dilute the brew with 4 parts of warm water before using.

◆ EASY DOES IT

The actual transplanting process is best done with a gentle touch. I squeeze plants out of their containers from the bottom, and sometimes use a table knife to pry them out if they're stuck. Quite often, I find that the roots have grown together into a tight mass at the bottom of the containers. Although it seems cruel and I can almost hear the little plants saying "Ouch" when I do it, I gently break apart the lowest inch of the root mass and spread it out, butterfly style. This little trick makes new roots grow out in different directions, which makes a big difference in the performance of the plants.

◆ GIVE 'EM A DRINK

Just before you're ready to transplant your vegetable seedlings, water them with a solution of 2 ounces of salt or baking soda per gallon of water. This will temporarily stop growth and increase their strength so they can stand right up and say "Boo" to the changing conditions they'll face outdoors.

Perennial Pleasures

To my way of thinking, flowering perennials are some of the greatest labor-savers in all of gardendom. Unlike annuals, which live for one year, set seed, and then die, perennials simply die back to the roots and go dormant in the winter. If you plant them right and give them just a little

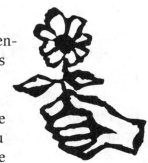

basic TLC, they'll keep coming back, filling your yard with color and fragrance year after year.

◆ WHEN, OH WHEN?

In early spring, all perennials wake up from their long winter's nap rarin' to grow. That's the best time to plant most of them in your garden, but some prefer fall planting. So how do you know when to plant what? The plant tag or catalog description will tell you. But when in doubt, just remember what Grandma Putt always said: "Great blooms come from great roots." In calendar terms, that translates into the following guidelines:

☞ Plant early bloomers in early fall. That will give them plenty of time to develop good, strong root structures before the first hard freeze sets in. Bleeding heart and coralbells like that head start. And poppies and peonies really need it—so don't even think of planting them in the spring.

☞ Plant later-blooming perennials in early spring, as soon as you can work the ground and the danger of freezing has passed. This roster includes such garden-variety favorites as asters, black-eyed Susans, chrysanthemums, and phlox. When you get them in early, they'll have all spring and early summer to put down roots before they launch their big floral display.

◆ THE PERENNIAL FOUNTAIN OF YOUTH

As most perennial plants age, the centers of the clumps become more woody and brittle. Happily, these sections are usually surrounded by younger, more vigorous crowns. So every 3 to 5 years, you need to dig and divide them. In the process, you'll get rid of the old dying parts and replant healthy, rooted crowns into fresh, fertile soil.

◆ DIVIDE AND CONQUER

In most climates, late winter to late spring is prime time for dividing clump-forming perennials to make sure they keep growing happily. (It's also one of my favorite times for getting out in the yard and working off all those calories I've consumed during the winter!) Most years I have more divisions than I can possibly use in my own yard, so I share the extras with friends, neighbors, and the folks who have flower beds in my town's community garden. Here's my simple 6-step division process:

Perennial Pointers

If early spring has come and gone, don't worry: You can still plant perennials that are actively growing. Just make sure they never dry out completely, and steer clear of strong fertilizers that can encourage top growth at the expense of root development. Remember, to perform like troupers over the long haul, your plants will need to spend the summer growing roots, not producing a blockbuster floral display.

1. With a digging fork, loosen the soil around the outside of the clump and try to lift it out so that it's intact.

2. Drop the clump soundly onto the ground so that it loosens up, or even breaks apart.

3. Pull or cut away the healthiest-looking pieces.

4. Spade a 3-inch layer of peat moss into the soil.

5. Set the divisions into their new homes.

6. Saturate the area with my Perennial Perk-Me-Up Tonic (at right).

◆ PLANTING POTTED PERENNIALS

Planting a perennial, shrub, or even a tree that's been grown in a pot is pretty straightforward. Here's how to do it in five easy steps:

1. Prepare a planting hole that's twice as deep and wide as the container, amend the soil with organic matter, and then refill the hole halfway.

2. Give the pot a few sound smacks to loosen the plant. If the soil and roots are nice and wet, the whole tangled mass should slide right out.

3. Now set the plant in the hole, spread out the roots as much as possible without breaking them, and place the plant so that it's about an inch higher than it grew in its container. That's the sweet spot, because as the soil settles (and you add mulch), it will sink down about an inch. (I like to lay the handle of my shovel over the top of the hole. When the thick side of the handle lines up with the soil in the container, I know the depth is just right.) If the plant is too low, take it out, put some more enriched soil under it, and check the depth again.

4. When you know you've got the depth right, start filling in soil around the plant, stopping to add water every few inches. Putting water right into the planting hole ensures that the roots will stay moist, and helps squeeze out big pockets of air that can leave roots thirsty.

5. Top off the surrounding soil with mulch, and you're done!

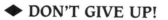

◆ **DON'T GIVE UP!**

If you order perennials by mail and they arrive looking dead in their pots, don't throw them out—and don't call customer service. Mail-order companies try to ship plants when they've just broken dormancy and are ready to be put into the ground. Your new arrivals may be brown and shriveled on the surface, but you can bet that by early summer, they'll be growing like gangbusters.

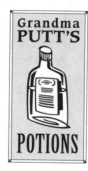

Grandma PUTT'S POTIONS

Perennial Perk-Me-Up Tonic

This excellent elixir will get your newly divided perennials back on their feet in no time at all.

1 can of beer
1 cup of ammonia
½ cup of dishwashing liquid
½ cup of liquid fertilizer
½ cup of corn syrup

Mix all of these ingredients in a 20 gallon hose-end sprayer, and saturate the ground around the perennials to the point of run-off.

◆ **THE STATE OF THE UNION**

Some roses, trees, and other woody plants are really two plants in one, because they are grafted. If you see a knobby bulge just above the soil line, you are probably looking at a graft union—the place where a cutting was grafted onto a rootstock, creating a plant that's prettier and more productive than its ungrafted counterpart. How you treat these plants when you put them into the ground depends on where you live. Here's a rundown:

In cool climates (USDA Zone 6 and below): the graft union should be right at the soil line, or, in the case of roses, even partially buried.

In warmer territory (Zone 7 and higher): set plants so that the graft union is an inch or two above the soil line. Otherwise, new stems may emerge from below the graft, and you'll end up with the plant used as the rootstock rather than the showier one that's been grafted onto it.

◆ GIVE 'EM ELBOW ROOM

Keep the mature size of a plant in mind when you're planting, and you won't end up with a crowded house of a garden. The tags that come on plants often suggest proper spacing, which is based on the mature size of the plant and how much root space it needs. Keep in mind that it often takes shrubs three to five years to fill out and grow, and trees can take a lifetime!

Know Your Terms

The words *variety* and *cultivar* are often used interchangeably in catalogs and books, but there's a subtle difference between the two. A variety can be grown from seed, but a cultivar is propagated vegetatively, usually by rooting stem cuttings or dividing and replanting pieces of root taken from the parent plant. When you buy a named cultivar, you know it will grow up to be exactly like its parent in size, leaf type, flower color, fragrance, and so forth. With a variety, all bets are off in a seed-grown plant—any or all of those characteristics can be a little different. Named cultivars often cost a little more than plants labeled simply by their species name, but if you want to be sure of what you're getting, they're worth the price.

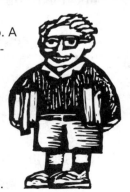

◆ TWO IN ONE

While you're waiting for slow-growing plants to reach full size, do what Grandma Putt did: Use the open space between them to grow annual flowers and spring-flowering bulbs, which make fine bedfellows for shrubs and perennials.

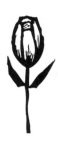

Bare-Root Babies

Some plants go into such a deep sleep when they become dormant that they can be pulled from the soil, washed clean, and sold with their roots as bare as a baby's bottom. Many of the plants that you order from catalogs come shipped bare-root. That's because plants with no heavy soil on their roots are easier and less expensive to ship from place to place, and because the plants are so clean, there is little chance of shipping soil-borne diseases along with them. Roses, raspberries, and other brambles are often sold with bare roots, as are many fruit trees and flowering vines. Bare-root plants are sold only in late winter and early spring. Look here for my tips on getting the most from your bare-root babies.

◆ HANDLE WITH CARE

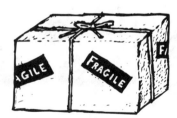

Like babies' bare bottoms, bare-root plants need delicate handling. If you can't plant them right away, lay them on the ground and pile about 4 inches of damp soil or compost over their roots so they won't freeze. (In gardeners' lingo, this process is called "heeling in.") Then, to get your babies off to a good, trouble-free start, give them a drink of Compost Tea (see page 292). When you lift out the plants a week or so later, don't be surprised if you see threadlike new roots—the first sign that the plants are emerging from their winter slumber.

◆ IT TAKES TWO TO TRANSPLANT

Recruit a helper when setting out bare-root plants. With two people on the job, it's fast work for one to gently pull and jiggle the plant to the correct depth, while the less fortunate one heaves in the soil alternated with sloppy slurps of water. As with container-grown plants, the goal is to have the plant sitting high in the soil, so that once the soil settles, the plant will be at the same depth at which it grew in the nursery field.

◆ UNTANGLE MANGLED ROOTS

From time to time, you may find that some roots on bare-root plants that arrived by mail are bent and broken in shipment. The fix is easy: Use clean, sharp pruning shears to trim off the injured roots. Then, as you plant, spread the remaining roots carefully to help the plant make a strong start.

Planting B-&-Bs

Long before there were bed-and-breakfast inns, B-&-B stood for balled-and-burlapped plants. Until the past decade or so, all shrubs and trees were sold with their roots tightly packed in soil, and the whole package was held in place with a snug wrapping of burlap. Larger trees and shrubs are still sold this way, so here's what you need to know.

◆ TOOLS OF THE TRADE

When setting out a B-&-B plant, use the claw end of a hammer to pull out the nails used to hold the burlap in place, along with strings of jute or wire. Set the plant in the planting hole, and then use scissors or shears to cut away most of the burlap. Because burlap is biodegradable, it's okay to leave a little bit under the plant, but I like to trim away as much as possible, so it won't become a barrier to new roots.

Before filling in soil around the root ball, thoroughly soak it with water. Add more water as you gradually fill in the planting hole, but don't worry about fertilizer at this point. Given sufficient root space and water, B-&-B shrubs and trees will get on with the first task before them, which is to grow new roots to replace the ones they lost when they were dug from the nursery field.

◆ DIG WIDE AND DEEP

When planting trees, dig a hole deep and wide enough for the roots. In the center, dig another hole as deep as you can with a post-hole digger. Fill this second hole with "Tree-mendous Planting Mix" (below). The roots of all trees, especially those with long tap roots, will benefit from this little bit of extra soil preparation.

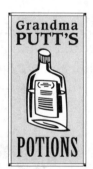

Tree-Mendous Planting Mix

Your newly planted trees will thank you when you start them off right with this super soil improver.

5 lbs. of compost
2 lbs. of gypsum
1 lb. of dry dog food
1 lb. of oatmeal

Mix all of the ingredients together, and use it to improve the soil when planting trees.

◆ YOUR ACHING BACK

Every day, gardeners suffer needless injuries to their backs (and other body parts, too) by lugging heavy plants to and fro all over their yards. So before you lift that tree or tote that shrub, keep these pointers in mind:

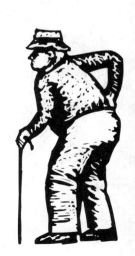

☞ If you'll be planting a number of shrubs or trees, invest in a wheeled dolly to move them.

☞ If you grow trees or other large plants in containers, keep those pots on rolling platforms so you can easily shift them from one place to another. You can buy special plant dol-

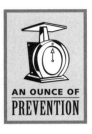

Foiled Again!

AN OUNCE OF PREVENTION

There's nothing mice and rabbits love more than newly planted trees. Protect your treasures with heavy-duty aluminum foil. Wrap it around the trunk from the top of the root ball up about 1 foot, and keep it there until the tree has established itself.

lies, or build your own from a board and heavy-duty casters.

☞ Before you put a heavy plant onto the ground by your planting hole, lay down an old blanket or piece of cardboard and use it to pull the plant into position.

☞ Last but not least, ask for help when you need it, because two people are always stronger than one!

◆ TATERS FOR TREES

Here's an old trick my Grandma Putt taught me. When planting a tree, line the planting hole with baking potatoes. They'll hold in moisture and provide nutrients to the tree as they decay.

Food, Water & Maintenance Magic

Just like us folks, plants have certain basic needs. Fortunately for those of us who can't (or don't care to) spend all our time tending our yards, most plants don't ask for much. Just give them a little food, a little water, and a little routine care, and they'll be happy as clams—and you will be even happier, because you'll head off problems before they start.

Plant Foods and Fertilizers

Some plants need little or no fertilizer at planting time, and others need a lot. Plants also differ in how often they like to be fed and the quantities of specific nutrients they need. Here's a look at the basics.

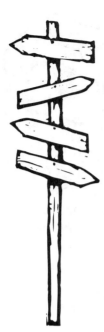

◆ WHICH WAY TO GO?

There are a lot of fertilizers on the market, but each falls into one of two basic categories: chemical/inorganic or natural/organic.

Chemical/inorganic fertilizers are manufactured using synthetic substances that contain highly concentrated amounts of specific nutrients plants need, primarily nitrogen, phosphorus, and potassium (see The Plant Food Pyramid on page 290). When you apply a chemical fertilizer, you see almost instant results, because the nutrients are immediately available to your plants. On the downside, this quick fix adds no nutrients to the soil itself. In fact, chemical fertilizers actually destroy the beneficial organisms that create the soil's natural nutrients. A pick-me-up dose now and then isn't likely to cause much harm, but used in large quantities over time, these chemicals build up in the soil and can actually hinder plant growth.

Organic/natural fertilizers, on the other hand, don't feed your plants at all. Rather, they add essential nutrients, major and minor, to the soil, where they become available to the plants. Organic fertilizers are made of naturally occurring substances, just like the ones I use in my tonics. When you shop for organic fertilizers, here are a few of the ingredients you may find on the label: nitrogen (found in cottonseed meal, alfalfa meal, and fish emulsion) phosphorus (found in poultry manure, rock phosphate, and bonemeal) and potassium (found in granite meal, kelp meal, and dairy manure).

> ### Don't Burn 'Em Up!
>
> If you use too much fertilizer or fail to mix it with the soil, plant roots can be destroyed and you'll see symptoms of fertilizer burn—leaves with brown, curled edges that look like they've been singed by a flame. Always err on the light side, blend fertilizer thoroughly into the soil, and follow up with a deep drench of water.

◆ WHAT'S IN THE BAG?

Fertilizer labels always include three hyphenated numbers, such as 10–5–5, which is called the guaranteed analysis. If you remember anything from high school chemistry, perhaps your brain will be willing to hold on to the letters N–P–K, which is what the guaranteed analysis is all about. The first number stands for nitrogen (N), the second one for phosphorus (P), and the last one represents potassium (K). Low numbers, like 6–2–4, mean that the fertilizer is not very concentrated, so the label will suggest using larger amounts than if the product had an analysis of 12–4–8, which contains twice as much actual fertilizer.

◆ EASY ON THE N!

All plants need some nitrogen in their diet, but don't overdo it. Too much of the Big N will make plants grow big and leafy, at the expense of blossoms, fruits, and seeds.

◆ THE PLANT FOOD PYRAMID

Plants make use of many nutrients, but nitrogen, phosphorus, and potassium are the biggies. Here's what each of them does for plants, nutritionally speaking:

Nitrogen: The main nutrient plants use to grow new leaves and stems. A high-nitrogen fertilizer will green up a lawn quickly and cause a lot of leafy growth in other plants.

Phosphorus: Promotes the growth of vigorous roots and the formation of flowers and seeds. Bulb fertilizers are often high in phosphorus, as are lawn fertilizers intended for use in the fall, because strong roots help these plants survive winter better.

Potassium: Supports all phases of plant growth and helps plants stand strong when insects and diseases attack.

◆ FIDO CAN'T BE WRONG

Here's a little secret I discovered years ago—believe it or not, dried dog food contains many of the same nutrients found in organic fertilizers such as bloodmeal and bonemeal! So grab a handful and work it into the soil for an added energy boost when planting, or sprinkle it around growing plants.

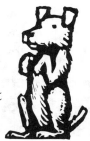

◆ MIRACLE MICRONUTRIENTS

Plants do not live on nitrogen, phosphorus, and potassium alone. They also need other nutrients, including calcium, magnesium, and sulfur. The best way I know to provide your plants with healthy, balanced nutrition is to give them regular doses of Grandma Putt's Compost Tea (page 292) and my All-Season Green-Up Tonic (at right). Believe me, if those green leafy guys in your yard could talk, they'd say, "Boy, that hits the spot!"

◆ PLEASE PASS THE CALCIUM

Your plants will usually find the calcium they need in soil that's been amended with organic matter that has a near-neutral pH, but it doesn't pay to take chances. To avoid calcium shortages, sprinkle on a little gypsum from time to time. Besides providing this necessary nutrient, gypsum helps dissolve salts that can build up in gardens and hinder plant growth.

Another great source of calcium is probably sitting in your refrigerator: eggshells. So why not do what Grandma Putt did? Every time you cook

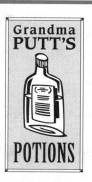

Grandma **PUTT'S**

POTIONS

All-Season Green-Up Tonic

Looking for a surefire way to help your yard and gardens sail through the growing season? Then serve them this sweet snack right up to the first hard frost, and they'll be lean, mean, and green growing machines!

1 can of beer
1 cup of ammonia
½ cup of dishwashing liquid
½ cup of liquid lawn food
½ cup of molasses or clear corn syrup

Mix all of these ingredients in a large bucket, pour into a 20 gallon hose-end sprayer, and saturate your lawn, trees, flowers, and vegetables every three weeks throughout the growing season.

some eggs, crush the shells, soak them in warm water overnight, and pour the water on your plants. They'll thank you by growing up to be big, strong, and beautiful.

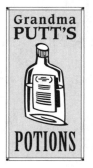

Compost Tea

Compost tea is the most healthful drink a plant could want. It delivers a well-balanced supply of important nutrients—major and minor—and fends off diseases at the same time. What more could a plant ask for?

1½ gal. of fresh compost
4½ gal. of warm water

Pour the water into a 5 gallon bucket. Scoop the compost into a cotton, burlap, or pantyhose sack, tie it closed, and put it into the water. Cover the bucket and let it steep for three to seven days. Pour the solution into a watering can or misting bottle, and give your plants a good spritzing with it every two to three weeks.

Note: You can make manure tea (another wonder drink) using this same recipe. Just substitute 1½ gallons of well-cured manure for the compost, and use the finished product in the same way.

◆ FERTILIZER FOR ALL

I'm often asked if there is any one fertilizer that's good for all flowers. The answer is yes—any garden food that's low in nitrogen and high in potash and phosphorus will do the trick. For bulbs and perennials, add some bonemeal to the soil. During the growing season, you can add liquefied table scraps (but not meats or fats) to your flower beds, as well.

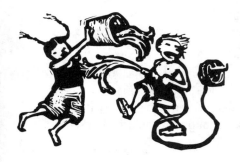

Getting Water Everywhere

I know I've been telling you to water just about everything you plant, but truth be told, I'm really worried about using too much water. You should be, too. Water is much too precious to waste, and in some places it's in dangerously short supply. All plants need water when they're young, but as they develop deep and extensive roots, you should have to water them less and less. Here are some of my tricks for keeping water use to a minimum.

◆ GO DEEP

To encourage deep roots, give plants deep water. By this I mean to really soak the soil so that water penetrates deeply, which usually takes some time. That's why soaker hoses are so handy. They release water slowly, so it has a chance to sink in and percolate down deep, where it belongs. Water that stays mostly near the surface encourages shallow roots to form, which makes plants need more water rather than less—and tends to make them weak and disease-prone, besides.

◆ SOCK IT TO 'EM

Here's a secret I learned long ago from my Grandma Putt, who never let anything go to waste. When your vegetable garden needs a drink, water it with the help of old socks. Put one sock inside the other, and use a short length of wire or a rubber band to attach the sock to the end of your garden hose. Now you've got a great soaker to lay over the mulch. Water for about an hour each day, three times a week.

◆ CATCH THE RAIN

Always provide a catch basin around your newly transplanted trees, shrubs, and evergreens. Since the main requirement of any new transplant is sufficient water, it is important to build a saucer around the base of each plant to catch and retain water, especially rainwater. Don't hill the soil around the base of a plant except in the fall, when you want the excess water to drain away.

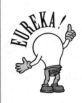

Water Jugs

It can take a l-o-n-g time to satisfy the thirst of a tree or a big shrub. Even if you have a soaker hose, it can't be every-place at once. That's where a big collection of plastic milk jugs comes in handy. Just use an ice pick or a big nail to poke small holes in the sides, about an inch above the bottom. Fill the jugs with water, place them all around the root zone, and let your plants drink up!

◆ WHEN TO SAY WHEN

How can you tell if you've soaked the soil long enough? Scoop up a handful of soil about 3 inches down. If you can shape it into a tight ball, chances are your soil is wet all the way down to the roots. If not, then you need to water some more.

◆ RAIN, RAIN COME MY WAY

My Grandma Putt sure knew what she was doing when she put sturdy oak barrels out to collect the rain. Of course, back then, rainwater was used for just about everything—from drinking and cooking to bathing and watering the garden.

Nowadays, there is no good reason why you can't collect rainwater for your garden plants. And now it's even easier to do because you have a choice of any number of containers in all shapes, sizes, and colors that you can easily slip under a downspout. Just use the old noggin—don't use anything so large that it's impossible to move once it's full!

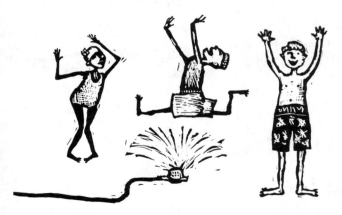

◆ BEAT THE HEAT

Keep your container plants happy through the long, hot summer by setting up this sim-ple automatic watering system. Here's all you need to do: Before you pot up each plant, run one end of a piece of cord or rope through the drainage hole and into the pot, leaving a long piece outside. Then fill a milk jug with water and set the other end of the cord into it. After that, all you need to do is keep the jug filled with water. This is an especially great trouble-saver if you're planning a summer vacation and won't be around to tend your plants!

Soak It to Me

Water soaks into the soil at different speeds, depending on the soil's composition. If you don't know your soil type, you can buy a soil test kit at garden centers, through catalogs, or at your local County Extension office. Once you know your basic soil type, use the table below as your handy-dandy guide to watering.

SOIL TYPE	SOAK RATE (IN. PER HR.)	SOAK TIME (PER IN.)
Sand	2.0	½ hr.
Sandy loam	1.0	1 hr.
Loam	0.5	2 hr.
Silt loam	0.4	2¼ hr.
Clay loam	0.3	3¼ hr.
Clay	0.2	5 hr.

Make Merry with Mulches

No matter what you are planting, the last step, the icing on the cake, is to apply some kind of mulch over the surface of the soil. Mulches help keep the soil moist, discourage weeds, and look nice, too. And, because mulches stop rainwater from splashing up into plant leaves, they also reduce problems with some kinds of diseases.

◆ WHICH MULCH FOR ME?

Every well-dressed landscape includes mulch, and you can choose mulches based on appearance for front-yard flower beds and shrub groupings. However, in other parts of your land-

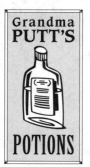

scape, it's smart to base your decisions on other mulch characteristics, such as their effects on soil temperature and plant growth. Here's a quick run-down on the most popular mulches and what they can and can't do for your plants:

Bark mulch: Long lasting and easy to apply, so it's ideal for mulching foundation shrubs and yard trees, and you can even use it to pave woodland pathways. I like small to medium-size chunks of bark better than larger ones, which tend to float away in heavy rains.

Chopped leaves: Free for the raking, and they're ideal for shady areas planted with azaleas, dog-woods, and other shallow-rooted plants that prefer acid soil (oak leaves are best). A leaf mulch keeps the soil cool, too, which is an extra asset in warm climates.

Gravel: Its light color, fine texture, and clean appearance make it a popular choice for mulching on soil next to houses. Gravel stops rainwater from splashing mud onto the house, and it's long lasting, too. However, weeds will push through pebbles unless you place weed barrier film over the ground before you start spreading your gravel. After a year or two, a few weeds invariably appear in gravel mulch, but any weeds will be easy to pull out or clean up with a glyphosate product if you get them when they're young.

Grandma PUTT'S POTIONS

Mulch Moisturizer Tonic

In the spring, whenever you add a fresh new layer of organic mulch to your bed, overspray it with this terrific tonic to give it a little extra kick.

1 can of regular cola (not diet)
½ cup of ammonia
½ cup of antiseptic mouthwash
½ cup of baby shampoo

Mix these ingredients in your 20 gallon hose-end sprayer, and give your mulch a nice, long, cool drink.

Wheat straw: Unsurpassed for controlling erosion on slopes planted with shrubs, or on gentle inclines that have been sown with grass seed. Wheat straw also makes a nice mulch for vegetable gardens, and, unlike hay, it contains no pesky weed seeds. When you purchase it in bales, you can easily peel off "books" of straw to lay down around your plants.

Wood chips: Work just like bark, and nowadays you can buy them dyed in colors like rust, red, and black.

Let Tomatoes See Red

If you grow tomatoes, treat your crop to a mulch of red, reflective plastic. Scientists have found that it improves the yield and health of America's favorite vegetable. The mulch warms the soil, which tomatoes really like, and the red color deters aphids and thrips, which are common vectors of some tomato diseases.

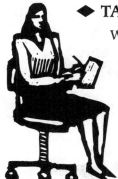

◆ TAKE NOTES

When you buy bark nuggets or any other type of bagged mulch to use in a shrub bed or around specific plantings, write down how much you use. That way, when it's time to renew your supply, you won't have to guess: You'll know exactly how much you need.

◆ ROLL-OUT THE BARRIERS

Would your mulch work better with a little underwear? You bet it would! Before you spread an organic mulch beneath shrubs and trees, cover the ground with a roll-out fabric weed barrier. Weed barrier fabrics, made from spunbound or woven polypropylene, block the light weeds need to germinate and grow. A few weeds may eventually appear from seeds that blow into the top layer of mulch or get dropped there by birds, but they will have scant roots, so you can yank them out with a gentle tug.

◆ LOCAL FAVORITES

If you want to see how dark brown cocoa shells work as mulch, visit Hershey Gardens, home of Hershey Chocolate in Hershey,

Pennsylvania. For a peek at pecan shell mulches, head on over to Mobile, Alabama. If peanut shell mulch interests you, take a trip to north Florida. All of these are examples of mulches that are locally abundant, and because they're all organic, they'll break down over time, adding valuable nutrients and structure to your soil.

◆ TAKE IT AWAY!

In every part of the country, there are terrific organic mulches that are just lying around somewhere, or that somebody needs to get rid of. Here are some good-looking and nutritious mulches:

- ✔ Chopped tobacco stalks
- ✔ Ground corncobs
- ✔ Mushroom compost
- ✔ Pine needles
- ✔ Seaweed
- ✔ Shredded bark
- ✔ Shredded oak leaves

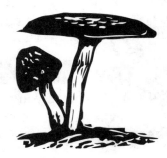

Support Your Plants!

Some plants can stand on their own just fine, but many need help staying on the up-and-up. That's important for reasons besides good looks: When a plant that's meant to grow upright lies down on the job, it becomes a prime target for all kinds of pesky pests and dastardly diseases—and that can mean big trouble for you.

◆ ALL TOGETHER

Grandma Putt liked to grow her tall plants in big masses. Instead of staking each individual plant, she'd install stakes in a random pattern among them. Then she'd weave jute or string among the stakes and stems to form a tangled network of gentle support.

◆ BEWARE THE TIES THAT BIND

No matter what kind of support you give your plants, always tie the stems in place with strips of soft cloth, old pantyhose, or some other material that won't chafe against tender stems as they tremble in the wind. Remember: A bruised or cut stem leaves any plant wide open to pests and diseases, so play it safe by keeping ties soft.

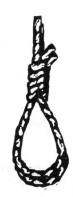

◆ TO EACH ITS OWN

The best way to support a plant depends on its natural growth habit. There are three major types of support:

1. Trellises, arbors, and arches. These not only support vines, but also add to their beauty and usefulness in your yard. Just bear in mind that the bigger and heavier a vine is, the sturdier its trellis needs to be.

2. Stakes. These work best with tall plants like delphiniums, lilies, and monkshood. There are more kinds of stakes than you can shake a stake at—bamboo, metal, plastic, and recycled prunings, to name just a few. Simply push the stake into the ground (very gently, so as not to damage the roots) and loosely fasten the stem to it.

3. Links, loops, and grids. These support systems are tailor-made for bushy perennial flowers that tend to flop over as soon as their tops become heavy with blooms. Peonies, tall garden phlox, and good, old black-eyed Susans all fall into this category. You can buy supports made of heavy wire that you simply stick into the ground around plants in the spring, so that the stems and leaves grow up through them. It doesn't get much easier than that!

Pruning: The Shape of Things to Come

You're probably reading this section because something in your yard has grown way too big. That's the usual reason people prune, but there are better reasons to thin stems and cut back limbs. Pruning helps direct plant growth to where you want it, so the best reason to use your pruning shears is to help plants grow taller, wider, or stronger by putting more energy into a few robust branches instead of spreading it thinly to a number of little stems.

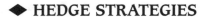

◆ HEDGE STRATEGIES

To keep from becoming a slave to a hedge, invest in rechargeable electric pruning shears. They're great timesavers! The next step is to time your pruning to coincide with your hedge's natural growth surges. Prune it in late spring, midsummer, and again in early fall. Stop pruning when winter is still at least six weeks away, because tender new growth is easily injured by cold. Hedges that wear brown tips until spring are always a sad sight—and are also prime targets for disease and pest invasions.

◆ THE FACTS OF LIFE

Whenever you cut back a stem, you encourage another to grow somewhere else. Usually, the new growth will emerge just below where you cut. This is a simple fact of plant life, and it's one you need to carry in your head before you ever touch a plant with a tool that cuts wood. If you shear back a plant by removing all the stem tips, crew cut style, the next growth spurt will consist of a number of small stems that sprout out all over. So the next time you prune, you'll be cutting through thicker growth than you encountered the time before. That's fine if the plant in question is a hedge plant that's meant to grow that way. But with most shrubs and all trees, it's better to follow the natural shape of the plant. First remove damaged or awkward stems, and then go back and shape them up just a little bit.

◆ PRUNE TO PROMOTE BLOOM

One excellent reason to prune is to help flowering plants bloom like crazy. When you "deadhead" marigolds, zinnias, and many other annual flowers by pinching or cutting off old blossoms, the plants respond by producing new stems laden with baby buds. Sometimes you can coax a second coming out of perennial flowers this way, too, or at least prolong the bloom time of those that bloom all in a rush, as peonies and chrysanthemums like to do.

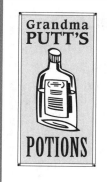

Grandma PUTT'S POTIONS

Tea Anyone?

To give her roses a post-pruning pick-me-up, Grandma Putt laid tea bags onto the soil underneath each bush. The tannic acid in the tea made the soil slightly acidic, which makes roses pleased as punch!

◆ PEP 'EM UP

Some plants wear themselves out if you don't discipline them a little with your pruning shears. For example, left to their own devices, hybrid tea roses will cover themselves with blossoms and then get so exhausted that they quit cold turkey. But if you remove some of their branches after the first flush of bloom, you give them the energy to flower again. More important, you help them fend off disease by allowing air to circulate freely through the branches—and as Grandma Putt used to say, trying to grow healthy roses without good air circulation is like trying to swim without water!

◆ 'TIS THE SEASON

To figure out when to prune any flowering plant, just think about when it blooms. To take the guesswork out of when to

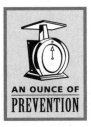

Oh, Deer!

Anytime you prune shrubs during the growing season, as you do with spring and early-summer bloomers, you stimulate new growth—and there's nothing deer like more than those tender young shoots. To keep the brown-eyed bruisers at bay, just tie up some mothballs in old pantyhose and hang the pouches from the branches of susceptible shrubs.

prune what, note which of your shrubs fall into which time slot and write the names on a calendar in the appropriate months. Then, bingo—you'll be a pruning wiz, and your shrubs will shower you with blossoms! Most popular landscape plants fit into one of these four categories:

Spring bloomers: include azaleas, forsythias, and lilacs. They develop their buds by the time they become dormant in the fall. If they need pruning (which they often don't), do your cutting in late spring or early summer, right after the flowers fade. The new wood that grows during the summer will have plenty of mature buds by the season's end.

Early summer bloomers: include many roses and spireas. These often benefit from light fall pruning to thin branches.

Shrubs that produce pretty berries: such as viburnums. These can be lightly pruned in the winter after birds have consumed the fall crop of fruit.

Mid- to late-summer bloomers: include buddleias and crepe myrtles. These are prunable anytime they are dormant, and often benefit from serious pruning in late winter or early spring. Vigorous new growth that follows on the heels of hard pruning usually leads to a heavy set of flowers.

◆ THE RIGHT STUFF

I've seen garages that have more pruning tools hanging on the walls than I've seen in some garden centers. That's fine if your aim is to own a record-breaking tool collection. But if all you want is a healthy, good-looking landscape, you don't need much in the way of hardware. These three see most of the action in my yard:

Hand clippers. A.k.a. pruners, shears, or snips. These are used for dead-heading flowers, cutting back annuals and perennials in the fall, harvesting herbs, and pruning roses and other shrubs.

Loppers. Heavy-duty pruners with extra-long handles. You need a pair of these if you have high shrubs or small trees.

Pruning saws. They come in various shapes and sizes, all designed to cut branches that are too thick for either hand clippers or loppers.

◆ THE MONSTERS ARE COMING!

If you have an older landscape, you may have evergreens that naturally want to grow into monster-sized specimens. In that case, pruning is the only way to keep them in line, but sometimes the cure is a killer. For example, broad-leafed evergreens (which grow mostly from Zone 6 southward) will often recover from radical pruning, but overgrown needle evergreens such as arborvitae, juniper, and hemlock never get over the shock of aggressive pruning. A haircut probably won't kill your plants, but your good intentions may lead to permanent brown "dead zones" where new growth will never appear. A better strategy is to get rid of seriously overgrown evergreens and replace them with something better—and permanently smaller!

◆ TIME TO RENEW

Thinning out old branches and topping off those that have grown long and leggy is called renewal pruning. If you remove about one-third of old growth in this way, the shrub will respond by producing a huge flush of energetic new growth. There is a definite rhyme and reason to renewal pruning, so here's how to go about it in 5 easy steps:

Step 1. Find any dead stems, which often have gray rather than brown bark, and cut them off as close to the ground as possible. Or cut off deadwood where it joins a healthy stem.

Step 2. Repeat Step 1 with any stems that show evidence of disease—dark cankers, nasty splits in the bark, or leaves that are covered with yellow spots or patches.

Step 3. Take two steps backward, and look for stems that cross each other or stick out in odd directions. then remove the weaker one, which is often the older branch.

Step 4. Trim off any very low branches that are spindly because they get so little sunlight.

Step 5. If a tall stem towers above all the others, reach down into the shrub and cut it off where it joins a larger stem.

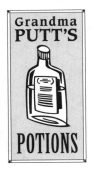

Super Shrub Restorer

1 can of beer
1 cup of ammonia
½ cup of dish-
 washing liquid
½ cup of molasses
 or clear corn syrup

Mix all of these ingredients in your 20 gallon hose-end sprayer. Drench shrubs thoroughly, including the undersides of leaves, where little critters often hide. If you have some left over, spray it on your trees and lawn, too.

◆ ON THE REBOUND

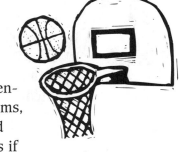

Because they have such exten-sive root systems, established old shrubs often become glorious specimens if you prune them thoughtfully, replace old mulches with new material, and give them a nice pick-me-up that cleans old stems and leaves and washes off little pests that may be hid-ing in the foliage. My Super Shrub Restorer (above) is just the ticket for perking up old shrubs and getting them started on their way to a robust new life.

CHAPTER 9

The Old Jalopy

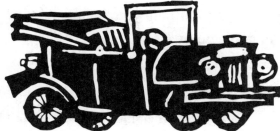

It seems these days that almost every family has at least one car—about half have two or more. As a matter of fact, every year about 15 million cars and trucks are manufactured and sold in the United States. Another 35 million automobiles are produced annually throughout the rest of the world. But not everyone drives a new car. Some 30 million used autos are resold each year in this country alone. (Come to think of it, I was behind most of them on my way to the beach last summer!)

So any way you slice it, it all adds up to a heck of a lot of vehicles to take care of! In this chapter, I'll give you some tips and tricks for maintaining your car—inside and out—whether it's one of the newly minted or an old faithful jalopy that you've had for years.

For instance, I'll reveal my top-secret tip for better vision when you drive at night (you won't believe it!). And I'll bet you don't know the difference between car wax and car polish—but after reading this chapter, you sure will. Did you put a scratch in your car's paint? Don't fret, I'll tell you about the product you probably already have in your bathroom or cosmetics case that will help you take care of that scratch.

There's loads of fun in this chapter, too. Case in point: Henry Ford invented the automobile, right? Nope! But you'll find out here who did. And if you're a commuter, you may be interested to know just how much of your lifespan you're spending in your car. The answer may surprise you! Read on for lots more auto advice.

Keeping It Safe and Sound

Americans drive more than anyone else—but then, we have a lot of places to go! Here are some good old-fashioned, commonsense tips to make your driving safe as can be, and to help you keep your car in good repair for as long as you own it.

Drive Safely

We all know the statistics—there are plenty of accidents every day on back roads and highways. So your best protection is to drive defensively, keep your car in good working order, and keep your wits about you when you're on the road. Here's how to do it.

> *Frequent naps prevent old age, especially if taken while driving.*

◆ BE PREPARED

Before you set out on a trip—especially in winter—make sure that all of your car's components are in good working order: your battery, brakes, defroster, heater, lights, and windshield wipers. And check all fluids, too: antifreeze, oil, and windshield wiper fluid. Once you've done that, you're ready to roll.

◆ CLEAN BEAMS

You want common sense? Here's some Grandma Putt-style common sense. Years ago, when I owned my second car, I remember complaining to Grandma Putt that my headlights seemed really dim and that I was thinking about replacing them. After all, bright headlights are vital to safe nighttime driving.

Well, a couple of nights later I got into my car to run an errand. I switched on the headlights and much to my surprise, the lights were bright—really bright. When I came home, I commented to Grandma how all of a sudden the lights were bright

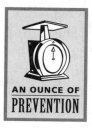

AN OUNCE OF
PREVENTION

A Car Safety Kit
Every Driver Should Have

You know how important it is to have a first-aid kit in your house and workshop. Well, it's just as important to have one for your car, too—only in this case, it's a safety kit that can come in handy in all kinds of emergency situations when you're on the road. So take a few minutes to gather up these items and put them into a sturdy container to store in your car.

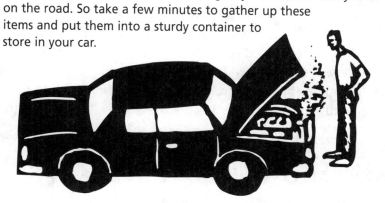

☑ **Gallon of water and snack food.** Just in case you're stuck in your car. Maybe you're stuck in snow or during a torrential rainstorm, or you're just waiting for your husband to return with a can of gas.

☑ **Warm blanket.** See above.

☑ **Flashlight with extra bulbs and batteries.** This sure comes in handy when you have to add windshield wiper fluid or change a tire on a dark night.

☑ **Ice scraper and a small broom.** (I use a whisk broom). For those of you who live in the north, you'll need these to remove ice and snow from your car.

☑ **Swiss army knife.** This is one item that's always handy to have, and not just for emergencies. The knife can cut your sandwich, the bottle opener can open your bottle of soda, and you can groom your nails (or open an envelope or unscrew a slotted screw) with the file.

again. I told her that it must have been a loose connection; that I had simply hit a bump and that had made the lights bright again. Grandma Putt couldn't contain herself and she started roaring with laughter. "Well," she said, "you can thank me for that."

I knew Grandma was good at many things, but I was fairly confident that she didn't know a stitch about changing headlights. "What did you do, Gram?" I asked. She shook her head and said with a laugh, "I cleaned them, Jerry. I just cleaned them."

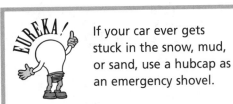

If your car ever gets stuck in the snow, mud, or sand, use a hubcap as an emergency shovel.

So now I give my headlights a good going over every time I gas up and each time I do, I can feel Grandma smiling down at me. And as a bonus, my headlights always give off bright, clear light.

◆ NICE KITTY!

There's one thing I never leave home without in the winter: cat litter. No, it's not for kitty accidents I might encounter on the road, but for traction. I can't tell you how many times a sprinkling of clay (not clumping) cat litter under my tires has helped me out of an icy parking space. It gives me just enough traction to send me on my way. As a plus, the weight of the bag in the trunk of your car helps you have better control of rear-wheel-drive vehicle in bad weather.

◆ KEEP YOUR DISTANCE

You know you're supposed to allow a safe distance between your car and the car in front of you when you're driving. But what exactly is a safe distance? One way to figure it out is to allow for one car length for every 10 miles an hour of speed. But that can be tricky to calculate, especially at my age. So here's an easier way to make sure that you're not driving too close to the car in front of you.

Pick out a landmark, such as a sign, in the distance. As soon as the car in front of you passes the landmark start counting, one one thousand, two one thousand, three one thousand. If you pass that same landmark before you get to three one thousand (3 seconds), you're too close to the car in front of you, so slow down. In good weather, allow at least 3 seconds between you and the car in front of you. If the driving conditions are poor, allow even more.

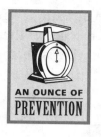

AN OUNCE OF PREVENTION

Arrive Alive

It's not unusual to get drowsy during a long drive. To combat fatigue, take frequent, scheduled rest stops. Plan on a 15-minute break for every two hours of driving during your trip. If you can, get out of the car and take a walk. Stretch your legs, arms, and neck muscles. Drink a cold soda or water or have some hot coffee. If you're hungry, have a light snack (a heavy meal may give you the snoozies). If you can't or don't want to get out of the car, recline the seat and stretch your arms and legs. Better to get there a little late than not at all!

Tire Talk

You don't need to be a car mechanic to change a tire, but you do need one to rotate them. And you should be tire-savvy enough to know when your tires need inflating. Read on, my friends, for some good advice.

◆ TIME FOR A CHANGE

Changing a tire is sort of like changing a baby: Nobody wants to do it, but it's got to be done. It can be intimidating (especially if you don't know what you're doing). And no matter how hard you try, you're most likely going to get dirty...and possibly wet.

The trickiest part of changing a tire is the fact that your car will be raised up in the air on a jack. At that point, your car is balanced quite precariously on a device whose design has remained virtually the same as it was when it supported your grandfather's 1940 Packard. That means you need to be extra careful—especially when you must change a tire on the side of the road. Here are some ways to keep your car (and you) safe and sound during the procedure.

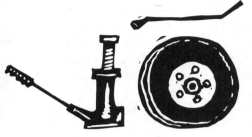

◆ KEEP A LEVEL HEAD

When you've got a flat tire and are looking for a place to pull off the road, try to find an area that is (1) level and on solid ground, (2) away from traffic and curves, and (3) in plain sight to other drivers. However, don't spend too much time searching for a perfect spot—driving on a flat can damage the tire's rim and possibly other parts of your car. When you do find a good spot, be sure to apply the hand brake to prevent the car from rolling.

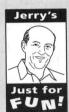

Jerry's Just for FUN!

He May Be More Famous, but...

Many folks think that Henry Ford invented the automobile, but in fact it was Carl Benz, in Munich, Germany. In 1885, he combined the internal combustion engine (invented by his fellow countryman Gottlieb Daimler) with a three-wheeled carriage. The next year, Daimler built the first four-wheeled, engine-powered vehicle.

Ford wasn't the first American car inventor, either. That distinction belongs to Andrew L. Riker, who in 1890 became the first American to build a battery-powered tricycle. Soon afterward, William Morrison's 1893 design of a six-passenger electric wagon was the first American auto to appear at a World's Fair. Also in 1893, the brothers Charles Edgar and J. Frank Duryea built the first gasoline-powered American car. In 1895, they won the first auto race held in the United States, with Frank driving. Talk about do-it-yourselfers!

Good ol' Henry Ford didn't get around to manufacturing cars until 1899. What a Johnny-come-lately!

◆ LIGHT IT UP

When you need to pull off the road at night or in bad weather, make sure you and your car are visible. Use your hazard lights and any reflectors or flares you have (that's why you carry them!). While you're working on the tire, leave your trunk open so that the trunk light stays on and illuminates the whole back of your car. And then turn on the dome light inside your car. In short, do whatever you need to do to be seen.

◆ BE STILL

Common sense tells you (or it ought to, anyway) that while your car is up on the jack, any car movement can be very dangerous. So be sure to follow these rules:

1. Don't leave your children inside the car while you jack it up.

2. Remove the spare tire and any other tools you need from the car *before* you jack it up.

3. Don't lean against the car or put your weight on it while operating the jack or while you're loosening or tightening the lug nuts. You may need to put a lot of oomph on the lug nuts to loosen them, so do it before you jack up the car. You don't have to completely remove them. Just loosen them a little to prevent your having to rock the car too much while it's up on the jack.

Xs and Os

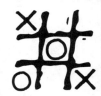

When you tighten the lug nuts on a spare tire, it's best to work in an X rather than an O pattern. What the heck does that mean? Well, think of the lug nuts as the numbers on a clock. Instead of tightening the nuts in a clockwise manner (12 o'clock, then 3 o'clock, then 6 o'clock, then 9 o'clock), tighten 12 o'clock, then 6 o'clock, then 3 o'clock, and then 9 o'clock.

◆ CUSHION THE BLOW

After you remove the flat tire, place it under the edge of the car while it's jacked up. That way, if the jack does slip or let go, the tire—not your body—will take the brunt of the fall. For the same reason, it's a good idea to place the spare tire under the edge of the car while you're removing the flat.

◆ DON'T BE SO UPTIGHT

After you place the spare tire on the car, tighten the lug nuts just enough to keep the tire in place. Don't tighten the nuts until you've lowered the car and brought it safely back to terra firma. (Remember the rule about not rocking the car while it's on the jack?)

◆ MAKE HASTE

When you finish changing a tire, don't bother to replace the hubcap or stow the jack neatly away. Throw the flat into your trunk and get the heck out of there. Don't spend any more time on the side of the road than you have to. You can take time to organize and neaten everything in your trunk later, perhaps at the service station while your flat is being repaired.

◆ THE QUARTER TEST

Having your tires properly inflated will help your car run more smoothly and keep the wheels in alignment. Here's how to tell whether your tires are under- or over-inflated, and it won't cost you a nickel, either, although you will need a quarter.

For each tire, insert a quarter into the tread at the inside, center, and outside of the tire. If the quarter fits deeper into the tread at the edges than in the center, the tire is over-inflated. If the tread is deeper in the center than at the edges, the tire needs more air.

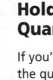

Hold That Quarter!

If you've just tried the quarter test and the tread is deeper on one side of the tire than the other, better use that quarter to call your mechanic. Your wheels could be out of alignment.

AN OUNCE OF PREVENTION

◆ WHY ROTATE?

Rotate your tires? Don't they rotate every time you drive? Seriously though, rotating your car tires means switching the tires from one side to the other and from front to back. No matter how new your car is or how well your steering is aligned, your tires don't wear evenly. There are many reasons for this: weight distribution in your car (are you usually the only occupant?), your driving habits, or taking more right turns than left, or vice versa. Taking the time to rotate your tires every 10,000 miles will help them wear evenly and extend their life. But don't do it yourself. Rotating the tires means removing them and balancing them, too, and that's a job best left for a pro.

If your annual mileage is around 10,000, have the service station that performs your yearly inspection rotate your tires during the same visit. It's a relatively easy and inexpensive procedure that will prolong the life of your tires.

Gas-Saving Techniques

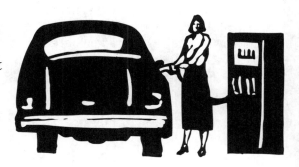

You know, when you make an effort to save gas, you're doing your part to help the environment, too. And that's a win-win situation in my book.

◆ PLAN AHEAD

Are you one of those folks who jumps in the car every single time you need something from the store? If so, shame on you! One of the easiest ways to save gas is to do a little planning. At the beginning of the week, sit down with the family and make a list of all the errands that need to be done. Organize those errands by location, and then tackle them all in one day. Not only will this little trick save you gas money, but it will save you time, too.

◆ TAKE THE BUS

Do you live in a university or college town? Call and find out if the school operates a free or reduced-cost shuttle around town. You may not need to be a student to use it. If you're lucky, you could save hundreds of dollars a year by using a shuttle service!

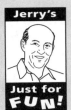

Electricity Killed the Electric Car

Gas-guzzling cars are pollution-spewing noise-makers, right? So why not switch to quiet and clean electric cars? You may think this is a recent option, but actually it's about as old as the automobile itself.

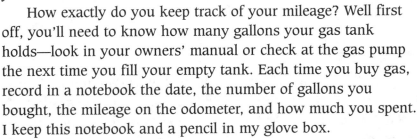

Back in the 1890s and early 1900s, electric cars were about as common as gas-powered ones. Gas-powered engines could run longer and appealed to those who enjoyed "touring" in their automobiles. But gas vehicles were dirty and hard to start because they needed to be cranked up first. Their silent electric cousins, on the other hand, were thought to be just the thing for city dwellers, ladies, and those who didn't want to get their hands and clothes soiled. In fact, many prominent folks at the time, such as President Woodrow Wilson, Andrew Carnegie, and even Henry and Clara Ford owned electric cars. It seemed as though both could co-exist. All that changed in 1912 when the people at Cadillac added an electric starter to their gasoline-powered cars. Soon anybody could drive, whether or not they could turn the crank. That made the gas-powered cars more popular. Unfortunately, due to its limited range, the electric car still hasn't caught on.

◆ MONITOR YOUR MILEAGE

One good way to monitor your spending on gas is to keep track of your mileage. Not only will it remind you just how much money you spend on gas, but it will clue you in to problems with your car, too. For instance, if you consistently get 28 miles per gallon and that number suddenly drops to 20, you'll know that something's wrong with your car and that it's time to visit your mechanic.

How exactly do you keep track of your mileage? Well first off, you'll need to know how many gallons your gas tank holds—look in your owners' manual or check at the gas pump the next time you fill your empty tank. Each time you buy gas, record in a notebook the date, the number of gallons you bought, the mileage on the odometer, and how much you spent. I keep this notebook and a pencil in my glove box.

Let's say your tank holds 12 gallons. One day you fill the car up and note that the odometer reads 15,000 miles. When the tank is half empty the mileage is 15,180. The difference is 6 gallons and 180 miles. Divide 180 miles by 6 gallons and you'll know that your car got 30 miles per gallon. Check the mileage at every half tank or so. This simple exercise will help you track your spending and make sure that nothing is wrong with your car.

◆ SKIP THE WARM-UP

Here's good news for the person in your family whose job is to warm up the car on a frigid winter morning— you're fired! Today's cars don't need to be warmed up before they're driven, and in fact, doing so can damage the car. So all you're doing is wasting gas. If you warm up the car just to get the heater going, skip it and treat yourself to a good hat, a pair of warm gloves, and a nice comfortable seat cushion.

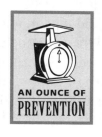

AN OUNCE OF PREVENTION

Don't Run in the Garage

If you're determined to warm up your car before you drive it, even though most times you don't need to, here's something very important to keep in mind.

Never, ever run the engine with the garage door closed. Always open it wide to allow the exhaust to escape. **Carbon monoxide can be deadly,** so you want it all to vent out, not accumulate in your garage. This is especially important if you have a garage that's attached to your house. To be really safe, back the car out of the garage and let it idle in the driveway. Otherwise, carbon monoxide can seep into your house and put everyone there— especially children and pets—at risk.

◆ A.C.? OK!

I love unexpected tips like this one. You probably think that using your air conditioner is bad for your gas mileage and you're right—but only up to 40 miles an hour. When you're driving faster than 40 mph, it's actually more fuel-efficient to use your air conditioner than it is to roll down your windows.

Why? When your windows are rolled up, your car is more aerodynamic. And while running the air conditioner does reduce your mileage, it's a smaller mileage reduction than what you lose from the drag caused by driving with open windows. Pretty neat, huh?

◆ DON'T TOP IT OFF

Here's an earth-friendly, money-saving tip that Grandma Putt would have loved. Are you one of those folks who tops off her gas tank by adding more gas even after the pump tells you it's full, just to get to an even dollar amount? Well, you're wasting gas and money, and hurting the environment—a triple whammy.

When you top off your tank, that gas doesn't get used by your car. It simply evaporates or spills out. Every gallon of spilled or evaporated gas adds the same amount of hydrocarbons to the air as the tailpipe of a car driving 7,500 miles. That's a heck of a lot of damage to the earth. So don't top it off.

A Clean Car Is a Happy Car

I've owned some real gas-guzzling, dinged-up relics in my time on the road (I don't believe in buying new cars—used ones are a much better value). Those cars may

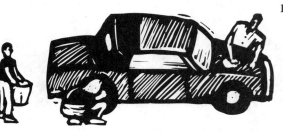

not have been beauties, but they've always been clean. I guess I was trying to fool myself into thinking that my 1973 Plymouth Valiant ran as well as it looked. And I believed that washing my 1975 Impala every other weekend made it more streamlined, cut down on wind resistance, and therefore saved me gas money. (Actually, washing your car DOES make it less wind-resistant and saves you gas money—read on to find out why.)

Down and Dirty

I've always kept my cars clean—and now that I own a car younger than the current presidential administration, I'm even better about cleaning it on a regular basis. Here are my hints and tips for having the cleanest car on the block.

◆ CLEAN CARS FINISH FIRST

...and keep their finish. You never know what good ol' Mother Nature has planned for your car. Be it acid rain, pollen, snow, road salt, or incontinent sea gulls and pigeons—the outside of your car takes a real beating. Substances such as road salt and bird droppings have very caustic properties and, when left on over time, can eat away at the painted surfaces of your car. Even a vehicle that spends most of its time in a garage can fall victim to a leaking roof or pipe. By washing your car on a regular basis, you can prevent damage to its finish and give it a longer life.

◆ I CAN SEE!

Wash your windshield regularly and you'll always see clearly. And if you keep your windshield clean, there's less dirt and grime to collect on the wiper blades, so they'll last longer. To clean the wiper blades, pull each wiper away from the windshield and apply ammonia to a rag or napkin and rub it down both sides of the blade.

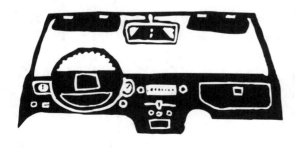

Window Washing 101

Don't leave your newly washed car windows full of streaks. Follow these simple rules for spotless auto glass.

☑ Wash your windows in the shade. Sunlight makes them dry too quickly and causes streaks.

☑ When you dry your windows, use a horizontal motion on one side and a vertical motion on the other. That way you'll know immediately which side the streaks are on.

☑ The best materials to use when you clean your windows are linen towels, chamois, or newspaper.

☑ You don't need to use harsh chemicals to wash your car windows. A mixture of 1 part vinegar and 1 part water will do the trick.

☑ If you smoke, clean the inside of your car windows with a mixture of 1 quart of water and 2 tablespoons of lemon juice. The juice will cut through the grime on the windows and also leave a pleasant scent.

◆ SIX CAR-CLEANING MUSTS

Here's what you need to wash your car the right way:

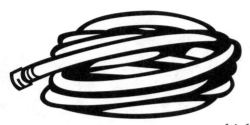

1. A hose with running water. There's nothing better than running water to rinse off the suds from your car. Pouring water from a bucket just doesn't work as well—there always seems to be a little grit left at the bottom. One thing to avoid, though, is a high-pressure nozzle on the hose. You don't want to blast the road grime off—it will damage the finish.

2. A large bucket. It should be large enough to rinse a large sponge several times without needing more clean water.

3. Soap. There are plenty of specially formulated carwash soaps on the shelves of auto parts stores. The one thing they all have in common is a neutral pH. That's so the detergent won't strip the paint's finish. Call me crazy, but I like to use a mild, pH-balanced baby shampoo. I buy a gallon of the store brand; it's a lot less expensive than automotive soap. (And I don't cry if I get some in my eyes.)

4. A large sponge. A natural sponge is my first choice. The dirt gets caught in all the nooks and crannies and it won't drag the grime across the surface of the paint, potentially scratching it, like a flat, synthetic sponge can.

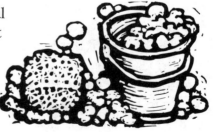

5. Several large towels. Old, clean bath towels work as well as the natural or synthetic chamois that you'll find in your local automotive supply store. In fact, I'm told that natural chamois contains oils that can prematurely wear down a car's finish, so you're better off saving those old bathroom discards.

6. A natural-bristle scrub brush. This is great for cleaning the tires without scratching up the wheel covers.

◆ MADE IN THE SHADE

The perfect carwash starts with choosing the perfect spot. Park the car in the shade and let it cool down before you start to wash it. By working in the shade, you avoid exposing your car to the dreaded thermo-shock. This happens when a hot car is suddenly sprayed with cold water, potentially causing hairline cracks in the paint's surface. You know how your toes curl up when you first step into cold water at the beach? It's kind of the same thing. For the same reason, you should also avoid using water that's too hot.

◆ GIVE MOTHER NATURE A HAND

When you wash your car, you remove highly toxic substances like auto emissions from its surface. If you wash your car on the street, those pollutants, as well as the soap you're using, can get washed down the storm drains in the street. Wash water that flows into storm drains doesn't necessarily feed into the local treatment plant (water that flows into sanitary sewers does), but it can possibly flow into local waterways such as creeks, lakes, and estuaries. By washing on grass or gravel, you give Mother Nature a better chance to filter those substances out of the water.

Of course, if you and your neighbors use well water, you'll want to wash your car where you know the runoff will go down a sanitary sewer. Staff at the local municipal utilities office should be able to confirm which sewers are which.

Inclined to Dry

EUREKA!

Park your just-washed and still wet car on a hill, and let gravity go to work for you. How? Simple—parking on an incline helps water run off your car more easily (and quickly, too).

◆ UN-BUCKLE FOR SAFETY

Before you start washing your car, make sure you're not wearing a large belt buckle, lots of gold chains, or a fancy wristwatch or jewelry. Why? Well, if you lean over the car to get at a hard-to-reach

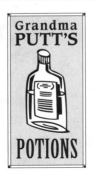

Air Fresheners Straight from the Kitchen

Whether it's the odor of a wet pooch or the lingering scent of cigarette smoke that you're trying to eliminate from your car, all you need are these few ingredients from your kitchen:

Vinegar. Of course, this is one of Grandma Putt's all-time favorite air fresheners for the house and the car. To rid your car of any unpleasant odor, pour a little vinegar into a shallow bowl and set it in your car overnight. Just remember to take it out before you go for a spin, or you'll have vinegar spinning all around your car's interior!

Cinnamon and cloves. To keep your car smelling fresh all the time, crush some cinnamon sticks and cloves, and put them in small cheesecloth bags that you make yourself. Stash the bags under the seats in your car. If cinnamon and cloves aren't to your liking, use any herbs or spices that are.

Vanilla. Soak a cotton ball with vanilla extract (the genuine article, not artificial vanilla flavoring), and put it under the front seat. Your car will smell delicious!

surface, you may end up leaving a scratch in the paint. (The same goes for when you wax or replace windshield wipers—any time you will be leaning over the car.) After a while, it can get expensive.

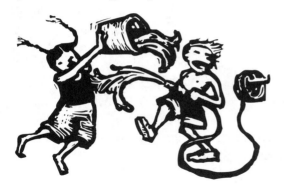

◆ WETTER IS BETTER

To start washing, wet the entire car with the hose before applying any soapy water. This pre-soak will loosen the grime on the car's surface, and that means less scrubbing for you.

◆ ALL THE CAR'S A STAGE

Plan to wash the car in stages. If you soap up the entire car, some parts may dry before you have a chance to scrub them. So instead of a dirty car, you'll have a soapy, dirty car.

◆ WORST THINGS FIRST

I like to start with the dirtiest part of the car—the tires. Use the scrub brush dipped in soapy water to give them a good scrub, then hose them down afterwards. Don't forget to wash under the wheel wells, as well as under the car itself.

I had a neighbor who was a fanatic about keeping his car clean. In fact, he placed his lawn sprinkler under the car to give it a good spraying! Of course, doing this will wet your brake lines (unless your vehicle has a closed bottom). That means you shouldn't go for a ride right away because you may have trouble stopping! Rather, let the underside of your car dry first.

◆ START AT THE TOP

Once you've conquered the tires, it's time to head for the roof. Wet the sponge with soapy, lukewarm water, and scrub the roof of the car. Then move down to the windows, trunk, and rear bumper. Before the soapy water dries, work quickly to hose it off with clear water.

Scrub the hood next. Rinse this section and move on to each side, working from front to back. After rinsing, finish up by washing the headlights, then the front bumper.

When you're done washing, give the entire car a rinse with the hose, allowing the water to cascade down from the top.

◆ IT'S DRYING TIME

Sure, your car will dry all by itself on a warm summer's day while you kick back with a tall, cold one. But due to the impervious nature of your car's finish, water tends to bead up. And those water droplets dry, leaving little spots. The result? Your freshly washed car looks like it has a case of the measles.

You've worked hard getting your car clean, so spend a few more minutes drying it off with those clean, old bath towels you've been saving. And, use more than one. Think of how wet a towel gets when you dry yourself off after a shower or bath—even a small car has more surfaces to dry than you do.

◆ SHOUT THEM OUT

Bugs will drive you crazy, especially when they're stuck all over your car. I have friends who live down south, and I tell you, this is a very annoying problem for them. Now, I know that lots of folks use oil, like WD-40, to remove bugs, but that leaves a slight residue.

Here's a trick that I think works much better. Go into your laundry room and grab that pre-wash stain treatment (like Shout). Spray a little onto the buggy bits (you don't need to use a lot because that stuff is concentrated anyway), and let it sit for a couple of minutes. Then wash it—and the bugs—right off.

◆ GIVE BUGS A WASH

I've also had good luck removing stuck-on dead bugs from my car with a mixture of 3 parts glass cleaner (the blue kind) with 1 part liquid dishwashing soap. Let it sit for a minute, and then gently wipe off the bugs with a sponge.

◆ SCOUR POWER

Of course, my all-time favorite bug-scouring solution is—you guessed it—baking soda! Just sprinkle some on a wet sponge and scrub off dead bugs (and any other dirt) from your car. The best part is that the baking soda is strong enough to make a good scouring powder, but gentle enough not to do any damage to your car's finish.

◆ DASHING DASHBOARD

Two items will clean pretty much anything inside your car: a can of Pledge furniture polish and a spray bottle containing vinegar and water. With these two concoctions you can clean any glass, chrome, vinyl, rubber, metal—even leather—in your car. After using the water-and-vinegar mix to remove the dirt and grime on leather or vinyl, use the Pledge furniture polish to restore the shine and luster to the seats, steering wheel, and dashboard (the lemon scent isn't bad, either).

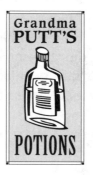

Chrome Cleaners

Here's an old-time solution for removing rust from any chrome on your car. Crumple up a piece of aluminum foil so that the shiny side is facing out, then just scrub the rusty spots. They'll disappear like magic!

Baby oil works well as a chrome polish, too, although it doesn't remove rust. Apply it with a soft clean cloth to make chrome shine.

Polishing and Waxing

If you've followed my advice so far, you have a spanking-clean car in front of you. But if the finish still looks dull instead of new-car glossy, then it's time to polish the car.

◆ WAX OR POLISH: WHAT'S THE DIFFERENCE?

Automotive supply stores sell plenty of products designed to restore, preserve, and protect your car's good looks; and this is no time to peer into the cupboard to find a frugal replacement. These surface solutions fall into two categories: wax and polish. Wax is just that, a substance, usually carnuba, used to put a finishing coat on your car to protect the paint.

Polish performs a similar function, while adding one more component—a small quantity of grit that removes some of the old finish and actually resurfaces it, removing light scratches, swirl marks, and dirt particles that have stuck to your car. Be aware that just like people, polishes come in varying degrees of abrasiveness. Some even contain clay and will remove a layer of paint, so read the labels carefully.

So how do you choose? Well, it depends on your car. Older

cars (20 years old or more) were painted with several thin layers of pigmented (colored) paint with a thin, glossy coat of lacquer on top. A hard wax finish was placed on top of this to protect the shine and give it depth. One way to protect an older car's factory paint job is to first polish it and then apply a layer of wax. Do this as often as possible, at least four times a year.

These days, cars get two layers of paint, a thin, pigmented base coat and a thick, glossy, clear topcoat. This finish is tougher and requires less waxing, although it still requires polishing from time to time, ideally at least twice a year.

Whether you wax or polish, remember that the finish is your car's first line of defense against corrosion, so treat it well.

◆ WAX ON, WAX OFF

Wax and polish are used in pretty much the same way. Start by working in a cool, shaded area. If the wax or polish dries too quickly, it can be hard work to remove it. Working in sections, apply the wax or polish with a damp, soft cloth. When the polish has dried somewhat and begins to haze, remove it with another clean soft cloth. But don't go around in circles. Using a circular polishing motion is often the cause of "swirl marks" in the finish. Instead, apply and remove the wax or polish with a gentle front-to-back (or back-to-front) motion, following the way air flows over the car. This method will buff out previous swirl marks and light scratches.

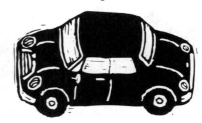

Jerry's **Just for** **FUN!**

Home Away from Home

The average commuter spends almost 400 hours in his or her automobile each year. WOW! Talk about time marching on—or should I say, rolling along?

Miscellaneous Car Tips

Well, we've covered a lot of ground on car safety, maintenance, and cleaning, but I do have more car tips to share with you. Here are some of my favorites.

◆ GIVE IT A MANICURE?

Uh, oh. You just got home from the grocery store and there's a big scratch on the door of your car. Panic time? Not at all. That is, not if you have some clear nail polish on hand. Wipe the scratch and dry it well, then give it a coat or two of nail polish. The polish will keep the scratch clean and dry and prevent rust from developing. Now remember, this is just a temporary solution. As soon as possible, you (or someone) should sand the scratch, then prime and paint it with matching touch-up paint from the auto supply store or your car dealer.

◆ PUT A NOTCH IN YOUR KEY

Don't you hate fumbling with your car keys in the dark? Let's see now, is that the key to the trunk, the door, or the ignition? Here's how I keep them straight. With my metal file, I put a notch in the head (not the jagged part) of my door key. That way I can get into my car quickly. Then I can use the interior light to see which key is which.

◆ UNSTICK STUCK BUMPER STICKERS

Of course you're proud of your daughter, but now that she's in medical school, maybe it's time to remove that bumper sticker from when she was in the high school color guard. For this and other sticky problems, try my gentle removal method. Use a hair dryer to soften the adhesive, then scrape the sticker off with an old credit card. If your bumper is painted, keep the heat low to prevent damage.

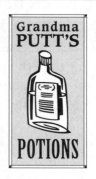

Another Sticky Situation

My Grandma Putt had a simple solution for removing bumper stickers—vinegar!

Bring some vinegar to a boil on the stove. Find a sponge and some heavy gloves. Take the pot of boiled vinegar, the sponge, and the gloves out to your car. Now put on the gloves and carefully saturate the sponge with the vinegar—don't burn yourself! Gently squeeze the sponge over the sticker to saturate it with the vinegar. If it's a stubborn adhesive, you may need to hold the sponge on the sticker for a minute. It should then come right off.

◆ DE-STICK DECALS

Old window decals and stickers can be tough to remove, but fortunately, the glass they're stuck to can withstand harsher treatment than the painted or chrome finish of a bumper. Soak the decal with lighter fluid or nail polish remover for a few minutes, then carefully scrape it away with a razor blade.

A safety note: Lighter fluid and nail polish remover are highly flammable. Don't use them around a hot engine or on a car that's been sitting in the sun.

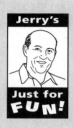

Jerry's Just for FUN!

Sticker Shock

The average price of an automobile today is four times higher than it was 20 years ago. Now, is your income four times higher, too? I didn't think so. OUCH!

◆ FOG ERASER

Here's a handy item to have when your car windows steam up on the inside. (It's a trick I picked up from an old friend who was a teacher.) Carry a felt blackboard eraser in your glove compartment during the cold seasons. A couple of wipes will quickly remove the condensation.

◆ ANTENNA ATTENTION

If your car has a radio antenna that slides up and down, but tends to get stuck, give it a little help. Take an old candle stub or piece of sealing wax and occasionally lubricate the antenna while it's fully extended. Waxed paper will work great, too.

◆ THE GREASY KEY OPENS THE LOCK

Put a drop or two of *synthetic* oil on your key and slide it in and out of the door lock a few times. The oil will coat the inside of the lock and prevent it from icing up in the winter. But don't try this with regular motor oil or household oil because it will thicken up in the cold and gum up the lock.

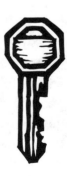

Jerry's Wild and Wonderful Uses for Household Stuff

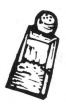

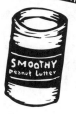

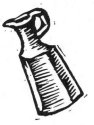

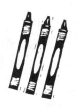

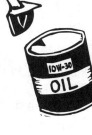

Welcome to my All Tips and Tricks—All of the Time section. It's a fascinating collection of all sorts of wild and wonderful uses for a wide variety of common household products. For convenience, I've arranged this section alphabetically so you can see at a glance what you can do with the stuff you already have on hand. So take your time as you flip through these next few pages—I'm sure you'll find more than a few tricks that'll help make your life a whole lot easier.

A Word of Warning: Whenever you are going to use one of these tips, tricks, or tonics, please be careful. Test a bit of the solution first on a hidden area, or for skin products, dab a little on a small patch of skin before you go whole hog. Above all else, exercise caution!

AMMONIA

If you think it's only for cleaning, read on!

◆ If you have squirrels living in your chimney, get them to leave by pouring a little ammonia in a pan and placing it in the hearth. Make sure that the flue is open and the fumes can travel up the chimney.

◆ To keep dogs and other critters from rummaging around in your garbage cans, soak a rag or old sock in full-strength ammonia, and tie it to the handle of the lid.

◆ For an effective homemade paint remover, mix one part turpentine with two parts ammonia. After brushing it on, let it sit for a few minutes, then wipe it off with a clean, damp cloth.

◆ Take the itch out of mosquito bites by dabbing a little bit of ammonia on them *before* you start scratching like crazy. If the skin is already broken, be prepared for some mighty painful stinging!

BABY OIL

It's not just for babies anymore!

◆ A drop or two of baby oil in your bath water will leave your skin feeling soft and fresh. But be careful getting out of the bath—the oil may make it slippery.

◆ Can't get that knot out of your jewelry chain? Put a drop of baby oil on the knot to loosen it, and then work it out with a couple of safety pins or sewing needles. (Magnifying eyeglasses sure come in handy for that job!)

◆ Keep soap scum from forming on your shower doors by giving them a good rubdown with a tiny bit of baby oil on a clean rag or sponge. Don't use too much, though, or you'll end up with a greasy mess.

◆ Out of makeup remover or cold cream? Put a little baby oil on a cotton ball and use that instead—but be careful around your eyes.

A Salute to Baby Oil

Jerry's Just for FUN!

Looking for a product with some veeery interesting uses? I nominate baby oil!

The Canadian Coast Guard highly recommends it for polishing chrome.

Or are you planning on showing off your prize chickens at the county fair? Then soften dry or rough skin on their feet with a little baby oil.

◆ Got a Band-Aid stuck on you? Baby oil (or mineral oil for that matter) will dissolve the adhesive. Soak it with a cotton ball and it'll come right off.

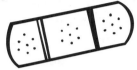

◆ Baby oil is a great chrome polish. Apply it with a soft, clean cloth to make all of the chrome on your car or around your home shine.

BAKING SODA

Thank goodness for that little yellow box!

◆ To clean and deodorize a wooden cutting board, mix equal parts baking soda and salt with enough water to make a paste. Scrub this concoction into the board, and leave it on for a few hours before rinsing thoroughly.

◆ Baking soda is a terrific, mild scouring powder. Sprinkle it on a damp sponge and use it

It's Not Just for Baking

Back in Grandma Putt's day, if you had indigestion, a fast solution was to take a little bicarb...baking soda. But the ancient Sumerians already knew that in 3500 B.C. They discovered that the alkaline properties of sodium bicarbonate did a great job of neutralizing the stomach's natural acids.

to clean your countertops, sinks, kitchen fixtures, appliances— almost anything!

◆ You know that an open box of baking soda keeps your refrigerator smelling fresh and sweet, but did you know it can do the same for your cupboards, too? Replace it every two months or so.

◆ Sprinkle a generous amount of baking soda in your cat's litter box before you add the litter. It will help control odors.

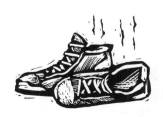

◆ Stinky sneakers? When you take them off,

sprinkle in some baking soda and let it sit overnight. In the morning, dump out the baking soda and enjoy the nice fresh smell.

◆ Clean your hairbrushes and combs in a solution of baking soda and hot water.

◆ Baking soda can keep your sinks from clogging. Once a week, pour in about ½ cup and rinse well with boiling water.

◆ Does your rug have an unpleasant smell? Sprinkle the area with baking soda. Let it sit for about a half hour and then vacuum. You may have to repeat the process more than once in order to get rid of strong odors.

Dry Doggie Shampoo

When it's too cold to give your dog a bath, rub some baking soda into his fur. Let it sit for awhile and then brush it out. The baking soda absorbs dirt and oils and will leave your pet smelling sweeter.

◆ To freshen and deodorize your laundry and boost the effectiveness of chlorine bleach, add about 1/2 cup of baking soda to each load of wash.

◆ Clean your outdoor lawn and deck furniture with a solution of 1 gallon of warm water and 2 cups of baking soda.

◆ Clean out that kiddie pool with a solution of 1 gallon of hot water and 4 cups of baking soda.

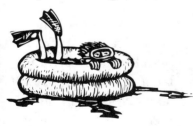

◆ When it's time to wash the inside of your refrigerator, sprinkle some baking soda on a damp sponge and use that to give it a good going over.

◆ Banish lingering odors from your thermos. Fill it with hot water, add 1/4 cup or so of baking soda, and let it sit overnight. (Don't put the lid on.) In the morning, wash and dry the thermos as usual.

◆ Use baking soda to clean your coffee pot. To a pot full of water, add 2 tablespoons of baking soda. Heat as if you're brewing a pot of coffee. When you're finished, run two more pots of water through it.

◆ Clean cement and linoleum floors with a baking soda and water solution. For greasy stains, sprinkle the bak-ing soda straight on the spot and scrub away.

◆ You can keep your dishwasher smelling fresh and clean by sprinkling some baking soda in the bottom between uses. Once a month, run the dishwasher empty with baking soda only (no soap) to clean it.

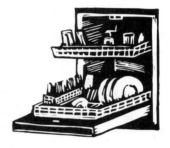

◆ Get rid of odors on your hands by adding baking soda to the soapy water when you scrub.

◆ Baking soda can soften your skin. Add 1 cup to your warm bath water the next time you decide to soak.

◆ Baking soda can relieve the itch and sting of insect bites and rashes such as poison ivy. Make a thin paste of baking soda and cool water, and apply it directly to the affected area. This also works well to relieve the burning and itching caused by mild sunburn.

◆ When you remove the box of baking soda from your refrigerator, pour it down your sink to eliminate odors there.

BLEACH

Out of the laundry room and into the rest of the house!

◆ Soak wooden clothespins in a bucket of warm water with a half cup of bleach. This

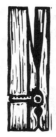 will prevent mildew from forming, and the clothespins won't stain your freshly cleaned laundry.

◆ Before you repaint your home's siding, wash it down with a solution of hot water and bleach (about 1 quart of bleach to 1 gallon of water) to kill mildew, which will affect the paint job.

◆ Here's a good home-made cleaning solution for wooden decks. Fill a bucket with a couple of gallons of hot water, about a quart of household bleach, and about $1/2$ cup of powdered laundry detergent. Scrub the deck with a brush (such as a push broom), and then rinse it well with water.

CAR WAX

Excuse me for waxing poetic about this handy substance!

◆ When the snow starts to fall, grab that car wax. Apply some to your snow shovel blade, and when you go out to shovel the driveway, the snow won't stick.

◆ Protect your metal outdoor furniture from the elements by applying a coat of car wax to it after you clean it.

◆ To make those bumper stickers easier to

Bleach Trivia

Household bleach is found in four out of five households in the United States. Here's what most of those folks probably don't know about this popular product:

Even though it's sometimes called chlorine bleach, there's no chlorine in household bleach! Chlorine is used to manufacture bleach, but the end product contains no chlorine.

Grandma Putt's favorite use for bleach was to put a drop of bleach in a quart of water and use that for fresh-cut flowers. The bleach keeps the water fresh and the flowers lively for days.

remove, apply them after you've applied a thin layer of car wax to the bumper. It also helps if you remove them within 4 to 6 weeks.

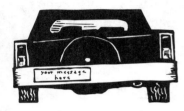

◆ To remove stubborn white rings left on your wood furniture by wet cups or glasses, try gently rubbing the rings with a little car wax.

◆ Hey, model airplane builders—car wax can come in handy for you, too. If you get model cement on the clear plastic pieces of your model, polish it away with a little car wax.

◆ Do you have any stained glass in your home? One way to keep the lead part around the glass looking beautiful is to shine it up with some light-duty car wax—just make sure to get any residue off.

CASTOR OIL

You don't have to ingest it to make this beany oil work for you!

◆ Mix 1 cup of castor oil with 3 gallons of water, and use it to drench the mole mounds in your yard. The critters will head for the hills!

◆ To ease laugh lines around your mouth and crow's feet around your eyes, gently rub castor oil into and around those areas just before bedtime. (Don't worry—it's odorless!)

◆ If your favorite leather shoes stiffened up because they got wet, soften them by washing them with warm water, and then thoroughly rubbing castor oil into the leather.

◆ Lubricate your scissors, tongs, and other kitchen utensils with a drop or two of castor oil.

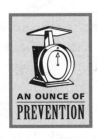

◆ To get rid of unsightly and bothersome warts on your hands, use castor oil once a day like a hand cream.

CAT LITTER

It's litter-ally one of my favorite substances!

◆ Keep a bag of clay (not clumping) cat litter in your car trunk. A sprinkling under your tires will help you out of an icy parking space; it gives just enough trac-

---

AN OUNCE OF PREVENTION

Wax Away Soap Scum

After you clean your bathroom wall tiles, give them a good going over with liquid car wax. The tiles will shine like mad, and soap scum will have a hard time taking hold, making cleaning a lot easier next time.

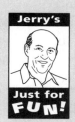

A Lotta Loot from Litter

Cat litter was "invented" in 1948 by a man named Ed Lowe from Cassopolis, Michigan. No big deal? Well, Mr. Lowe's idea went on to become Tidy Cat brand litter—a business that earns $210 million annually. That's a whole lotta litter!

tion to get you out of a slick spot.

◆ Sprinkle plain, unscented clay (not clumping) cat litter, ground to a rough powder, on oily upholstery stains. Let it sit, then vacuum up.

◆ Keep some unscented clay (not clumping) cat litter on hand in the garage to absorb spilled motor oil during your next oil change.

◆ Cat litter makes a great large-scale deodorizer—simply sprinkle it in garbage cans, in the fireplace, and in open boxes in musty rooms. The air should clear up overnight.

◆ Put cat litter as filler material in beanbag toys, dolls, or old socks that can be stitched together and used as draft sealers along the bottoms of doorways.

◆ To improve traction on an icy sidewalk, sprinkle clay (not clumping) cat litter on the area. It won't harm the sidewalk or the lawn.

CHALK

Chalk one up for—chalk!

◆ Rub white blackboard chalk into a stained collar before you wash it. The chalk will absorb some of the stain.

◆ If you place several pieces of chalk in a toolbox, they will absorb moisture and help pre-

vent rust from developing on the tools.

◆ Clean your marble with a damp, soft cloth that has been dipped in powdered chalk. Once you're done, clean the surface with clear water to remove the chalk, and then dry thoroughly.

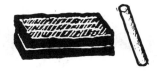

◆ Chalk can be used to polish metal. Simply sprinkle powdered chalk on a damp cloth, and rub the tarnished piece until it's shiny again.

◆ To keep ants and slugs out of your garden, scatter powdered chalk around the edges. The insect invaders won't dare cross the line!

CHARCOAL

When you're done barbecuing, put the charcoal to good use.

◆ Good old barbecuing charcoal (not the kind infused with lighter

Show Me the Charcoal!

Most of the charcoal used in the United States is made in the "Show Me" state of Missouri. Besides being the prime ingredient for our backyard barbecues, charcoal is used for:

☑ making gunpowder   ☑ manufacturing glass

☑ filtering water   ☑ feeding poultry

☑ curing tobacco   ☑ making high chrome steel

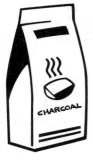

fluid) is terrific at absorbing moisture. Keep a briquette or two in your toolbox to keep your tools from rusting. Put a few in boxes of books to keep them from taking on musty odors. Put one or two in your tackle box, too.

◆ Place a bowl of activated charcoal (available from pet and health food stores) on a shelf in the back of a closet or in an old trunk to absorb smells and musty odors.

◆ To eliminate freezer odors, spread activated charcoal in a shallow pan, and set it in the freezer overnight.

◆ Place a piece of charcoal in a closed bookcase to absorb moisture and help keep the books dry.

CLUB SODA/ SELTZER

It can quench your thirst and solve household dilemmas, too.

◆ Served cold, club soda is the first thing to try on most spills, right after they happen, to keep them from staining.

◆ Instead of drinking it, pour some club soda on a sponge and polish stainless steel appliances with it.

◆ Some folks swear that club soda is the perfect solution for keeping linoleum floors sparkling and looking new.

◆ Club soda is also a great rust remover—simply pour some over rusty nuts, bolts, and screws and give them a couple of minutes to loosen up.

COOKING OILS

Oil's well that ends well!

◆ Olive oil can make your patent leather bags and shoes shine! First, clean the patent leather with a damp cloth, then use a clean cloth to apply just a little olive oil. Buff until it shines.

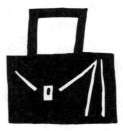

◆ Rub a little olive oil into your leather shoes to moisturize and shine the leather.

An old-time concoction to keep hair from falling out is a mixture of olive oil and a raw egg. Apply it to your hair and scalp, and rinse it out with warm water.

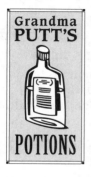

A few drops of vegetable oil rubbed into leather gloves will soften and revive them. (This trick works really well on baseball gloves, too!)

Here's a homemade ointment for bumps and bruises. Steep some mullein flowers in a little warmed olive oil, and rub it on the painful spot.

Before you fill a plastic storage container with tomato sauce or any other tomato-based food, wipe the inside with a thin coat of vegetable oil. This'll keep the sauce from staining the container.

Here's a recipe for a wood floor polish, right out of your cupboard. Mix a solution of vegetable oil and white vinegar in equal amounts in a spray bottle. Apply a thin mist to the floor, and rub it in well using cotton rags or a wax applicator from the hardware store. Remove the excess polish with clean cotton rags, and then buff to a shine. Be careful—the floor will be a bit slippery at first.

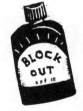

A dab of vegetable (or motor or suntan) oil will help you remove a tick. Cover it with some oil—the oil will loosen the tick's grip on you. Then carefully, with tweezers, remove the tick—all of it—and wash the area well.

CORNSTARCH

It's not just for cooking anymore!

Use a sprinkle or two of cornstarch to untie a really tough knot.

Mix a pinch or two of cornstarch in with your ammonia-and-water solution to get your windows and walls deep-down clean.

Is Rover dirty, but you don't have time to give him a bath? Rub some cornstarch into his coat, brush it out, and then fluff him up good as new.

To send roaches off to that great roach coach

Wipe Away Makeup

Grandma Putt didn't wear makeup very often, but when she did (for a very special occasion), she didn't remove it with fancy cold creams. No sirree, her makeup remover came right out of the pantry—she used cooking oil on a piece of cotton, which worked like a charm!

Grandma PUTT'S POTIONS

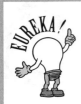

Easy Off

Sprinkle a little cornstarch on your hands *before* putting on your latex dishwashing gloves, and they'll be a cinch to remove when you're done.

in the sky, mix equal parts of cornstarch and plaster of paris, and sprinkle it behind your appliances and cupboards.

◆ To help prevent chafing and eliminate diaper rash, bathe sensitive areas with baking soda water, dry well, and then dust with cornstarch.

CRAYONS

Draw upon these clever ideas!

◆ Use an appropriately colored crayon on your leather shoes instead of shoe polish when you don't want to get your hands dirty—or when you're out of polish. Draw a few lines around the whole shoe,

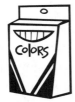

or cover up scuffed areas, and finish by buffing with a cloth or shoe brush.

◆ Cover a scratch in stained wood furniture with a matching crayon.

◆ Save your old, broken crayons, and melt them down to use to seal envelopes. Or mix them with a little paraffin to make brightly colored candles.

DENTURE CLEANING TABLETS

Even if you don't have dentures, get yourself some effervescent denture cleaning tablets for lots of odd jobs around the house.

◆ Denture cleaning tablets are great for

cleaning your coffeemaker. Drop the tablet in the coffeemaker, add hot water, and run it through as you would a regular pot of coffee. Follow that up with a pot or two of clear water.

◆ Don't have time to scrub the toilet bowl? Drop a couple of denture cleaning tablets in the bowl. Come back later, give it a quick brush, and you're all done!

◆ You don't need me to tell you how tea can stain your cup and teapot. What you may need me to tell you is that a denture cleaning tablet can clean them. Drop one or two in your pot and cup, add water, and let them do the job.

◆ Use denture cleaning tablets to get rid of the gunk that collects in the bottom of your vases. Pour in some water, add two tablets, and let stand. Then rinse the gunk away. Not sure this really works? Well, it just so happens that the folks at Waterford Crystal recommend cleaning tough stains from crystal decanters and vases with…you guessed it, denture cleaning tablets!

◆ Here's how to clean your thermos. Fill it with hot water, and drop in two denture cleaning tablets. *Don't* put the top on. Just let it sit for a couple of hours, and then rinse it out.

FABRIC SOFTENER SHEETS

They've softened your clothes, so it's time to throw them away, right? Wrong! Make those used fabric softener sheets do double-duty.

◆ Keep your suitcases smelling fresh and sweet when you're not traveling by keeping a used fabric softener sheet in each one.

◆ You might not be able to get back that new car smell, but you can at least help your jalopy smell better by tucking a fabric softener sheet or two under the front and back seats of your car. Just replace them when they lose their air-freshening ability.

◆ Is your television screen so dusty that you can't see what's on tonight? Just grab a used fabric softener sheet and lightly rub the screen with it. The sheet will lift the dust right off. And guess what? This works on your computer screen, too!

◆ Used fabric softener sheets make good dusting rags for all sorts of surfaces—the coffee table, blinds, lamp shades, windowsills… you name it.

◆ Not only can fabric softener sheets make your clean laundry soft and fresh, but they can help your waiting-to-get-washed laundry smell a bit better. When you pull the used sheet out of the dryer, throw it right in the hamper.

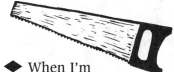

◆ When I'm doing some sawing or woodworking and I don't have a tack cloth (or the ingredients to make my own tack cloth), I pull up the dust with a used fabric softener sheet. It works pretty good, in a pinch.

Don't Throw it Out!

Even after you've used and reused that fabric softener sheet, try to get one more use out of it: Tear it into strips and use it to tie up your tomato plants!

◆ Are your shoes a little, um, ripe? Well, if you have some used fabric softener sheets lying around, you have a solution. When you take your shoes off, put the used fabric softener sheets in. They'll help reduce odor. This is most effective for brand-new shoes that you don't wear often. It keeps them smelling fresh a little longer.

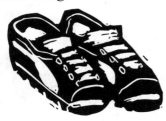

◆ Grandma Putt always had a bar of sweet-smelling soap in her closet. These days, I just spear a used fabric softener sheet on a wire hanger, and hang it in my closet. It always smells fresh. (You can put a sheet in each of your dresser drawers, too!)

HAIR SPRAY

Use it to solve some sticky problems!

◆ My favorite way to get rid of ink stains on clothing is to spray the spot with hair spray before laundering as usual. (Make sure to test this on a hidden area of the garment first.)

◆ Keep your favorite greeting cards around a lot longer by spraying them with a light coat of hair spray.

◆ For you sewing buffs, it's easier to thread your needle if you stiffen the end of the thread with a little hair spray first.

◆ A light coat of hair spray will keep newly polished pieces of brass from tarnishing.

◆ You can make inexpensive wrapping paper by spraying the Sunday comics with hair spray. It seals in the ink while giving the paper a nice, bright sheen. And kids love it!

◆ Keep those runs in your nylons from getting out of control by spraying them immediately with hair spray.

HONEY

Try these sweet, syrupy solutions.

◆ A drop of honey on a bee sting will keep it from itching.

◆ Honey is the prime ingredient in a home-made facial masque! Add 2 tablespoons of

---

Sew Soft

Here's a great tip a friend told me about. When you're getting ready to do some hand sewing, run the thread and needle through a used (or new) fabric softener sheet. It will keep the thread from clinging to the fabric, and that will keep it from getting tangled.

Baking Booster

Thinking of substituting honey for sugar in a recipe? Go ahead, but don't forget the baking soda! For every cup (8 ounces) of honey you use in a baking recipe, add $1/2$ teaspoon of baking soda. Why? There are two good reasons. One, the baking soda is a leavening agent that lightens the weight of the honey. And two, it acts as a base that counteracts the acidity of the honey.

honey to 1 cup of warm water, and mix well. Apply the honey-water to your face, let it sit for about a half hour, then rinse it off.

◆ Tickle in your throat? Put a tablespoon or two of honey into a cup of hot water, and add a teaspoon of lemon juice. Drink this throughout the day for sore throat relief.

HYDROGEN PEROXIDE

Bubble, bubble, less toil and trouble. Let hydrogen peroxide help you around the house.

◆ Here's a bath solution that will eliminate the smell the next time your dog tangles with a

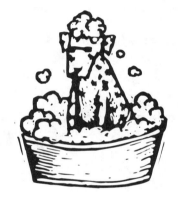

skunk. Mix 2 cups of fresh hydrogen peroxide, $1/4$ to $1/2$ cup of household baking soda, and 1 tablespoon of mild dishwashing detergent. This shampoo is mild enough to use anytime your pet smells a little strong— just be sure not to get any in his eyes.

◆ If your store-bought, scratchless scrubbing powder doesn't do the trick on tough stains, give it a boost with

something from the medicine chest. Make a paste out of the cleanser and some fresh hydrogen peroxide. Add a pinch of cream of tartar to it. Leave this poultice on the stain for a half hour, then scrub off with a brush or kitchen pad. *Caution:* Do this only with non-chlorine scrubbing powders. Combining chlorine with any other chemical can be dangerous.

◆ Wash toxic chemicals from fruits and vegetables with hydrogen peroxide. Rinse with water.

◆ Pre-treat grass and dirt stains on white cotton socks with hydrogen peroxide before laundering. It's gentler on cotton fibers than bleach.

◆ Hydrogen peroxide is great for removing blood stains from light-colored fabrics. Pre-treat the stain before laundering.

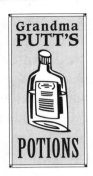

Halitosis Helper

Of course you've heard of brushing your teeth with a mixture of hydrogen peroxide and baking soda, but good old peroxide is great for curing bad breath, too. When my breath was a bit offensive, Grandma Putt mixed up a mouth rinse of peroxide and water. It worked like a charm!

◆ Freshen up and clean your toothbrush by letting it soak in ½ cup (or enough to cover the bristles) of hydrogen peroxide.

◆ Clean stains in your bathtub or shower with hydrogen peroxide and cream of tartar. Make a thin paste of the two, and spread it on the stains. When the paste dries, the stain will be gone. Just wipe it up with a sponge and rinse well.

◆ Linens that have been stored for a long time can become yellowed with age. But don't use bleach to clean them. Sponge the spots with hydrogen peroxide.

If the whole piece is yellowed, submerge it in the peroxide for an hour or so, then rinse with cold water, and wash as usual.

◆ To brighten your smile, brush your teeth with a little hydrogen peroxide after your regular brushing routine.

IODINE

It takes care of all kinds of boo-boos.

◆ Use iodine to hide scratches in your dark wood furniture.

◆ Can't find that darn splinter? Apply a drop of iodine to the area to quickly and easily locate the painful offender.

◆ If you're camping and find yourself without a safe water supply, thoroughly mix 6 to 8 drops of iodine per quart of water, then wait 30 minutes before drinking it.

LEMONS AND LEMON JUICE

Pucker up with these practical pointers!

◆ If you smoke (heck, even if you don't), clean the inside of your windows with a mixture of 2 tablespoons of lemon juice (fresh or bottled) and 1 quart of water. They'll shine like mad.

◆ Dab a little lemon juice (fresh or bottled) on a soft, clean cloth and rub it onto dark-colored leather shoes, then buff to shine.

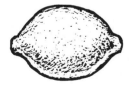

◆ Here's a garden-fresh mild, astringent for your face. Boil a few sprigs of fresh thyme in

2 cups of water. Take the pot off the heat and leave the thyme to steep in the water for 5 to 7 minutes. When the mixture cools down, remove the thyme (discard it), and add a teaspoon or so of lemon juice (fresh or bottled). Pour this concoction into a glass bottle with a top and store it in the refrigerator. Apply it after you wash your face.

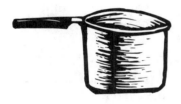

◆ To relieve almost any kind of itching, make a paste of lemon juice (fresh or bottled) and cornstarch, and apply that to the itchy area.

◆ Throat a little hoarse? Put a tablespoon or two of honey into a cup of hot water and add a teaspoon of lemon juice (fresh or bottled). Drink this throughout the day for relief from the sore throat.

◆ Here's an old-time hiccup remedy that really works: Cut a small slice of lemon and put it under your tongue. Suck it once and hold the juice in your mouth for 10 seconds. Swallow the lemon juice and your hiccups will be gone.

◆ After you squeeze a lemon, cut it in big chunks, and run it through your garbage disposal to keep it smelling fresh.

◆ If you find mildew spots on a piece of cotton clothing, make a solution of lemon juice (bottled or fresh) and

salt, and rub it on the stains. They should disappear in a jiffy.

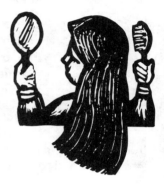

◆ Lemon juice (fresh or bottled) can help reduce dandruff and make your hair shinier. After you shampoo, mix a little lemon juice in water and rinse with that. Then rinse again with clear water. The juice cuts through the residue left behind by your shampoo and conditioner.

◆ Lemon juice can clean the copper bottoms of your pots and pans. Pour the juice (bottled or fresh) on the pot bottom or rub a cut slice of lemon on the pot, and it will remove the tarnish.

◆ Rust stains in your bathtub or shower? Make a thin paste by

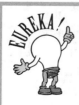

Lemony Fresh

Put a few drops of lemon juice (fresh or bottled) in your vacuum cleaner's dust bag to freshen the air as you vacuum.

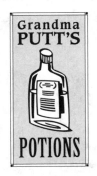

Grandma Putt's Old-Fashioned Lemonade

Did someone say lemonade? Here's the recipe Grandma Putt used!

2 cups of water
½ cup of sugar
½ cup of lemon juice (fresh-squeezed is best, but you can use the bottled kind—just don't tell Grandma Putt!)
Lots of ice

In a saucepan, bring the water to a boil. Stir in the sugar, reduce the heat, and continue to stir until the sugar dissolves completely. Remove from the heat and let cool. Add the lemon juice, stir well, and refrigerate until cold. Pour into glasses, add cold water and ice to taste—and enjoy!

mixing lemon juice (fresh or bottled) and borax. Spread that on the stains and scrub a bit. When the paste dries, the stains should be gone.

MEAT TENDERIZER

You won't believe what this concoction can do!

◆ Meat tenderizer relieves the pain and itch of insect bites because it breaks down the protein in the poison. Make a paste of tenderizer and water, and spread it on the bite or sting.

◆ For organic, protein-based clothing stains like milk, egg, and blood, make a paste of meat tenderizer mixed with a few drops of water. Work it into the stain and then launder as usual.

◆ Bring a shaker of meat tenderizer with you when you're enjoying the great outdoors. At the beach, meat tenderizer soothes the sting of a jellyfish. Just rub the stung area with meat tenderizer for quick relief. And anytime you're outdoors and get stung by a bee, make a paste of meat tenderizer and water, and apply to the sting site to numb the pain.

MILK

Milk moo juice for all it's worth!

◆ Milk can actually get rid of ballpoint pen ink on cotton and synthetic fabrics. Dampen a sponge with milk and dab it on the stain. But be patient; it may take a while. Then launder as usual.

◆ Shine up your leather purses and shoes with milk. Pour a little milk on a clean, soft rag and rub it into the leather.

◆ If you accidentally get pepper in your eye, flush it with a few drops of milk. The same applies if cayenne pepper gets too hot on your skin. Wash it off with a cloth dipped in milk.

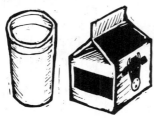

◆ For a milk-and-honey facial cleanser, mix 2 tablespoons of whole milk with 2 teaspoons of warmed (not hot) honey. This mixture doesn't keep very well, so make it as you need it. Rinse your face, massage the cleanser in for a couple of minutes, then rinse it off and pat your face dry.

◆ Having some spicy food? You can put out the fire by drinking a glass of milk, which will neutralize the heat.

MOTOR OIL (SYNTHETIC)

It's not just for your car!

◆ Prevent locks from icing up in the winter by putting a drop or two of synthetic oil on your key, and sliding it in and out of the door lock a few times. The oil will coat the inside of the lock. Don't try this with regular motor oil or household oil, though. Unless it's synthetic, the oil will thicken in the cold and gum up the lock.

◆ To prevent your yard and garden tools from rusting, store them in a box filled with sand that has a little motor oil added to it.

◆ For all you do-it-yourself cement guys, brush motor oil onto your wooden frame before pouring in the concrete, and you'll end up with cleaner forms and neater concrete.

NAIL POLISH

Sure, it makes your nails look nice, but there's so much more that nail polish can do.

◆ Clear nail polish can stop a run in hosiery in its tracks. While the run is still small, brush some nail polish on it. When the polish dries, the run will be stopped.

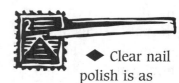 ◆ Clear nail polish is as cheap as can be, so you should always keep some around. I use it as a glue for stamps that I take off envelopes.

◆ A temporary solution to a scratch in your car's finish is as close as your makeup kit. Give

When Buttermilk's Better Milk

Here's a notation I found in one of Grandma Putt's old-time books: "To whiten yellowed bed or table linen, soak it for about a week in buttermilk, and it will wash out as white as snow."

the scratch a coat or two of clear nail polish. This'll keep the scratch clean and dry, and prevent rust from developing until you get matching touch-up paint from the auto-supply store.

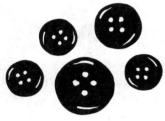

◆ Don't you just hate losing buttons? I sure do! Here's a trick that Grandma Putt taught me. The next time you sew one on, put just a drop of clear nail polish on top of the button, over the thread. Then when the polish dries, it will fasten the thread to the button and make the button a bit more secure.

NAIL POLISH REMOVER

Sure, it removes nail polish, but here are some other neat ways to use this fluid.

◆ Use nail polish remover to get rid of scuff marks on a linoleum floor. *Caution:* Test this method on a hidden part of the floor first, and rinse it well so that no polish remover remains. It could damage the floor.

◆ Here's an easy way to remove an old decal from your car's windshield. Soak the decal with nail polish remover for a few minutes, then carefully scrape it away with a razor blade.

◆ To remove grease stains from white shoes, gently rub with nail polish remover. Just be careful not to remove any of the finish.

◆ If you've got ink stains on your best shirt, saturate the spot with nail polish remover, then blot dry with a clean cloth. Repeat if necessary, then launder as usual.

◆ Self-adhesive hooks can be removed from unpainted surfaces by dribbling a little nail polish remover over them.

ONION

And you thought they were only for warding off vampires!

◆ Rub a cut onion on the inside of your car's windshield. This will keep it from fogging up.

◆ If you're feeling faint, hold a cut onion under your nose until you come around.

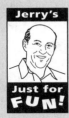

Now That's Old!

Nail polish was invented in China 5,000 years ago. Today's nail polish is actually a kind of automotive paint—think about that the next time you are getting a manicure!

Jerry's Just for FUN!

Cut Out Rust

Need to clean a rusty knife? Here's a great tip: Use it to slice up an onion or two, and it will be as good as new.

◆ Slice an onion in half and put it in a just-painted cabinet to get rid of that obnoxious paint smell.

◆ Onion juice, applied twice a day, is just the thing to get rid of the itch and burn of athlete's foot.

◆ Eliminate unsightly warts by rubbing them with half an onion that's been dipped in salt.

PEANUT BUTTER

It sticks to the roof of your mouth—and gets rid of gum!

◆ Gum in your child's hair? Slather it with peanut butter. The oils in it will break down the gum and after you work on it for awhile, the gum should slide right out.

◆ Use peanut butter to unstick the stuck—remove those darn little pieces of price tags on pots, pans, and other metal or plastic products by rubbing them with peanut butter until they slide right off.

◆ Peanut butter works great on removing road tar from your car, shoes, pants, etc. Simply rub it in to work off the tar.

PENCIL

Here's where we get to the point!

◆ Rub the point of a pencil on the teeth of a zipper to keep it zipping and unzipping smoothly.

◆ Rub a pencil along the edges of a key to keep it from sticking in the lock.

◆ Use pencils as plant stakes for young house-plants. Simply tie the plant to the pencil with bits of soft string.

◆ Recycle your pencil shaving by stuffing sachets full of them. Stick the sachets in drawers or closets where they'll repel clothes moths. You can also use pencil shavings to get rid of whatever's bugging your houseplants. Sprinkle the shavings on the soil, and the bugs will soon be gone!

PETROLEUM JELLY

It's slippery, it's gooey, it's cheap—and it sure comes in handy for all sorts of uses.

◆ Rub a little petroleum jelly into the palm of a new baseball glove when you're breaking it in to help soften it up.

◆ A cotton ball soaked in petroleum jelly makes a great emergency fire starter when you're out camping.

◆ Did a little birdie leave a "present" on your leather jacket? Remove the stain by rubbing it with some petroleum jelly.

◆ Put a little petroleum jelly on your lips before applying lipstick. It'll help the lipstick go on more evenly. Apply a little afterwards for extra sheen.

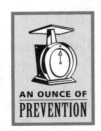

◆ Use petroleum jelly to soften your cuticles. Gently rub a dab into each nail base.

◆ Before going out on a cold day, apply some petroleum jelly to your lips and nose to prevent them from chapping.

◆ Rub some petroleum jelly on your forehead and neck before you dye your hair or give your-

---

Not Here You Don't!

Do you have birdhouses or bird boxes in your yard? You can keep wasps out of them by smearing a coat of petroleum jelly on the inside top of the box.

AN OUNCE OF PREVENTION

---

self a permanent. The jelly will keep the dye from staining your skin.

◆ Skin feeling a little dry? Rub on some petroleum jelly. Turn on your shower and let the bathroom get good and steamy. Then go sit in the "steam bath" for 15 minutes or so while the jelly works its magic.

◆ A dab of petroleum jelly on an old door hinge will quiet a squeak.

◆ Petroleum jelly will help heal a minor cut or scrape—all by itself.

◆ Tired of your candles getting stuck in your good candleholders? Try this trick. Use a cotton swab to dab some petroleum jelly inside the candle holder before you put

---

the candle in. Even if the wax drips, you'll be able to get it off easily and you can get the candle out easily, too.

◆ Does it drive you crazy when you can't get the lid off of the Krazy Glue? When you get a new tube of glue, smear just a little petroleum jelly inside the cap or around the rim. Then the next time you need the glue, the lid will come right off!

◆ You finished your painting project, but now you've got a bigger project— getting the paint off of your hands. Next time, make it easy on yourself. Rub your hands all over with just a

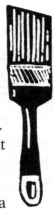

little petroleum jelly before you start painting. That way, when it's time to clean up, the paint will come right off.

◆ Those patent leather shoes looking a little dull? Not to worry—grab a soft cotton cloth and a little petroleum jelly. Make sure the shoes are clean and dry, and then rub a bit of the jelly into the leather. In no time they'll be shiny as new.

POTATOES

Gotta love those spuds!

◆ Got some mud on cotton or synthetic clothing? Try rubbing out the spots with a slice of raw potato, then launder as usual.

◆ To make your hair color darker, brush your hair several times with a brush or comb that's been dipped in boiled potato water. To set the color, sit in the sun.

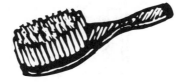

◆ Potatoes can take away some food stains on your skin. Rub a potato slice on strawberry or blueberry stains, and rinse well with water.

◆ Potatoes hold heat and cold well, so boil one and use it as a warm compress, or stick one in the refrigerator to use to keep an area cold.

◆ If you've been bitten by a bug, rub a sliced potato on the insect bite for instant itch relief.

◆ If your scuffed shoes just won't take a shine, rub 'em with a raw potato, then polish them. They'll look like new!

RUBBING ALCOHOL

It cleans, it disinfects, it shines, and more!

◆ After mopping, disinfect your bucket by wiping it out with a little rubbing alcohol on a rag.

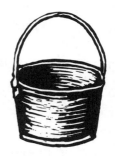

◆ Blot an ink stain with rubbing alcohol before laundering. It will help the stain come out more easily.

◆ Before cleaning your windowsills, wipe them with a cloth dipped in

---

Soften Hands While You Sleep

Before you retire for the evening, coat your hands with petroleum jelly. Put on a pair of white cotton gloves, and in the morning your hands will be as soft as a baby's. (This works for your feet, too. Slip on a pair of white cotton socks, and wake up with baby-soft feet.)

rubbing alcohol. The alcohol should dissolve the dirt enough for the detergent to clean better.

◆ In a spray bottle, mix ½ cup of rubbing alcohol, 3 cups of water and 1 tablespoon of liquid laundry detergent, and use as an after-shower spray for your tiled bathroom walls.

◆ Before breaking a blister with a needle, wipe them both with some rubbing alcohol to kill germs and prevent infection.

◆ Two tablespoons of rubbing alcohol mixed in a pint of water makes an inexpensive weed killer.

◆ When you clean your bathroom, give the sink fixtures a final rubdown with a little rubbing

alcohol. It will kill germs and shine the chrome. It will also shine the mirror in your bathroom and remove deodorant, hair spray, and perfume residue, too.

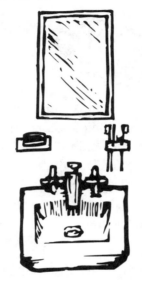

◆ Is the plastic case on your computer looking dingy? Grab some cotton balls, cotton swabs, and rubbing alcohol. Rubbing alcohol will clean

up the keyboard, mouse, and casing. It removes almost all ink stains and grime, too.

◆ Once a week, clean your telephone with a little rubbing alcohol. It will remove oils, grease, fingerprints, and ink stains, plus it kills germs.

◆ Make your own reusable ice pack. You'll need a heavy-duty freezer baggie. Mix up 1 part rubbing alcohol with 2 parts water. Put it in the bag and squeeze out all of the air. (Don't fill the bag too full.) Put the pack in the freezer. Since alcohol won't freeze, it will make the contents of the bag slushy rather than rock hard.

SALT

Salt of the earth. And the kitchen. And the laundry room. And...

◆ If new dentures or braces are a little uncomfortable, gargle with a mix of salt and

Rub Out Sap

Have you ever parked your car under a pine tree? Uh-oh, that could mean your nice clean car is covered with drops of sap. Here's how to remove it. Dampen a soft cotton cloth with rubbing alcohol and buff the sap away. And next time? Park in the garage!

warm water to toughen up your gums.

◆ A bottle with "shoulders" can be difficult to clean. Extend your reach by putting a little salt into the bottle to act as a mild scouring agent. Swirl it around to clean out all of the nooks and crannies.

◆ Dried food spills on stove tops can be scoured away with a dash of salt and a little water. Dampen the stain first, then add the salt. It acts as a mild abrasive.

◆ Try this all-purpose gargle for a sore throat: warm, salty water with a pinch of cayenne and a crushed clove of garlic added in. Okay, it may not taste great, but it works wonders!

◆ Unclog a drain blocked with grease by mixing up a solution of 1 cup of salt and 1 cup of baking soda.

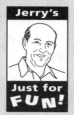

And They Salted it Away, Too!

Did you ever say: "Back to the salt mines," when you had a job to complete? Well you may not really rely on salt for your living, but ancient Roman soldiers were paid a special stipend for salt rations called *salarium,* or salt money. This is where we get our word salary. And if a soldier wasn't doing his job, they said he was "not worth his salt." Now you know!

Sprinkle the mixture into the drain, then pour in several cups of boiling water. Your drain should be as good as new.

◆ Damp laundry that sits too long in hot weather may develop spots of mold or mildew. Here's how to get rid of them. Mix up a paste of lemon juice and salt. Then, with a cotton swab or your finger, rub the mixture into the spots.

◆ Here's an old trick to help your stockings and panty hose last longer. Make up a solution of 2 cups of table salt in 1 gallon of water. Stir until the salt dissolves, then immerse the stockings in the solution for 3 or 4 hours. Wring them out and let them dry.

◆ Don't clean your fish tank or goldfish bowl with soap—it could leave behind residue that's harmful to your fish. Instead, clean your tank with hot water, a sponge, and table salt. Use the salt as a scouring powder. When the tank is clean, rinse it out very well with clean water.

◆ Here's a salty solution from Grandma Putt. When you wash a new pair of blue jeans for the first time, add a quarter cup of table salt to the wash cycle. The salt will keep the jeans from bleeding too much and at the same time, will soften them up.

◆ Perspiration stains on your clothing mean that you've been working hard, but they're not very pretty. To remove them from cotton fabric, make up a bucket of salty water—a cup or two of salt to each gallon of water. Soak the clothing in the water for an hour or so, wring them out, then launder as usual.

◆ The next time something messy drips in the oven, grab the salt and pour some on the stain. Make sure to do that while the oven is still hot. The next morning, when the oven has cooled, just wipe up the stain with a damp sponge.

> *...it is an interesting biological fact that all of us have, in our veins, the exact same percentage of salt in our blood that exists in the ocean, and therefore, we have salt in our blood, in our sweat, in our tears. We are tied to the ocean. And when we go back to the sea—whether it is to sail or to watch it—we are going back from whence we came.*
>
> JOHN F. KENNEDY

SUGAR AND SPICE AND EVERYTHING NICE

Some tips on how to use the ingredients from your baking and spice cabinets—you might be surprised at what you find here!

◆ The next time hiccups have you gulping for air, swallow a teaspoon of sugar. It works like a charm.

◆ White flour sprinkled on a dry rag makes an excellent (and scratchless) chrome polish.

◆ Cayenne pepper can make your houseplants a little less appetizing to your pets. Mix a teaspoon of cayenne pepper into a cup of water. Pour this mixture into a clean spray bottle and spray the leaves on your houseplants with it. The smell alone may deter pets from nibbling.

◆ Dry mustard will remove onion odors

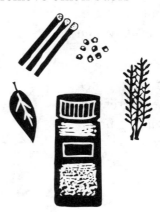

from your hands or cutting board. Rub it in, then rinse it off.

◆ An old trick to keep ants out of the cupboard was to sprinkle some cloves around the inside.

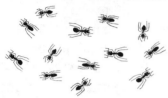

◆ Temporary relief from toothache is as close as your cupboard. Mix allspice powder in a cup of boiling water. Steep it for 10 to 20 minutes and strain. While the tea is still warm, swish it around your mouth.

◆ Here's a old-fashioned cure for athlete's foot. Steep 15 or 20 broken cinnamon sticks in about 8 cups of boiling water. Remove the pot from the heat, and let the mixture steep for about an hour. Put this "tea" in a bucket, and soak your feet in it for 15 minutes or so. When you're done, rinse your feet.

◆ Cream of tartar not only makes meringue fluffy, but it can help eliminate bathroom stains. Mix up a paste made of cream of tartar and peroxide, and spread it on the stain. Scrub a bit, then let it sit until it dries, and wipe it away.

◆ The next time you clean the fridge, add a few drops of vanilla extract to the soapy water. It will help the fridge smell fresh.

TALCUM POWDER

Get that powder off the bathroom shelf and put it to good use around the house.

◆ Squeaky wood floor? Sprinkle some talcum powder around the area of the squeak. Gently sweep it into the cracks between the floorboards. Use a damp mop to pick up the excess powder, so the floor won't be slippery. Don't use a vacuum, though, or it'll suck up the talc right out of the cracks.

◆ If your zipper sticks or is hard to close, sprinkle some talcum powder on it.

◆ To locate a mouse hole, sprinkle a little talcum powder along

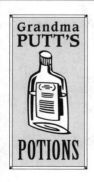

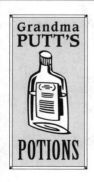

Homemade Furniture Polish

Here's Grandma Putt's secret recipe: Mix about ¹/₂ cup each of malt vinegar and linseed oil in clean jelly jar with a lid. Add 1¹/₂ teaspoons of lemon or lavender oil for scent. She'd use this concoction to clean and polish all of her wood furniture.

Grandma **PUTT'S** POTIONS

the baseboards. The mice will walk through it and leave a powdery trail all the way to where they're getting in.

◆ Here's a way for gentlemen to get an extra-smooth shave. Pat your face and neck with a little talcum powder before you shave, whether you lather up or use an electric razor.

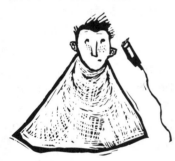

TEA (HERBAL AND BLACK)

Who knew that brewed tea, tea bags, and tea leaves could do so much!

◆ If your feet are sweaty and tend to smell, try this home remedy: Brew up a couple of quarts of extra-strong black tea, then when it's cooled sufficiently, soak your feet in

it for about 10 minutes. The tannins in the tea will dry out your feet after the soak is done, and the odor will be gone as well.

◆ You forgot to put on a hat and now your scalp is all sunburned? Make up a pot of green tea. Let it cool off (you can even pop it into the refrigerator for a while), and then rinse your hair with it after you shampoo. It will relieve the pain.

◆ Use tea sachets to cure stinky shoes. Grab a pair of old stockings and cut them off at the knees. Put 2 or 3 tablespoons of tea leaves (either loose tea or from

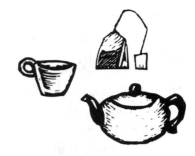

cut-open tea bags) into each foot stocking. Tie off the top and put one sachet in each shoe. Use the shoe sachets between wearings to keep shoes smelling sweet.

◆ Want to refinish that yard-sale find? After you strip off the old paint, try staining the wood with strong tea. *Caution:* This stain is permanent, so make sure to test this method on an inconspicuous spot first and don't

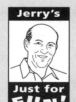

The First Tea Time

According to legend, the first person to brew tea was the Chinese emperor Shen Nung. The story goes that in 2737 B.C., he was boiling water when leaves from a tea plant accidentally dropped into the pot. He didn't notice until he brought his cup to his mouth, but decided to drink anyway because the aroma was so enticing. He later wrote that the drink "gladdens and cheers the heart." I guess he liked it!

Jerry's
Just for FUN!

try it on an expensive piece of furniture.

◆ Soothe itchy skin with fresh mint tea. Brew up a cup and allow it to cool for a minute or two. Then take a soft cloth or cotton ball, dip it into the tea, and apply it as a compress to the affected skin.

◆ Grandma Putt made her own insect repellent from pennyroyal tea, and you can, too. Make 2 or 3 cups of tea. Then into that, put a drop or two of eucalyptus oil. Put that mixture in a small spray bottle and apply it whenever you go outside.

◆ Got bad breath? Drink some peppermint tea to sweeten it up.

◆ Ease the discomfort of corns by applying a compress of very strong chamomile tea. Soak a cotton ball in the tea, and apply it frequently throughout the day.

> *Thank God for tea! What would the world do without tea? How did it exist? I am glad I was not born before tea.*
>
> SYDNEY SMITH

◆ Control dandruff with a strong tea of yarrow and chaparral (available in health food stores.) After you wash your hair, apply the tea, let it sit for a minute, then rinse it out. Another old-time cure for dry scalp is to make a tea of water, sage, and rosemary—it has a delightful fragrance, and it soothes scalp irritation.

◆ A tea made from parsley, taken often throughout the day, will help reduce a fever. Place a teaspoonful of dried parsley in a tea ball and steep it in a cup of hot water for about 7 minutes.

◆ Chamomile tea, available in most health food stores and Mediterranean food markets, is known to bring on sleepiness. Have a cup before bedtime to fight mild insomnia.

◆ Giving up smoking is really tough. Give yourself a helping hand by helping yourself to a cup of herbal tea. Choose one containing catnip, chamomile, hops, lobelia, peppermint, skullcap, or valerian. Each of these herbs is known to lessen the urge for nicotine and help you relax.

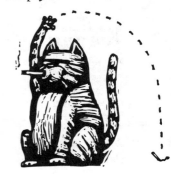

◆ Chamomile tea, cooled sufficiently, makes a great facial toner. Apply it after you've washed your face. Brew an extra cup of chamomile tea and set it aside for the next time you wash your hair. After you shampoo, rinse your hair with the tea to add shine.

TOOTHPASTE

It cleans your teeth—and so much more!

◆ Use toothpaste as a mild abrasive to remove minor scratches in glass.

◆ Here's a trick for you divers: use toothpaste to clean salt deposits on masks and other diving equipment.

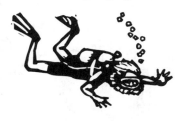

◆ Has your little Picasso been drawing on your painted walls? Spread some toothpaste on the spot and let it sit for 30 minutes. Then wipe clean.

◆ Use toothpaste as an emergency jewelry cleaner. Work it into the piece with an old toothbrush, then rinse it well with water. Polish to a shine.

◆ Restore a scratched plastic surface to like-new condition by covering it with toothpaste, then buffing with a clean, dry cloth.

VINEGAR

Sure, it makes great salad dressing. But have you heard about all the other wondrous things that vinegar can do?

◆ Mix white vinegar and water, and use to remove the dirt from leather or vinyl.

◆ Treat your dust mop with a solution of two parts white vinegar and one part vegetable oil.

◆ Sponge a perspiration stain with a solution of 1 tablespoon of white vinegar and 1 cup of water, then launder as usual.

◆ Get rid of grime on kitchen appliances by wiping them with a solution of 2 tablespoons of white vinegar to 3 cups of hot water.

◆ Clean and freshen the inside of your refrigerator by wiping it down with ½ cup of white vinegar added to a small bucket of hot water.

◆ Been in the sun too long? Put white vinegar

Very Vinegar

Vinegar was one of the world's first medicines. It's even mentioned in the Bible for its healing properties. And doctors used it during WWI to treat wounds.

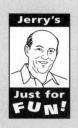

Old Wine, New Uses

Vinegar was discovered more than 10,000 years ago by someone who found that his wine, though past the point of drinking, was terrific for all sorts of other uses!

in a spray bottle and keep it in the refrigerator. Spritz it on to cool and soothe the pain of sunburn. This also works well for minor burns from the stove or a hot iron.

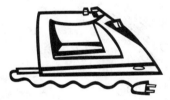

◆ White vinegar will help kill the fungus that causes athlete's foot. Sponge it on before you get out of the shower, then rinse and dry your toes well.

◆ Pat white vinegar on insect bites to ease that annoying itching.

◆ Vinegar is one of Grandma Putt's all-time favorite air fresheners

for the house and the car. To get rid of unpleasant odors, pour a little white vinegar into a shallow bowl and set it out overnight.

◆ To get salt stains off of leather (not suede) shoes and boots, dampen a sponge or a rag with some vinegar, and wipe it right off. Now wear those shoes with pride!

◆ If you have ants coming into your home in the summertime, give this a try. Dampen a sponge with some vinegar and wipe your countertops with it. That ought to keep the ants off your counters. Some folks tell me it repels cockroaches, too.

◆ Cloudy vases and drinking glasses? Here's

how to get rid of that film, which can be caused by hard water. Fill a saucepan with vinegar and heat it until it's almost too hot to put your finger in. Soak your vases and glasses in the hot vinegar for about 3 hours, and then wash as usual (you may have to scrub with a plastic scouring pad). The cloudiness should disappear.

◆ When you run out of chrome or stainless steel polish, reach for the vinegar. Dampen a sponge or paper towel with vinegar, and use that to clean and shine all of your sink fixtures.

◆ Want to get rid of mold, mildew, and their odors in your bathroom? Wipe down tiled walls once a week or so with a sponge doused with straight vinegar.

◆ You can clean all of the windows and mirrors in your house with a 50-50 solution of vinegar and water. (Use black-and-white newsprint to dry them.)

A Nicer De-Icer

Mix up a batch of windshield de-icer by combining 3 parts white vinegar with 1 part water. Spray it on your windshield and car windows before you go to bed. In the morning, they should all be ice-free.

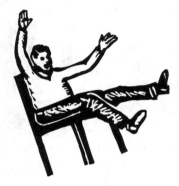

◆ Are the seats of your cane chairs sagging? Don't go on a diet. Rather, wash down the seats with a 50-50 solution of vinegar and water. Set the chairs outside to dry on a hot day. As the cane dries, it will tighten right up.

◆ Here's how to clean and soften those paint-saturated paintbrushes that have been left out all night. First, pour enough vinegar into a saucepan to cover the bristles of the brushes, and then bring the vinegar to a simmer. Hold the bristles in the simmering vinegar until they soften. Then wash the brushes as usual.

◆ You know that vinegar makes a good cleaner, but did you know that it can boost the cleaning power of an inexpensive liquid dish-washing detergent, too? When you fill up the sink, add an ounce or two of vinegar along with the dishwashing soap. The vinegar cuts grease.

◆ Are hard-water deposits clogging up your shower head? Remove the head and soak it in some hot vinegar for an hour or two. Then wash the head and replace it.

Index